Perspectives on **Disability** & **Rehabilitation**

With deep appreciation,
this book is dedicated to my parents,
Roma and Harry Whalley and to my husband,
Ike Hammell.

Commissioning Editor: Susan Young
Development Editor: Catherine Jackson
Project Manager: Joannah Duncan
Designer: Stewart Larking

Perspectives
on **Disability**
& **Rehabilitation**
Contesting assumptions; challenging practice

Karen Whalley Hammell PhD, MSc, OT(C), DipCOT
Researcher and writer, Oxbow, Saskatchewan, Canada

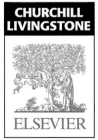

CHURCHILL
LIVINGSTONE

ELSEVIER

EDINBURGH   LONDON   NEW YORK   OXFORD   PHILADELPHIA   ST LOUIS   SYDNEY   TORONTO   2006

CHURCHILL
LIVINGSTONE

First published 2006

ISBN 0 443 10059 4

British Library Cataloguing in Publication Data
A catalogue record for this book is available from the British Library

Library of Congress Cataloging in Publication Data
A catalog record for this book is available from the Library of Congress

---

Notice

Knowledge and best practice in this field are constantly changing. As new research and experience broaden our knowledge, changes in practice, treatment and drug therapy may become necessary or appropriate. Readers are advised to check the most current information provided (i) on procedures featured or (ii) by the manufacturer of each product to be administered, to verify the recommended dose or formula, the method and duration of administration, and contraindications. It is the responsibility of the practitioner, relying on their own experience and knowledge of the patient, to make diagnoses, to determine dosages and the best treatment for each individual patient, and to take all appropriate safety precautions. To the fullest extent of the law, neither the publisher nor the author assumes any liability for any injury and/or damage.

Working together to grow
libraries in developing countries

www.elsevier.com | www.bookaid.org | www.sabre.org

ELSEVIER   BOOK AID
            International   Sabre Foundation

ELSEVIER   your source for books,
            journals and multimedia
            in the health sciences
www.elsevierhealth.com

The
Publisher's
policy is to use
**paper manufactured
from sustainable forests**

The Publisher

Printed in China

Contents

Chapter 11

Author information

Karen Whalley Hammell is an occupational therapist with a Master of Science degree (with Distinction) in Rehabilitation Studies from the University of Southampton, UK and a Doctor of Philosophy degree in Interdisciplinary Studies (Rehabilitation Sciences, Anthropology, Sociology) from the University of British Columbia, Canada. She has worked as a clinician in both the UK and Canada, and in a variety of hospitals, rehabilitation centres and urban and rural communities.

Dr Hammell is the author of many peer-reviewed papers and of chapters contributed to several occupational and physical therapy texts published in Canada, the UK and USA. She is also the author of *Spinal cord injury rehabilitation* (1995) and an editor and author of *Using qualitative research: a practical introduction for occupational and physical therapists* (2000) and of *Qualitative research in evidence-based rehabilitation* (2004).

Preface

Despite a recent explosion of publications emanating from the social sciences, humanities – and particularly from within Disability Studies – that contest, critique and challenge the way in which disability is understood and "managed", this burgeoning literature has been virtually unnoticed by those professional and academic disciplines that rely upon the presence of disability in society, such as nursing, occupational therapy and physiotherapy. Thus immune from alternative views, rehabilitation practitioners fail to question the premise that their professional assumptions are either benevolent or "right".

The aim of *Perspectives on Disability and Rehabilitation: Contesting assumptions; challenging practice* is to provide an accessible introduction to many different theoretical perspectives, using these insights to contest prevailing assumptions about disability, to explore issues of power and professional dominance and to unmask and challenge the paradigms, practice and ideologies of rehabilitation.

The book encourages readers to question the taken-for-granted nature of traditional knowledge and assumptions within the rehabilitation, health and community care industries, and aims to stimulate a more critical approach both to the nature of rehabilitation following injury or illness and to the "problem" of physical difference and disability. It relates eclectic theoretical view-points to practical examples to suggest ways in which a renewed understanding of both disability and rehabilitation might contribute to a more equitable and productive relationship between disabled people and those who work in the fields of health and social care.

Through its interrogation and exploration of different theoretical perspectives on disability and rehabilitation, this book provides a unique text for students and practitioners of nursing, occupational therapy, physiotherapy and social work and for educators and researchers in these fields.

The meaning ascribed to the concept of disability determines its response. Drawing upon diverse perspectives this book provides different ways of thinking about disability and suggests new directions for rehabilitation research, theory, practice and service delivery.

Karen Whalley Hammell,
Oxbow, Saskatchewan, Canada, 2006

Chapter 1

Exploring the assumptions underpinning rehabilitation

Central to the problem of rehabilitation is the failure to address the issue of power and to acknowledge the existence of ideology.
(Oliver 1996a p 104)

INTRODUCTION: CONTESTING ASSUMPTIONS AND CHALLENGING PRACTICE

The rehabilitation professions are maturing disciplines, with many members pursuing advanced academic studies to the master and doctoral levels. It would seem reasonable to expect that these intellectual advances would lead to a critical interrogation of taken-for-granted ways of thinking about both disability and rehabilitation and a continual challenging of 'common sense' assumptions. Acceptance of received wisdom – perhaps formerly excusable – is no longer permissible.

Every profession relies, to a greater or lesser degree, on shared assumptions. Among the rehabilitation professions, these beliefs concern the nature of their work (apolitical, relevant and useful), the nature of their goals (increasing function, performance and independence to enhance quality of life) and the calibre of their relationships with their patients and clients (benevolent, client-centred and helpful). To determine whether these theories and assumptions enjoy a supportive evidence base requires a critical exploration of literatures pertaining both to rehabilitation and to disability.

To *explore* is to travel into a territory in order to examine it thoroughly and learn more about it. An exploration of the assumptions that underpin rehabilitation – and of the evidence that supports or contests these assumptions – will contribute to a renewed understanding of both disability and rehabilitation. New perspectives have the potential to suggest new directions for rehabilitation research, theory, practice and service delivery, and for the education of future rehabilitation practitioners.

This chapter lays the foundation for those that follow. It explains the use of various terms and devices and begins to construct an argument for the importance of theoretical perspectives that will be developed throughout subsequent chapters. Acknowledging that many of the contentions and arguments in this book challenge both traditional rehabilitation dogma and professional dominance, research and experiential literature will be used liberally to demonstrate the evidence bases that support the book's contentions. A glossary outlines particular words and theories with which rehabilitation therapists might not be familiar.

WHAT IS THE RELEVANCE OF THEORY?

This is a book about ideas: a book about theories. A *theory* is a framework of ideas that is formulated to explain something; a system of explanatory principles. By definition, theories are speculative in nature and vary in the degree to which they are supported by substantive evidence.

However, because theories – even when unacknowledged or unstated – inform professional actions, theories are more than sets of formalized ideas, taken-for-granted assumptions or systems of beliefs: how we think determines how we act. Within the rehabilitation industry, the ways in which 'disability' and 'rehabilitation' are theorized determine professional actions and the nature of the response to disability. As students, clinicians, theorists, researchers or educators, we therefore need to develop an acute sensitivity to the imbedded values and assumptions in society, in our professions and in current theories and cultivate an acute self-awareness of our personal values, perspectives and biases (Field & Morse 1985). Because theories about disability have consequences for disabled people, they must be exposed to rigorous critical analysis and demonstrated to be able to withstand the challenge of alternative perspectives (failing which, they must be revised). This book is a contribution to this process.

EXPLORING THEORIES AND ASSUMPTIONS: THE INTELLECTUAL IMPERATIVE

Historically, disability as a subject of inquiry was surrendered to the medical and healthcare professions, with few researchers in other intellectual fields demonstrating an interest in – or awareness of – this minority group. In addition, prohibitive barriers to higher education guaranteed that few disabled people had the opportunity to penetrate academia or influence the agendas of researchers. In the absence of contesting evidence, contrasting viewpoints or informed critiques, the rehabilitation professions were able to cling to their traditional assumptions without fear of challenge. This is no longer the case.

Within the past decade, disability has been subjected to critical interrogation by theorists from many academic disciplines. Throughout the social sciences and humanities, disability is increasingly being explored as a category of difference, like gender, that is defined according to specific social, cultural and historic contexts. In addition, in the same way that many universities have embraced departments of gender (or women's) studies and of gay and lesbian studies to facilitate scholarly research and thinking around issues of difference, so they are developing departments dedicated to disability studies.

Publications taking a critical stance toward the concept of disability began in the mid-1960s with the writings of a few disabled activists, such as Paul Hunt (1966). With the advent of a course pertaining to disability, created in the mid-1970s by the British Open University, there began a small trickle of literature that explored disability from an analytical perspective (e.g. Boswell & Wingrove 1974, Brechin et al 1981). This was augmented, in 1986, by an international journal, *Disability, Handicap and Society* (subsequently renamed *Disability and Society*). From about 1993, the trickle turned into a veritable tidal wave, with over 50 influential books arising in Australia, Canada, France, the UK and USA, and from diverse academic departments that have included sociology, social policy, anthropology, cultural studies, philosophy, gender studies, critical "race" studies, gay and lesbian studies, disability studies, law, development studies, literary studies, education, political science, history and geography. Formerly comprising a few anecdotal autobiographies, the disability literature now constitutes a broad-ranging, critical and contested field of study.

That this voluminous literature has been largely ignored by the rehabilitation professions is nothing short of extraordinary. Yet examination of the reference lists in professional journals and rehabilitation texts demonstrates that few theorists, therapists or nurses have elected to engage with the critiques and issues that arise from this parallel literature.

Further, despite the large number of books being published in the area of disability studies, these are rarely reviewed in the official journals of the rehabilitation professions. This has perpetuated the ignorance of alternative perspectives and limited the potential for exposure to a range of ideas.

In light of current political imperatives for client-centred practice, for consumer involvement and for evidence-informed practice, this lack of engagement with intellectual challenges must be both acknowledged and addressed. Because it is apparent that few rehabilitation professionals have kept pace with developments in the field of disability studies, this book is intended to introduce the ideas, theories, controversies and challenges that are arising from multiple perspectives. Contemporary theorists raise important questions, for example, about concepts of normality, independence and the physical body – issues central to rehabilitation – as well as to the role of cultural and social environments in producing prejudice and creating disadvantage; and to issues of power and privilege and of the systemic oppression of disabled people with which rehabilitation professionals are perceived to collude (Northway 1997).

Seeking to combat the traditional insularity of rehabilitation ideologies, this book argues for a cross-fertilisation of ideas. It also challenges hierarchies of power through which rehabilitation professionals privilege their own assumptions, perspectives and knowledge while overlooking or ignoring the perspectives both of disabled people and of other researchers and theorists.

KNOWLEDGE AND POWER

It has been observed that the more powerful ideas become and the greater their longevity, the greater their ability to survive contact with contesting evidence (Childs & Williams 1997). Clearly, if contesting evidence is overlooked, ignored or excluded, professional ideas, assumptions and dogma will survive indefinitely.

Recent critiques from disability theorists challenge those rehabilitation assumptions cited at the opening of this chapter, suggesting instead that the rehabilitation professions are not apolitical and that the rehabilitation process is often irrelevant, meaningless and useless (Abberley 1995, Morris 1991). The correlation between increased function and independence with perceptions of enhanced quality of life is challenged (Hammell 2004a) and the relationships between professionals and their patients and clients is perceived not as benevolent, client-centred and helpful, but as hierarchical and disempowering (Abberley 1995, Barnes & Mercer 2003, Dalley 1999, Johnson 1993, Jorgensen 2000, Morris 1991), with therapists perceived as sharing a pessimistic, deflating ethos (Cant 1997). At worst, the rehabilitation and healthcare professions are believed to constitute part of the problem of living with impairments (Barnes & Mercer 2003, French & Swain 2001, Oliver 1996a).

The dominance of one theory over another reflects particular alignments – or collusions – of power and knowledge. It is appropriate that professions espousing a client-centred orientation acknowledge the work of those about whom we theorize, determining the degree to which 'our' theories correspond to 'theirs'. There is also a need to explore disability from a wider perspective than that enabled through one disciplinary discourse. (*Discourses* are specific ways of thinking and speaking about the world.) An openness to, and respect for, others requires an appreciation of diverse intellectual positions and experiences (Williams 2001).

'There is no single *right* way to look at disability in society – but I would argue there is a wrong way. The wrong way is to mistake one's own disciplinary training as the only approach to understanding disability' (Groce 1999a p 291). Academic disciplines are arbitrary constructs with unstable boundaries. Postmodern theorists have criticized the production of knowledge within traditional axes of power such as specialized, compartmentalized 'disciplines' (Best & Kellner 1991, Foucault 1980). Real lives – and the worlds in which these lives are lived – cannot be neatly compartmentalized and demarcated into separate areas of disciplinary interest. A range of perspectives is required that traverses disciplinary boundaries and ideological frameworks in order to critique the foundations for claims to knowledge within the rehabilitation business.

EXPLORING THEORIES: THE IMPERATIVE OF EVIDENCE-BASED PRACTICE

In many countries, government policies and professional guidelines insist that healthcare practice should be 'evidence based' (Gomm & Davis 2000). Willingly embraced by the rehabilitation professions, since the mid-1990s evidence-based practice (see Chapter 10) has emerged as one of the most influential concepts in rehabilitation (Carpenter 2004a). Evidence-based medicine is said to integrate the '*best research evidence* with *clinical expertise* and *patient values*' (Sackett et al 2000 p 1). It is claimed that as evidence-based practice is incorporated into 'the practitioner's repertoire, the professions will see a shift to a more analytical, certain, and ultimately effective clinical practice in health care' (Law 2002 p 8). Thus, evidence-based practice is a foundation for professional competence (Hammell & Carpenter 2004).

As might be expected, the requisites for sound evidence-based practice are almost precisely reflected in the requirements for sound clinical reasoning. There is recognition among the rehabilitation professions that clinical expertise reflects a complex equation that includes *theoretical knowledge* in a process of clinical reasoning (see Chapter 8) that is informed by research evidence and the experiences of the therapist and the client; with an overall client-centred focus to ensure relevance (Hammell 2004a, Higgs & Bithell 2001). However, Carpenter (2004a p 8) observed that 'the role of theory in guiding clinical practice and research inquiry, and thus informing how rehabilitation professionals respond to individual client circumstances, has rarely been made explicit'. This lack of attention to the role of theory makes claims of allegiance to evidence-based practice both problematic and contestable.

Theories guide all professional actions, informing what we believe should be done in various situations (Hammell & Carpenter 2000). Recent focus on evidence-based practice has exposed the paucity of research evidence that either informs or supports occupational therapy theories (Hammell 2004b, Suto 2004, Walker et al 2000), a situation that is not unique to this one profession. Clearly, if theory informs rehabilitation practice (as it should), then research evidence must inform rehabilitation theory (Hammell 2004c). Providing research is undertaken in a rigorous and ethical manner, no good argument can be made for restricting the sources of such evidence.

EPISTEMOLOGY: WHOSE KNOWLEDGE AND PERSPECTIVES COUNT?

Any discussion of the multiple viewpoints from which a given issue can be interpreted or understood demands consideration of epistemology. *Epistemology* is the branch of philosophy concerned with theories of knowledge: beliefs about the nature of knowledge, how knowledge can be acquired and the reliability of claims to knowledge.

Knowledge is generated, in a formal way, through rigorous research. Many researchers in the health and social sciences believe that it is impossible to be objective, detached or devoid of values and that all researchers – whether using qualitative or quantitative methodologies – make interpretations of data according to their backgrounds and experience (Hammell 2002a, Holman 1993). These are epistemological assumptions.

Epistemological considerations include such issues as: Whose knowledge 'counts'? Do the theoretical perspectives of the rehabilitation professions have more merit than those of social scientists or of disability activists? If this is our belief, on what basis might such claims to superiority be made? Do the conjectures of therapists 'trump' those of their clients? Do rehabilitation professionals assume that they possess 'knowledge' (superior), whereas clients have 'beliefs' (inferior)? (Good 1994). On what basis? Whose theories inform how we act? Are dissenting perspectives permitted or ignored? This book aims to broaden the range of perspectives and theories that are permitted to penetrate the rehabilitation agenda. Clearly, issues of epistemology are also issues of power.

CONTENTIOUS TERMINOLOGY: "SCARE" QUOTES

Throughout this book, double quotation marks "..." will be used as scare quotes to indicate contentious and contested terms about which I have reservations. Single quotes are reserved for citations of the writings or comments of others. I use [*sic*] within quoted passages when I am uncomfortable with a word or expression utilized by the original author.

Scientific advances such as DNA analysis have demonstrated, for example, that the concept of race has no scientific basis (Davis 2002a, Thomas 1999). Davis (2001) explained that the very concept of "race" must be understood as the product of a particular period of history. Theories of race were central to the project of imperialism; indeed "race" was a construction of colonialism, used to justify "race"-based political rights, occupational allocation and income (Balibar & Wallerstein 1996). Cast adrift from its presumed foundation in biology, "race" can therefore be understood as a socially constructed phenomenon: an invention that provides the justification for inequalities and racism. Thus "race" is a contentious and contested term.

Similarly, the term "expert" is a problematic one for rehabilitation therapists. If a therapist applies specific, technical treatments for minor, short-term orthopaedic problems, for example, claims to expertise might be justifiable. However, this is not rehabilitation; it is treatment. Rehabilitation, by definition, is a process of enabling someone to live well with an impairment in the context of his or her environment and, as such, requires a complex, individually tailored approach (Hammell 2004a), making claims to "expert" status suspect. Indeed, it is rarely clear on what basis claims to expertise are made by rehabilitation therapists: whether, for example, this is on the basis of published peer-reviewed research, attainment of a doctoral degree, the esteem of one's peers, or from a perception that competence somehow accrues with 'patient miles' – the number of clients/patients treated over many years (Richardson 1999, Sumsion 1998). The latter proposition is particularly problematic in light of early research suggesting that misperceptions of clients' problems by rehabilitation professionals might actually worsen with the length of clinical experience (e.g. Bodenhamer et al 1983, Ernst 1987). It is important to note that 'experience' is not necessarily a positive term and is not a synonym for 'expertise'. Indeed, many clinicians who have years of experience demonstrate less expertise than recent graduates.

Some researchers have elected to refer to 'élite' therapists (Craik & Rappolt 2003), a term that is so unabashedly élitist as to be unable to withstand even the most tentative critique of client/professional power imbalances or of hierarchical, disempowering relationships with clients.

The term "expert" implies the superiority of certain sorts of knowledge. It privileges the therapist's knowledge and experience over the client's experiential knowledge and serves to reinforce and entrench professional dominance (see Chapter 9). Indeed, because 'adopting the position of the expert is immediately to adopt a position of power' (Childs & Williams 1997 p 22), the very notion of professional expertise must be deconstructed (Fook 2000). It is intriguing that claims to expertise are generally made without reference to the views of clients, who have noted instead that therapists demonstrate very little knowledge of what it means to live as a disabled person in the community (Hammell 1995) and whose interventions are therefore often perceived to be irrelevant (Abberley 1995). This is not to suggest a devaluing of professional expertise but to propose a form of practice in which the expertise of therapists is not privileged but viewed alongside the knowledge and experience (expertise) of others. Thus, whereas therapists might make legitimate claims to possessing specific, clinical expertise, the term 'expert' must be broadened to respect the knowledge of people who have different positions and perspectives based on their experiences as users of health care and as experts concerning their own problems, needs and perceptions of life's quality (Hammell 2004c).

CONTENTIOUS TERMINOLOGY: DISABLED PEOPLE

The use of the term 'disabled people' throughout this book rather than 'people with disabilities' is controversial but intentional. Oliver (1993 p 261) observed: 'it has been suggested that the term "people with disabilities" should be used in preference to "disabled people". This fits with the world view of liberal professionals who prefer to think about people first who just happen to have disabilities'. However, 'disabled people' is the preferred terminology of those within the disability movement who use it to make a political statement: they are not people 'with' disabilities, rather, they are people who are disabled (disadvantaged) by society's response to their differences (e.g. Coleridge 1993, DePoy & Gilson 2004, Driedger 1989, Morris 1993a, Oliver 1990).

Many disability theorists view disability as a social, cultural, economic and political phenomenon, claiming that environmental barriers disable people who have mental, intellectual or physical impairments (Oliver 1996a). They contend that referring to a 'person with a disability' implies that disability is something that an individual 'has', like a headache (DePoy & Gilson 2004, Oliver & Barnes 1998), arguing that 'this sidesteps the need for social and environmental change and explicitly denies the political nature of disability' (Swain et al 2003 p 14). Neufeldt (1999 p 32) explains: 'disability results when a person with an impairment encounters an inaccessible environment. It is therefore the environment which disables the person and so the term "person with a disability" is incorrect'. As subsequent chapters will demonstrate, an understanding of disability that is informed by critical disability theory recognizes that people with impairments might be disabled people, but renders the term 'people with disabilities' completely meaningless. To demonstrate their rejection of a term they regard as both incorrect and inane, some disability theorists refer to ablebodied people as 'people with abilities' (e.g. Finkelstein 1999a), because obviously if 'they' are 'people with disabilities', then 'we' must be 'people with abilities'. Thus, far from asserting politically correct, 'people first' terminology, this particular mode of semantics affirms the "inferiority" of some people and the "superiority" of others.

Further, 'the term "disabled people" is the choice of the major representative organizations of disabled people throughout the world and to use other terminology is to deny authenticity to the collective voice of disabled people' (Oliver 1993 p 261–2). For example, it has been the choice of Disabled Peoples' International, the global, 'grassroots' and cross-disability coalition of disabled people that is recognized by the United Nations as 'the representative voice of disabled people internationally' (Swain et al 2003 p 154).

Oliver (1990 p xiii) explained that disability is not something one 'has', indeed, 'far from being an appendage, disability is an essential part of the self'; just as being black is more fundamental to identity and experience than being a person 'with' black skin (Coleridge 1993). As Biko (1978 p 48) observed, 'being black is not a matter of pigmentation'.

Long preferred by disabled theorists and rights activists in the UK, the term 'disabled people' is increasing in usage among theorists in North America (Linton 1998). Further, as S. Miles (1996 p 515) has observed, 'parents have argued that they are disabled by virtue of being the full-time carers of severely disabled children and that, together with their children, they are affected by the stigma of disability'. Acknowledging that disability is something imposed on those who are impacted by impairments enables consideration of families who have an impaired member: they might all be disabled by their interactions with environments that are exclusionary and designed only for certain sorts of people and their families.

However, the stigma that attaches to the word 'disability' and its cultural connotations of ab-normality and in-validity, means that it is not embraced by all disabled people. Katbamna et al (2000) suggest that 'explanations for the persistence of negative perceptions of disability are located in the social construction of "normality" and "abnormality"' (see Chapter 2). Parents, in particular, might reject a description of their 'disabled child', believing this to connote an inadequacy in their child rather than inadequacies in the child's environment.

Nonetheless, if we are to begin to see disability in a new way, incorporate the perspectives of disability theorists, acknowledge the political nature of disability issues (Law 2004) and privilege the theories devised by disabled people rather than rehabilitation 'élites', the term 'disabled people' might be a useful place to start. 'The debate is not merely an academic one, or one of "political correctness". At the heart of it is the question of how one sees the impairment as distinct from the disability' (Neufeldt 1999 p 32). It also affects how one understands the concept of rehabilitation (see Chapter 4).

Using the term 'able-bodied' as a binary opposite to 'disabled' is inappropriate and will be avoided wherever possible. Binary opposites reflect a specific, Western ideology that has no equivalent within Eastern thought and that is contested by contemporary theorists. The tendency to name dualistic categories such as man/woman, white/black, straight/gay, able/disabled rightly locates social power with the privileged (left) label but is an unstable practice with little basis in reality (see Chapter 3). McRuer (2002) observed that able-bodiedness is defined by the Oxford English Dictionary in terms of the ability to work. Originating in the nineteenth century and the rise of industrial capitalism, this is a term that betrays its political roots: to be able-bodied is to be available to participate in particular systems of labour. Further, although 'able-bodiedness' can be differentiated from physical impairment, it obscures or ignores those with learning difficulties or mental illnesses, who might experience functional impairments and disability in the absence of physical 'imperfections' (Chappell 1998).

The term 'disability' is therefore used in this book to connote the physical, political, economic, legal, social and cultural experience of living with an impairment. Because the largest proportion of impairments are acquired in adulthood, many of the book's arguments and examples are structured around acquired rather than congenital impairments. Further, because the body and mind are indivisible, the word 'body' is generally employed as a more convenient way of denoting the body/mind.

CONTENTIOUS TERMINOLOGY: DISABILITY THEORY

Several universities have taken the term 'disability studies' and used it to describe programmes they have developed for studying people with impairments from a traditional, problem-oriented perspective that explores the ways in which disabled people might be "managed". Their focus is on service provision designed, delivered and evaluated by service providers, frequently underpinned by an agenda of cost containment.

Throughout this book, the terms 'disability studies', 'disability theory' (or 'theorists') or 'critical disability theory' are used to identify those pro-grammes of study, theorists or theoretical perspectives that take a *critical* approach to disability, in line with a commitment to advancing the social and political rights of disabled people (Thomas 1999). 'Critical theories' challenge conventional ideologies, identify oppressive social structures and promote social change. Critical theorists recognize 'that ideas possess a dual-edged capacity to both control and liberate' (Thomas 1993 p 20). Acknowledging that no theory can be objective or politically neutral, critical theory is explicitly focused on a goal of social justice.

CONTENTIOUS TERMINOLOGY: PATIENTS OR CLIENTS?

As an occupational therapist, I am accustomed to using the term 'client' and shall do so throughout this book. I recognize that this is a contentious term that often constitutes little more than lip-service to the notions of choice and empowerment that the word implies. Calling people 'clients' does not lead automatically to affording them the choice, or treating them with the respect, this term invokes.

Davis (1993) has argued that the term 'client' implies a degree of choice that is rarely available to disabled people. Rather than being able to select the therapist of one's choice (as one might a lawyer or a plumber), disabled people find instead that they are assigned their service providers. Further, Hugman (1991) observed that because health professionals are agents of the State (or private companies), it is the State or employer that tends to be viewed as the client, rather than the service user. This tension leads to the perception that those 'in the disability industry are the gatekeepers to the services we need' (Davis 1993 p 197): that therapists are accountable to their employer (or the State) in preference to their clients.

Davis (1993) also claimed that the decision to adopt the word 'client' reflects a pattern of practice in which professionals choose and define the nature of their relationship with disabled people. Indeed, the decision to adopt client-centred language arose from therapists themselves and was not the consequence of consultation with clients. It is worth noting that although occupational therapists, for example, have long defined what they mean by 'client-centred practice' (e.g. Canadian Association of Occupational Therapists (CAOT) 1983), more than 15 years passed before occupational ther-apy researchers asked clients what client-centred practice meant to them (Bibyk et al 1999, Corring 1999, Corring & Cook 1999; see Chapter 9).

In reality, Davis (1993 p 198) claimed that use of the term 'client' is 'a very neat bit of professional sleight of speech, [falsely] suggesting equivalence in choice and control'. I recognize, also, that the term 'patient' is a more apt description of one's powerless status in an emergency department, or in an acute-care or intensive-care situation and that 'client' is an inappropriate descriptor in certain circumstances.

However, 'patient' has historically been used to connote passivity and to reify power imbalances between people who are ill or injured and their professional caregivers, and for this reason alone it is less than satisfactory. It is also an overused term, such that researchers studying the experience of living with a diagnosed impairment for a period of many years will often refer to autonomous adults (who might not have sought medical care for considerable time) as 'patients' rather than 'people'. Further, because impairment can impact the lives of partners, parents and others, rehabilitation professionals might be involved with multiple family members (Oliver 1981); thus 'patient' is an artificially restrictive concept. In the absence of a more appropriate term, 'client' will have to suffice.

The term 'consumer' is also rejected because it reinforces the idea that professionals produce and clients consume (McKnight 1981), thus supporting, rather than challenging, notions of professional superiority and client dependency. Indeed, when a Swedish man with high tetraplegia informed me that he 'consumes three nurses a day' I realized that the term is completely untenable!

For convenience and readability, the term 'therapists' will be used in its original Greek sense, as a broad concept that includes all rehabilitation professionals who provide specialized intervention or care for disabled people. When specific therapists (such as physiotherapists) are discussed, this will be made clear.

CHALLENGING ASSUMPTIONS; CONTESTING POWER

I support the contention that the role of intellectuals in any discipline is to challenge the *paradigms* (sets of basic beliefs or assumptions) inherent in their field, raise questions, confront dogma and unmask conventional and accepted ideas (Said 1996). The cultural critic and literary theorist, Edward Said (1979) advocated for rigorous intellectual engagement that would contest the uncritical acceptance of authoritative ideas. Said called for a sceptical approach to orthodoxy, proposing that: 'The intellectual must be involved in a lifelong dispute with all the guardians of sacred vision or text' (Said 1996 p 88–9). As the rehabilitation professions aspire to intellectual maturity, there can be no 'sacred texts' but, rather, a reflexive interrogation of our theories and a resistance to the colonizing effects of powerful dogma. Importantly, 'this does not mean opposition for opposition's sake. But it does mean asking questions . . . [during] the rush to collective judgment and action' (Said 1996 p 33).

Said advocated a sensitivity to the ways in which other people are studied (1979) and a sceptical and engaged analysis of the ways in which humanity is 'thrust into pigeonholes' (1976 p 41) that categorize how 'others' are different from 'us'. If for no other reason, this makes his observations relevant to those professions centrally concerned with people categorized as 'different'.

I suggest that because the rehabilitation professions are engaged not solely with ideas but with people – because our ideas have implications – the act of challenging paradigms, raising questions, confronting dogma and unmasking conventional and accepted ideas is too important to leave to our intellectuals. Rather, this must be the obligation of all students, clinicians, researchers, educators and theorists.

This book therefore aims to provide an accessible introduction to many of the perspectives on disability and rehabilitation that are being generated by disabled and disability theorists outside the rehabilitation professions. My intent is not to weigh the relative merits of different perspectives to provide "right" answers but to provoke a more questioning and intellectually rigorous stance towards the assumptions, beliefs and knowledge that inform our professional actions. I aim to demonstrate that different perspectives exist, that our beliefs are not unchallenged, and that many of the taken-for-granted assumptions that underpin the rehabilitation professions lack a supportive evidence base.

CRITICISM OR CRITIQUE?

Hasselkus (2002 p 53) observed: 'If we are brave enough to step outside our world of rehabilitation and health care, we find examples of very harsh criticism indeed, aimed at what may be described as the self-serving nature of what we do'. Our professions have rarely stepped outside the literature, theories and assumptions of our world of rehabilitation and health care. In so doing, the intent of this book is not to criticize and disparage healthcare workers or the rehabilitation professions, whose intentions, for the most part, are unimpeachable (although recognizing that positive intentions do not guarantee positive outcomes). Rather, it is to encourage a critical appraisal – a critique – of the assumptions that underpin these professions and their intentions. In this spirit, I encourage readers to approach the book with an enquiring mind rather than a defensive stance. This exploration will begin at the beginning, with an examination of the ways in which disability is habitually defined and classified.

Chapter 2

Normality and the classification of difference

It is not just important what we speak about, but how and why we speak.
(hooks 1990 p 151)

INTRODUCTION: CLASSIFYING DIFFERENCE

This chapter begins an exploration of one of the cornerstones of rehabilitation: the classification and categorization of physical, cognitive and mental deviations from an assumed norm.

Since 1980, the World Health Organization's systems for classifying impairments and disabilities have been embraced, largely uncritically, by the rehabilitation professions. Disability theorists have been less complacent, critiquing the premise of normality against which judgements of deviance are made, challenging the privilege or right of powerful "experts" to make such judgements and contesting the belief that the outcome of being classified as deviant is necessarily benign or benevolent (Hammell 2004d). Far from being mere differences of interpretation, these issues concern the way in which disabled people are perceived, the allocation of healthcare resources and, in some instances, survival itself.

The focus of this chapter will be upon the ideology of *normality*. The chapter that follows will explore the idea of deviance and the consequences of being defined as deviant from the norm.

THE ICIDH AND ICF: TOOLS FOR CLASSIFICATION

The World Health Organization (WHO) developed the International Classification of Impairments, Disabilities and Handicaps (ICIDH; WHO 1980) and, later, the International Classification of Functioning, Disability and Health (ICF; WHO 2001) to try to provide a framework for classifying the consequences of injuries and diseases. The ICIDH identified 'the consequences of diseases and disorders at the level of the body (impairment), the person (disability), and the person as a social being (handicap)' (Badley 1993 p 161). Impairments were deemed to be the cause of both disability and handicap, thus any problems encountered in daily living, including discrimination, were attributed to personal flaws.

The ICF (also known as 'ICIDH-2') represents an attempt to acknowledge that people interact with their environments, identifying 'impairments' (perceived problems in body function or structure), 'activity limitations' (difficulties in executing a task or action) and 'participation restrictions' (problems in functioning at the societal level; WHO 2001). The ICF model requires consideration both of personal factors that impact an individual's ability to act and to participate and of environmental factors. These include the physical contexts, social and cultural contexts (attitudes, values), economic contexts (social systems and services), political contexts (policies, rules) and legal contexts in which impairments are experienced.

Although the ICF approach might appear to hold considerable promise, it is not without problems. For example, there is no possibility within the model for contemplating the role of environments in the creation of impairments. The environment is depicted as impacting the individual but specifically not the disease or 'disorder', despite the reality that many diseases, illnesses and injuries are produced by wars, violence, abuse, landmines, poverty, malnutrition, unsafe work practices, pollution and through the unequal distribution of resources. Indeed, Pfeiffer (1998 p 519) has argued: 'when half the world goes to sleep hungry and hundreds of thousands of people face death every day, the ICIDH-2 [ICF] is pointless'.

Further, while the minutiae of individual differences are coded by the ICF, there is no equivalent capacity for classifying and coding the discriminatory dimensions of societies, the performance of governments or the effects of their policies (Baylies 2002). Despite rhetoric suggesting that the ICF acknowledges the interaction of people and environments, it is clearly a tool that explores the environment only in regard to how it impacts individual lives. There is no capacity to examine broader social, political, legal or economic impacts upon the production of wide-spread impairments; or the impact of environments on the social disadvantage, oppression and marginalization experienced by populations of disabled people. In addition, the ICF fosters a view of disabled people as catalogues of deficits and deprivations rather than as people with various abilities and resources.

Goffman (1963a p 11) noted that 'society establishes the means of categorising persons and the complement of attributes felt to be ordinary and natural for members of each of these categories'. This also provides a means by which to categorize the "unnatural".

The classification and coding of people with impairments has been something of a preoccupation for the WHO, which spent two decades and some considerable effort honing its taxonomies in an attempt to identify the consequences of impairments for everyday life. Although the intent of the ICF is undoubtedly sincere, Hurst (2000) observed that no other minority group has been subjected to such sustained appraisal, such that an in-depth classification of individual differences is seen as necessary for analysis of their status, for provision of health or community services or for the implementation of policies to assure their rights; nor would this be deemed acceptable for people from ethnic minorities, women, or any other minority group. However, classification of the differences of disabled people remains largely unchallenged, as if this is somehow both inevitable and necessary (Hammell 2004d).

Globally, it is acknowledged that, in comparison to boys, girls are allocated less medical care, experience lower rates of education and suffer higher rates of exploitation, sexual abuse and violence (Ear-Dupuy 2004). In parts of Sudan, for example, only 1% of girls go to school (Guardian Weekly 2005). Most people would probably acknowledge that this widespread inequality arises not from biological differences but from cultural practices, discrimination and patriarchy. It is also obvious that coding and classifying the ways in which girls differ physically from boys would provide no helpful information with which to assure equality of opportunity for girls. Rather, this requires political will (Hammell 2004g).

It will be interesting to observe whether – and how – use of the ICF classification will actually shift the focus of policy makers and researchers from individuals to environments (physical, social, cultural, economic, political, legal) to enable the coding, classification and *change* both of social policies and of the distribution of resources and opportunities within societies.

QUALIFYING CONSENSUS

Due to their broad acceptance and uncritical adoption by the rehabilitation professions (e.g. Crouch 2003), it is unnecessary to make a case here for why one might choose to subscribe to the WHO's systems of classification. Indeed, throughout the medical and rehabilitation literatures the WHO classifications tend to be used automatically and without reference to alternative models or theories, reflecting an apparently unchallenged assumption that this model, or way of thinking, is correct or "right" (Northway 1997). Achieving publication within the disability studies literature requires that authors 'demonstrate an awareness of the contested nature' of the ICF (Disability and Society 2004). However, the professional rehabilitation journals do not demand the same degree of intellectual rigour. This might, perhaps, reflect a reluctance to challenge a tool that has been developed and accepted by more dominant and powerful professional groups: the triumph of power over probity.

The opposition expressed by disabled people to the ICIDH and ICF classifications has been in stark contrast to their almost universal and uncritical acceptance by researchers (Barnes & Mercer 1996). Pfeiffer (2000) observed that the WHO classifications have been ridiculed by disabled people and argued that the ICF should be dropped and 'more fruitful' activities undertaken by its adherents (p 1080).

Four years before the original ICIDH was published, disabled theorists had already articulated their own model of impairment and disability (see Chapter 4). Regrettably, the perspectives of disabled people are rarely permitted to influence or infiltrate professional theories (Hammell 2004b). Without apparent irony, Brättemark (1996 p 4) reported that a workshop, entitled 'The usefulness of the ICIDH' enabled the 'subjects of classification' to meet the "experts" involved in revising the ICIDH. Such statements reveal much about who holds the power to classify whom. Indeed, disregard of the views of disabled people concerning the ICF is regarded by Pfeiffer (2000 p 1079) as 'proof' that healthcare professionals 'are a part of the advantaged class' who will never pay attention to disabled people's views.

Critics contend that the ICF perpetuates a view of disability as a medical issue and that this legitimates the unwelcome and inappropriate control of disabled people's lives by various medical and healthcare professions. Although acknowledging the importance of healthcare professionals to healthcare needs, they challenge the power of these professionals to make decisions that have nothing to do with medicine, such as measuring the quality of life of disabled people, determining where they can park their cars (through their role as gatekeepers to disabled parking permits) and whether they are capable of working (Pfeiffer 1998). However, Finkelstein (1999b p 23) claimed that 'the obsession with assessing and labelling us [with tools such as the ICF] will be vigorously defended by people with abilities whose careers are shaped within the framework of able-bodied chauvinism'.

CONSTRUCTING THE NORM

Within the WHO's models, 'impairments' are defined as deviations from socially defined norms (Bickenbach 1993); thus one of the authors of the original ICIDH asserted that 'the assessment of disability requires a judgement of what is normal' (Badley 1998 p 21). Importantly, this requires a *judgement* – an opinion – because norms do not exist outside the human ideas that create them (Hammell 2004d). Thus, classifying an impairment first requires the construction of "norms" against which deviations can be judged.

Badley (1998 p 21) further claimed that 'departure from the norm can be in the direction of both deficiencies and excesses of expected activity performance and behaviour'. More than just establishing a norm, or desirable standard, this constructs a sort of 'bell-curve' of expected or acceptable performance.

Disability theorists have noted that the concept of the "norm" only entered the European languages in the nineteenth century, hand in hand with the development of statistics (Davis 1995, Priestley 2003). The concept of the normal body had been preceded through history by that of the 'ideal': a set of mythical coordinates to which all might aspire but none conform (Hammell 2004d). Development of the mathematical concept of 'the norm' and of the 'normal (bell) curve' created both the concept of the norm and of *deviance* from the norm (Davis 1995). Thus, Davis (2002b p 101) observed that 'people in the past 150 years have been encouraged to strive to be normal, to huddle under the main part of the curve'. I use the unpleasant term 'deviance' in this book to draw particular attention to the way in which deviation results directly from the use of statistical techniques that differentiate people, one from another: classifying some as normal and others as deviant from the norm. Indeed, Dijkers et al (2000 p S67) observe that 'deviation is central to the concept of disability'.

However, researchers are always obliged to return to the original sources of ideas, and if one does so in this instance, one discovers that statisticians are more careful in their terminology than are their mimics, referring to 'deviations *from the assumption of normality*' (Bland 1991 p 179, emphasis added). Statisticians recognize, therefore, that norms do not represent biological realities but are human creations: assumptions. It is through the collection of specific sorts of data and the use of statistical techniques that '"norms" are created against which individuals can be judged and classified' (Twigg 2000 p 12). These statistical concepts have been uncritically appropriated and applied to all arenas of human activity, appearance and experience (Davis 1995, DePoy & Gilson 2004) in a process that Davis (1995 p 29) has described as the 'tyranny of the norm'.

"Norms" are neither neutral nor objective (Thomson 1997a). They are not universal concepts but are the creation of cultural judgements: 'In any society, what constitutes "normality" is fluid and flexible, according to how the dominant value systems change and develop' (Corbett 1997 p 94). The linkage here between 'dominance' and 'values' is especially important. Dominant groups hold the power to legitimate their own values, portraying these as neutral, natural and objective while determining which differences are inferior and abnormal. 'Because it is the dominant population who defines the rules governing life in the society, for any socially significant human characteristic it is the dominant attribute [white, heterosexual, able-bodied] which provides the positive value standard against which subordinate differences are judged as inferior' (Kallen 2004 p 33).

Medical historians have demonstrated that the criteria for normality have changed through time and have been subject to social and cultural forces (Bickenbach 1993). The male body, for example, was traditionally viewed as the norm by those who wielded the most social power. (Indeed, the ability to define social norms is dependent upon wielding social power.) Those who held this social power and whose views therefore 'counted' (i.e. men) judged the female form to be deviant and inferior (Thomson 1997a). Even today, most anatomy textbooks illustrate the male form as the 'gold standard', whereas the female body is of interest for the ways in which it deviates from this valued "norm". Indeed, Pfeiffer's (1999 p 107) contention that the ICIDH 'definition of "normal" is Western, white, male, middle-class behaviour' supports the premise that social power dictates the delineation of social norms.

Through its systems of classification, the WHO reifies the idea of normality without acknowledging that ideas of what is "normal" depend on culture and situation (Oliver 1990). Indeed, disability theorists argue that the ICF is constructed on specific, Western notions of "normality" (Barnes 2003). Because ideas about "normal behaviour" are culturally dependent, the WHO's definition of impairment enables the labelling of political dissent and homosexuality as biomedical impairments (Dickson 1996). This 'dangerous nonsense' (Dickson 1996 p 53) would permit the incarceration of political dissidents, through labelling unconventional behaviour (e.g. dissent) as insanity.

It is evident that disabled people are represented in the WHO's taxonomies not as different but as defective, deviant, subnormal and inferior (Bickenbach 1993); but why should this matter? It matters because the logical outcome of establishing "norms" and "non-norms" is the attempt to norm the non-standard – the aim not only of rehabilitation, but of eugenics (Davis 1995). Indeed, many early statisticians were closely allied to the eugenic movement (Barnes & Mercer 2003, Davis 1995). Disability theorists claim that both the ICIDH and ICF facilitate the type of thinking that leads to eugenics (Pfeiffer 1998). The fatal consequences of being judged to be deviant from the "norm" will be explored in depth in Chapter 3.

The normalizing judgement

The process by which "norms" are established and the actions or attributes of individuals are judged, classified, assessed, measured and compared was described by the influential French philosopher Michel Foucault (1977) as the *normalizing judgement*. Foucault challenged the belief that knowledge is independent of power, arguing that knowledge is tied to power because of the ways it is used to classify and normalize individuals (Danaher et al 2000). Foucault exposed the classificatory practices by which "experts" elaborate norms and define populations as deviant (Twigg 2000). He demonstrated that powerful people judge "normality" and then strive to achieve conformity through various interventions (Nettleton 1994). Foucault claimed that the normalizing judgement 'hierarchizes in terms of value the abilities, the level, the "nature" of individuals' (Foucault 1984 p 195). Thus, a normalizing judgement is a value judgement.

The process of revising the ICF has taken several years and has occupied academics from many disciplines in over 60 countries. The attempt to redefine the classifications, utilize non-stigmatizing language and produce an interactive (rather than linear) model has been meticulous and painstaking. However, one cannot help but recall Foucault and his depiction of the normalizing judgement as an instrument of power wherein the actions, participation, indeed value of each individual are assessed, measured and compared. A normalizing judgement is always a value judgement.

JUDGING "NORMALITY": THE EXERCISE OF POWER

One of the most powerful tools wielded by the dominant group in a society is the power to define people. 'Those with the most power are able to wield that power by imposing inferiorizing and *invalidating* labels on those with less power' (Kallen 2004 p 34). Despite being scientifically erroneous, 'once invalidating labels are imposed, dominant authorities can *justify injustice*' (Kallen 2004 p 35). Within rehabilitation, those who wield power – doctors, nurses, therapists – are socially privileged to judge the ways in which people deviate from valued cultural norms. Indeed, the process of defining "normality" and "abnormality" is inevitably a process by which the powerful define the powerless. Pfeiffer (1999 p 107) observed that disabled people do 'not get to decide what is "normal" nor even who is to decide what is "normal"', rather, medical "experts" are empowered to judge the people they define as abnormal, deviant or impaired (Pfeiffer 2000).

The ICF accords "experts" the authority to identify "normality", draw a distinction between the "normal" and the "abnormal" and assess the desirability of certain forms of performance (Douard 1995). Non-impaired "normality" is the yardstick against which disabled people are measured (Hurst 2000).

Advocates of systems that classify (other) people contend that they possess the expertise to judge the normal and the abnormal, the valued and the deviant, and that they have the right to do so. Clearly, they also hold the power to do so (Foucault 1977). Implicit within this exercise of power is the assessment of the 'expectations for usual functioning in physical, psychological and social terms' (Badley 1998 p 21) and the 'reasons' for any failures to achieve levels of performance deemed to be normal (Douard 1995). As Douard (1995) observed, this can never be an objective exercise. Although it is recognized that an individual's assessment of his or her situation is unavoidably 'subjective', it is less commonly acknowledged that assessments undertaken by "experts" are also subjective: '"objectivity" is not bestowed upon a measure merely because another person makes it' (Mor & Guadagnoli 1988 p 1056). Noting that the process of designating norms is inevitably value-laden and subjective, Baylies (2002 p 729) argued that: 'Claims to scientific objectivity through engaging expert practitioners to establish "anchor points" (i.e. of "normality") [are] somewhat spurious'. Every assessment reflects the values of those undertaking the assessment. This is not a politically neutral enterprise (Douard 1995), rather, 'power is veiled by a rhetoric of neutrality that creates the illusion of meritocracy' (Thomson 1997a p 40).

Duckett and Pratt (2001) contend that psychologists have contributed to the oppression of minority populations through their use of various classificatory tools. 'Disabled people, women, ethnic minority groups, lesbian women, gay men and low-income groups have all found themselves brutalised by psychological discourse ... This has been achieved through, among other tactics, the construction and use of tools such as Intelligence Quotient (IQ) tests and the mental health Diagnostic Statistical Manual (DSM). Both are riddled with disabilist, racist, sexist, homophobic and middle-class ideologies'.

Although classificatory tools might appear to be objective, neutral and scientific, critics contend that this is an illusion that masks the specific values and ideologies that support the status quo. For example, breaking the taboos of culturally accepted behaviour constitutes a deviation from the norm, but the manner in which this is classified is subject to class bias: 'if you are poor, then you are a misfit. If you are rich, then you are an eccentric' (Pfeiffer 1998 p 520). In nineteenth century America a category of dementia known as 'drapetomania' was identified among those slaves who demonstrated an uncontrollable urge to escape from slavery (Davis 1997). This provides further evidence of the social power underlying the designation of social norms; and the collusion between the classificatory practices of the medical professions and the sociopolitical status quo.

Disability theorists contest the power of "experts" to reserve for themselves the privilege of classifying other people and challenge the suggestion that every problem experienced by those deemed 'different' should be blamed on their differences (Douard 1995, Hammell 2003a, Pfeiffer 1998). They also reject the premise that impairment is the sole determining force in disabled people's lives or that an impairment is more salient than other dimensions of identity such as social role or economic status: a "master" status (Barnes & Mercer 1996). Importantly, they contest those rehabilitation practices that strive to norm the non-standard.

STRIVING FOR NORMALITY

Rehabilitation enforces 'a version of normalcy that pressures disabled persons to fit in by appearing and functioning as much like non-disabled persons as possible' (Kielhofner 2004 p 241).

The ideology of normality has tended to be accepted uncritically by rehabilitation professionals (French 1994a, Oliver 1996a). Indeed, the rehabilitation professions have created their own norms; for example, "normal" posture, "normal" gait, "normal" handwriting. Jarman et al (2002 p 561) suggest that each rehabilitation profession 'must foster society's ongoing acceptance of its norms [e.g. "normal" gait, "normal" speech] in order to perpetuate its viability and gain access to new economic niches'. Thus the ideology of normality serves to reinforce professional power.

Once norms have been established, these easily become the goals towards which everyone 'ought' to aspire and strive (Pfeiffer 1998). Indeed, the actions of therapists are said to be 'implicitly designed to make individuals more "normal"' (Stalker & Jones 1998 p 180). From their experiences as rehabilitation clients, disabled people have criticized the emphasis that is placed on efforts to appear "normal", claiming that pursuit of this particular ideology is often undertaken at the expense of function, comfort or expediency (French 1994a, Meekosha 1998). They argue that the goal of "normality" reflects dominant standards and values of ableist societies and might not be in the best interest of disabled people. (*Ableism* refers to social practices that assume and privilege [physical] ability.) Goffman (1963a) noted that repeated and often painful medical and surgical procedures are frequently undertaken solely with the goal of making an individual appear more "normal".

Tara (cited in Miller et al 2004 p 31) complained that she and other disabled children: 'were told that we must be as "normal" as possible'. Indeed, disability scholars contend that the pressure placed on disabled children to strive for "normality" and conformity could constitute serious abuse (Middleton 1999, Priestley 2003, Swain et al 2003). A former rehabilitation client exclaimed: 'I couldn't see the point of all those agonizing exercises' (Begum 1994 p 48); and another reported that physiotherapy 'was painful and demoralising' (Middleton 1999 p 18). Although disabled people are encouraged in Western cultures to strive for 'functional improvement' through rigorous physiotherapy, Sandahl (2003) suggests this might be to achieve physiotherapy's normalizing goals rather than its supposed therapeutic ones: an effort to induce conformity rather than enhance function.

The rehabilitation enterprise, Kielhofner (2004) suggests, can be seen as reinforcing social control and maintaining social norms: 'therapy aims to eliminate clients' characteristics and traits that threaten the legitimacy of mainstream values, ideals, practices and rules' (p 241). Thus, rehabilitation is a political practice. It should not be surprising that disability theorists contend that "normality" is 'the illusion at the heart of the oppression of disabled people' (Drake 1998 p 183).

THE FUNCTIONS OF CLASSIFYING IMPAIRMENTS AND FUNCTIONS

The WHO's classifications were ostensibly designed to enable the identification of unmet needs among disabled people (although the difficulty in identifying needs from a system designed to classify individuals was evident even in the original ICIDH). Perhaps this best illustrates the degree to which disabled people are viewed as deviant from the norm – from 'us' – such that their needs for clean water, health care, homes, families, education, gainful employment opportunities, transportation and other basic rights cannot, apparently, be predicted or anticipated (Frost 1999, Hammell 2004d). As Shakespeare (1997a p 9) observed: 'disabled people do not have special needs. We have the same needs as anyone else'.

David, a resident of Vancouver, Canada who is paralysed below the neck following a fall explained, 'We just want what everyone wants – a home, family, a job – this isn't rocket science!'. Jomo, who also has a spinal cord injury (but with some residual arm function), and who lives in a remote village in Malawi, identified similar concerns, 'I would like to have a small grinding mill to serve the local farmers, so I would have more money to pay the friend who helps me with everything; money for food, soap and to educate my children and to construct a suitable house' (personal communication). The difficulties Jomo experiences in attaining basic medical supplies and in living in a hut with a doorway that is narrower than his wheelchair, in one of the world's poorest countries, precisely replicate those of Native Americans living on reservations in South Dakota, USA (Stillman 1994), in the world's wealthiest country. People who have impairments have "normal" needs, but Abberley (1993 p 111) argued that it is on the basis 'of having an abnormal number of our needs unmet [for education, housing, employment, transportation, etc.], that I think it is right to speak of disabled people as not being normal'. However, 'the idea that disabled people's needs are special has become part of the uncritical dogma that informs service provision' (Finkelstein & Stuart 1996 p 172–3).

Although many potential benefits were ascribed to the ICIDH and, later, to the ICF, the primary use of these classifications is for compiling statistics, filing and retrieving case records (according to the specified categories), assessing deviations from "normality" and determining eligibility for services and programmes (Badley 1998, Gray & Hendershot 2000). Clearly, such systems of classification are tools to assist professionals and bureaucrats in their work; they do not have any inherent benefit for those being coded and classified (Hammell 1998a).

Peters (1995) suggested that any progress towards the sort of broad understanding of disability outlined by the ICIDH requires an examination of the disablement experience from the perspectives of the insider. This apparently innovative notion – of asking people about their experience of disability and thus about their needs – has been the cornerstone of the Spinal Injuries Association (SIA) in Britain and has been the basis on which it has planned programmes and delivered services. Without recourse to a system to classify the consequences of injury, the SIA polled its membership (people with spinal cord lesions) and asked what they needed. From this database the SIA established peer counselling services; organized a personal care assistant scheme; lobbied for legislative changes pertaining to transportation, medical supplies, equipment and human rights; and bought wheelchair-accessible, affordable holiday accommodation (Campbell & Oliver 1996, d'Aboville 1991, Oliver & Hasler 1987). Notably, SIA was the first such organization in the UK run by, instead of for, disabled people and it developed workable, relevant models of service delivery 'in the teeth of opposition from professionals' (Campbell & Oliver 1996 p 187).

IMPLICATIONS FOR REHABILITATION

The ICF, like its predecessor the ICIDH, has been enthusiastically embraced by the rehabilitation professions (e.g. Crouch 2003, Stewart 2002), who posit all manner of benefits of their use to therapists, despite simultaneously noting that the ICF is 'a classification system' (Stewart 2002 p 17), 'a scientific coding system' (Crouch 2003 p 19). It is important to bear in mind that this is all it is. Although advocates claim, for example, that the ICF can inform service delivery, illuminate the experience of disability, structure outcome measurements or enable health promotion, this is not its purpose. The purpose of the ICF is to *classify* differences and deviations from assumed norms in every area of human life. The WHO taxonomies are not needs assessments but systems for classifying and documenting deviations from an assumed norm (Law 1992). This is their intent, clearly stated in their titles.

In addition, if therapists are to address outcomes that are relevant to individuals who have impairments then problems with 'activities' or 'participation' must be determined from the perspective of each client – not a self-defined "expert" – yet the ICF is neither a person-centred assessment tool nor one that incorporates people's appraisals of their own quality of life (Wade & Haligan 2003).

In Chapter 1 it was suggested that there is no one 'right' way to think about the issues to be discussed in this book. However, exposure to different perspectives requires that we do, at the very least, *think* about these issues; and that we think about them in a critical manner. Clearly, the use of the ICF is not 'wrong', but neither is it 'right'. Rather, its latent ideology, assumptions and implications must be critically appraised and cautiously applied whenever it is employed. Use of the ICF – or any system of classification – should not be inevitable.

Attempts will doubtless be made to try to find ways of making current rehabilitation models and theories fit the powerful ideology of the ICF. In particular, one can anticipate efforts to squeeze occupational therapy's theories of activity and participation ('occupation') into the WHO's more influential ICF framework (Hammell 2004d). However, intellectual rigour requires a critical stance, and an unwillingness to accept easy formulae or the conventional, received ideas of the powerful (Said 1996).

ALLOCATING RESOURCES

Discrimination against disabled people is often claimed to stem from superstitions, religious and cultural prejudices; however, the WHO's classifications have spawned two measures – the 'QALY' and the 'DALY' – that are used for global policy-making and serve to legitimate and institutionalize discrimination against disabled people by justifying the inequitable distribution of social and economic resources. Despite (or because of) this, these measures are enthusiastically embraced by many economists (Murray & Acharya 1997).

The quality-adjusted life year (QALY) and the disability-adjusted life year (DALY) are complementary concepts: 'QALYs are years of healthy life lived; DALYs are years of healthy life lost' (Arnesen & Nord 1999 p 1423). The QALY and DALY are both informed by the belief that the value of a life is determined solely by health status (Arnesen & Nord 1999) and they share some basic assumptions: 'First, that an individual or group's life quality can be described in a rigorous manner based solely on the presence or absence of physical conditions deviating from those of the normal population. Secondly, that future life quality can be accurately predicted solely on the basis of current physical condition, irrespective of social values or context. Finally, predictive instruments assume that positive life quality cannot be achieved in the presence of physical deficits' (Koch 2000 p 422). In summary, both these instruments are based on the premise that people who deviate from a set of physical "norms" cannot attain a positive life quality under any circumstances.

The quality-adjusted life year

The QALY is a quasi-scientific measure designed to prioritize health and social services (French 2004a). The QALY method entails multiplying each year of life of a person who survives an illness or injury by a fraction that expresses the impairment of quality of life believed to be experienced by that person (Walsh 1993).

Williams (1985), who designed the QALY, assessed quality of life by correlating degree of disability (based on physical mobility) with level of distress (as imagined by an "expert" panel). The rationale for this was that without freedom of mobility people are unable to perform daily living activities or engage in normal social interactions and are thus prohibited from enjoying both the ordinary pleasures of everyday life and the more subtle aspects of high-quality living. However, sociologists have observed that Williams does not enable consideration of the *reason* for impaired mobility: his primary quality of life indicator (Mulkay et al 1987). Is mobility impaired because of an impairment, because no suitable wheelchair is provided, because housing is not accessible or because no means of affordable transportation is available?

The outcome of QALY calculations will be dependent on who determines the quality of life rating (Gomm 2000). Perversely, the QALY determines this by "expert" consensus: quality of life is derived by asking a cross-section of people to imagine what life with a particular impairment might be like (Drummond 1987). This is an imaginative task and one that depends entirely on value judgements. It is also an enterprise that lacks evidence-based support. The profound discrepancy between imagination and the reality of living with an impairment has been demonstrated by many researchers (e.g. Bach & Barnett 1996, Basnett 2001, Menzel et al 2002, Woodend et al 1997). (The oppressive construct of 'the "expert"' has already been outlined in Chapter 1.)

QALYs are not just about defining options but about establishing the 'value frame' within which options are considered (Hodge 1994 p 53). Disabled people fall outside this value frame. Rather than attempting 'to equalize the physical and psychological disparities of the human condition, in attempts to give everyone a fair chance to live a decent life' (Dougherty 1994 p 65), the QALY is a tool that justifies and facilitates the inequitable distribution of healthcare resources.

Quality of life judgements reflect particular values, such that members of a society who do not embody valued cultural norms will be judged to have a low quality of life (Wolfensberger 1994). Singer and colleagues (1995 p 144) claimed that 'QALY thinking' places all disabled people on a lower ranking of quality of life than people in the majority population, thus the QALY gives a lower value to preserving the lives of people who have a permanent impairment than to preserving the lives of those who are not disabled.

Rawles (1989) contested the fundamental premise underpinning the QALY, arguing that to equate the value of human life with the absence of impairment is to undervalue human existence. He contended that 'life is valued for infinitely more reasons than absence of suffering' (p 146). The assumption that life is more valuable with a 'perfect' body is one manifestation of a specific, Western, materialistic frame of reference (Dijkers 1999). Indeed, although many Western theorists appear to equate any degree of suffering with a life that is inferior and one that ought to be avoided (or eliminated), this is not a universal ideology. Existential and Buddhist philosophies, for example, view suffering as an integral – indeed, inevitable – part of life (Kupperman 2001, Lavine 1984).

It is difficult to reconcile the logic of the QALY model with evidence that perceptions of quality of life are not dependent on physical function and that suicide rates are actually higher among people with 'marginal' impairments than among those with more profound functional deficits (e.g. DeVivo & Stover 1995, Hartkopp et al 1998). A growing body of research literature has failed to find a correlation between the severity of an impairment or degree of function and either distress (emotional suffering) or life satisfaction (e.g. Dallmeijer & van der Woude 2001, Elfström et al 2002, Macleod & Macleod 1998, Putzke et al 2002). Nonetheless, once it has been decided that the quality of life of people who have impairments must, by definition, be 'worse than death', it is a short, "logical" step to eugenics (Pfeiffer 1998; see Chapter 3).

The disability–adjusted life year

The DALY was invented as a tool for policy making for the WHO and, rather revealingly, the World Bank (Anand & Hanson 1997, Hahn 2002). Ostensibly providing a measure of the burden of disease, the DALY views time lived with an impairment as time lost (Priestley 2003). To obtain a DALY score, time lived with an impairment is converted into a 'time loss' by using a set of weights that reflect reductions in functional capacity. Adjustments are made through use of a set of value judgements.

Within the DALY, life is of value solely as a consequence of health status, thus burden of suffering is directly equated with functional limitation. This logic places greater emphasis on physical dysfunction than upon mental anguish (for example, depression) and cannot consider individuals' different abilities to live well with physical dysfunction (Anand & Hanson 1997). Further, suffering is perceived to be due to physical limitations rather than pain, for example. This is particularly problematic given substantial research evidence demonstrating that perceptions of quality of life are not positively correlated with proximity to "normality"; and that pain has a greater negative impact upon the experience of quality of life than does extent of physical impairment, level of function or degree of independence (e.g. Ville et al 2001, Vogel et al 1998, Westgren & Levi 1998). Further, the DALY 'inaccurately equates disability with ill health' (Metts 2001 p 449), irrespective of the reality that it is possible to have a significant degree of impairment and to be perfectly healthy (Hahn 2002).

Within the DALY, tetraplegia ('quadriplegia') is accorded a severity weighting of 1.0, which is the same score accorded death (Metts 2001). (The QALY rates tetraplegia as a state worse than death; Gomm 2000.) Indeed, the weighting system dictates that the value of one year of life for someone without an impairment is of equivalent worth to the lives of 9.524 people with tetraplegia (Arnesen & Nord 1999). Yet researchers have found high perceptions of quality of life even among people who have the highest levels of tetraplegia (Hall et al 1997, Hammell 2004f) and low perceptions of quality of life among people deemed "normal". This illustrates the DALY's lack of a supportive evidence base and demonstrates the tendency for "experts" to parrot cultural beliefs that people would be 'better off dead' than disabled. It also highlights problems that arose because the DALY's creators relied too heavily on the opinions of medical "experts" and failed to incorporate meaningful input from people who actually live with impairments (Metts 2001).

Reflecting pervasive cultural assumptions that disabled peoples' lives are not worth living (Abu-Habib 1997, Zandrow 2001) and that disabled people are worth less than those deemed to be "normal", the DALY dictates that for any given illness, fewer resources ought to be allocated to disabled people. Because the DALY approach explicitly assumes that the lives of disabled people have less value than those of "normates", it attaches lower value to life-extending measures for disabled people than their peers (Arensen & Nord 1999). Anand & Hanson (1997) argued that resource allocation decisions that are based on the DALY serve to entrench disadvantage among disabled people. It could thus be argued that by providing assessments for the DALY, therapists and physicians collude in the process of reinforcing inequality and in limiting resources to those most in need of their services.

Arnesen & Nord (1999) observe that valuing human beings solely for their functional capacity is contrary to the values entrenched in the United Nations' Universal Declaration of Human Rights, which recognizes: 'the inherent dignity and . . . the equal and inalienable rights of all members of the human family' (UN 1948, Resolution 217A III). This seems to have been overlooked by the creators and users of the QALY and DALY.

Metts (2001 p 452) argues that the DALY is 'fatally flawed' and is 'inappropriate for use by scholars or policy makers'. His argument centres on the failure of the DALY to recognize that the burden of living with an impairment is not a direct consequence of that impairment but is a complex function of personal, social and environmental factors. Metts notes, for example, that paraplegia could result in more than the hypothesized 50–70% decrease in quality of life for a member of a nomadic tribe yet in far less than this imagined percentage for a Western university professor. This observation is supported by research evidence that the consequences of paraplegia are affected by contextual factors: culture and development, socioeconomic status and gender and 'to ignore this in the measurement of the burden of disease is to avert one's gaze from reality' (Allotey et al 2003 p 956).

Impairments are experienced disproportionately among people who are socially disadvantaged (Albrecht 1992, Coleridge 1993, Ghai 2001, New Internationalist 1992). 'In the USA, UK and Canada about two-thirds of disabled people live below the poverty line. In many developing countries, the proportion is much greater and the poverty line itself far lower' (Turmusami 2001 p 195). Disabled people are among the poorest of the poor in every country (Groce 1999a, Stone 1999); thus, by asserting that disabled people are less entitled to scarce health resources, the DALY sanctions the diversion of resources towards the dominant, wealthy population and away from those who are poor and disabled (Anand & Hanson 1997). Indeed, it might not be too cynical to observe that those who have the power to design and use the QALY and DALY are engaged in a process of diverting resources to those who are comparatively affluent, physically and cognitively able and mentally stable: people who are most like themselves.

In many societies, boys and men are more valued than girls and women. In some, this leads to gender-based abortions, infanticide and abandonments (Ghai 2002). If social policies were to be based on these particular values, systems of classification and tools for resource allocation would weigh female lives as worth only a fraction of those of males, thereby justifying the denial of healthcare resources to women and girls that are extended to men and boys. Indeed, this is the situation for many of the world's girls and women (Ear-Dupuy 2004). The sort of international condemnation that arises from such injustices against women is virtually absent for the injustices against disabled people currently perpetrated and sanctioned by the DALY (Hahn 2002).

It is a small step from devaluing a condition to devaluing a person (Dijkers 1999). Through its various systems of classification, the WHO accords the life of a disabled person less value than that of someone whose body more closely adheres to social norms, irrespective of past, present or potential contributions to society. (Indeed, the DALY model assumes that people with impairments are unable to make any contribution to their communities; Groce 1999b.) Thus healthcare resources in both resource-rich and resource-poor countries are allocated according to ableist value judgements. The World Bank tells countries appealing for financial assistance that they must reduce their numbers of DALYs. 'The easiest way to reduce the DALYs is, of course, to reduce the number of people with disabilities [sic]' (Pfeiffer 2000 p 1081). Although the DALY lays claim to being an 'objective' measure of population health, the energy and enthusiasm with which its developers have advocated and promoted the DALY, obscuring in the process 'important scientific issues' makes such claims questionable (Allotey et al 2003).

Allocating resources: ethics and equality

We live in a world of finite resources and one in which existing resources are unequally distributed. Clearly, this produces tensions for policy makers and healthcare providers who seek to provide services with limited resources and competing demands. However, to reject on principle the distribution of resources based on constructions of physical "inferiority" (e.g. gender or ability) is also to reject the logic of the QALY and the DALY. Harris (1987 p 117) argued that because the QALY is ageist, racist and sexist, it is 'fatally flawed as a way of priority setting in health care and of dealing with the problem of scarce resources'.

Healthcare professionals have been perceived by their clients as the 'gate-keepers of scarce resources' (Swain et al 2003), which contradicts certain dimensions of the Codes of Ethics of the rehabilitation professions, such as: 'Services should be client centred and needs led' (College of Occupational Therapists (COT) 2000 para 3.3). Although the various professional organizations clearly recognize that resources are finite and that this demands certain choices (COT 2000), there has been little dialogue to determine how priorities can be made in a just and equitable manner. Quiet acquiescence to the role of resource gatekeeper appears to demonstrate accountability to structures of power rather than to disabled people.

REHABILITATION, IDEOLOGY AND POWER

An ideology is a system of ideas, beliefs and assumptions that operates below one's level of conscious awareness; thus an ideology constitutes 'the ideas and prejudices that are contained in what appear to be the basic assumptions of normal life' (Kingwell 1998 p 173). Kingwell (1998 p 173) contends that 'the ideas we blithely accept may often be, in fact, political ideas only masquerading as facts about the world', and indeed, ideologies play an important role in reinforcing and exercising power (Swain & French 2004).

Many of the critics cited in this chapter have alluded to the ideological underpinnings of the WHO's enterprises and the ways in which systems of classification are employed to reinforce specific relations of power. Rehabilitation therapists are not accustomed to thinking about their location within axes of power, having been socialized to view themselves as 'powerless' (relative to the dominant medical profession). Neither are they accustomed to thinking about their values and assumptions in terms of 'ideologies', having been absorbed into a professional culture where these ideas and beliefs are made to appear not only 'natural' and self-evident but benevolent and beneficial. Social theorists explain that this precisely characterizes a *dominant ideology*: an ideology that is taken for granted, that appears to be a 'natural' way of thinking (Barnes 1996a) and that operates by legitimizing social inequalities and power relations. Dominant ideologies establish what is "normal" (and therefore what is "abnormal") and define cultural values (Thompson 1997). However, because 'ideas do not descend fully formed from the heavens, but are always social products' (Thomas 1999 p 16), all ideas and beliefs require critical scrutiny.

The ideology of normality is regarded by some critics as the foundation of rehabilitation (Oliver 1996a). The primary aim of rehabilitation, it is argued, is to restore a disabled person to "normality" (whatever normality is understood to mean within a given social and cultural environment); and failing this, to restore the person to a state that is as close to "normality" as possible. In pursuit of this objective, 'surgical intervention and physical rehabilitation, whatever its cost in terms of the pain and suffering of disabled individuals, is always justified and justifiable' (Oliver 1996a p 37). Because "norms" reflect specific ideals of function and behaviour, Stiker (1999) has posited a relationship between the demands of social conformity and those of rehabilitation.

It is clear that the rehabilitation professions must challenge the ideology of normality and acknowledge that this is a social construction and not a factual reality. Imrie (1997) contends that rehabilitation supports the status quo and reproduces many of the values of ableism in that professionals shape the meaning of impairments around purely medical concerns with the objective of achieving social conformity and deflecting attention away from questions of power and status.

The critiques that have been outlined in this chapter suggest that the ideology of normality, the practice of classifying people, the hierarchical power relations between those who classify and those who are classified, and the justification for resource allocation based on constructions of superiority and inferiority cannot be unexamined. Wendell (1996) argued that classifying people on the basis of perceived deviancy is a social practice that involves the unequal exercise of power and that this has major economic, social, and psychological consequences for some people's lives.

Rehabilitation professionals cannot, unthinkingly, collude in the institutionalized discrimination of disabled people. As rehabilitation therapists, we are part of the social structure that identifies ab-normality and perpetuates inequality; we are not neutral players. Wendell (1996 p 23) claimed that 'to understand how the power of definition is exercised and experienced, we have to ask who does the defining in practice, for what purposes and with what consequences for those who are deemed to fit the definitions'. Positive intentions do not guarantee positive outcomes. Instead of classifying deviations from assumed norms in every dimension of human activity and participation it might be more fruitful to ascertain how people who have illnesses, injuries and impairments manage their everyday lives in a world designed to meet the needs of "normals" (Hammell 2004g).

This chapter has argued that rehabilitation is grounded in an ideology of normality and attempts to "norm" non-standard performance and behaviour. (Indeed, to be "normal" is to conform to what is usual or standard). Far from being a benevolent and scientific enterprise, the pursuit of "normality" was seen to be the pursuit of a human invention, culturally specific and value laden: an ideology with oppressive consequences for those who do not conform to its standards.

It has been proposed that all theory should be judged on the grounds of its political usefulness (Harris 1996, Kitzinger 1994): that theories should be evaluated not in terms of their utility, but of their consequences. The consequences of being classified as deviant to an assumed norm will be explored in the next chapter.

Chapter 3

Disability and deviance from the norm

What is 'normal' but another stereotype?
(Hockenberry 1995 p 89)

INTRODUCTION: DISABILITY AND DEVIANCE FROM THE NORM

The previous chapter explored the ideology of "normality", demonstrating that norms do not represent biological realities; norms reflect historically and culturally specific values. Nonetheless, the ideology of normality underpins much of the rehabilitation enterprise, with clients exhorted to strive to conform to a world that has been constructed to meet the needs of "normals".

The idea of normality requires a comparison; for how might "normality" be claimed in the absence of *ab*normality? Drawing on the work of post-colonial, feminist and queer theorists, this chapter explores the idea of abnormality: of deviance from an assumed and privileged norm. It examines the consequences for those who are judged to be deviant and challenges the belief that the outcome of being classified as deviant is necessarily benign or benevolent.

CONSTRUCTING IMPAIRMENTS

The ideology of normality has been largely uncontested by rehabilitation theorists, yet the work of anthropologists and historians shows that because normality is an ideological construction and not a biological "truth", the parameters of both normality *and abnormality* are subject to social and cultural variations (Ahmad 2000). Impairments thus reflect deviations from culturally defined norms and values rather than constituting consistent biomedical "facts" (Corker 1998a, Leavitt 1999a, Scheer 1994).

Cultures hold the power both to decide what is "normal" and to construct what constitutes an impairment. For example, severe facial scarring – a deviation from dominant ideals of "normality" or acceptability – might constitute an impairment yet have no inherent physical or functional consequences. Such scarring might, however, have significant social consequences in terms of stigma and prejudice that limit life opportunities (Wendell 1996). *Stigma* is a form of social branding of those individuals who transgress the norms and values of society (Goffman 1963a). The dominant, powerful social group determines which human differences are desirable or undesirable, thus stigmas reflect the value judgements of the dominant group (Coleman 1997).

Although the criteria that define an impairment will be obvious to those within a given culture, what 'counts' as an impairment will vary between cultures, as will the response to impairment and the value attributed to the person perceived to have an impairment. In some cultures, impairments of a severity to prohibit engagement in normal roles include having excessive freckles, flabby buttocks or illegitimate birth. In others, blindness has been admired as a sign of wisdom and insight rather than disparaged as a physical flaw (Scheer & Groce 1988). Cultures imbue 'individual variations of the human condition with significance more far-reaching than the simple ability to perform a given activity' (Whyte & Ingstad 1995 p 7). Because what counts as "normal" varies, what counts as deviant also varies. Neither is this a very scientific enterprise. Wilson & Beresford (2002) note that because there are no definitive laboratory tests for any specific mental illnesses, psychiatrists must resort to subjective judgements of behaviours and symptoms in labelling psychopathology.

Impairment can be seen to be a cultural and social issue rather than a purely medical one (Whyte 1995), thus Thomson (1997a p 5) argues that physical impairments might usefully be viewed 'as another culture-bound, physically justified difference to consider along with race, gender, class, ethnicity, and sexuality'. However, unlike the concepts of "race", gender, class, ethnicity and sexuality, which have been the focus of critical interrogation by theorists, impairment has been uncritically accepted as an abnormality by rehabilitation theorists, clinicians and researchers.

This perception is challenged by many deaf people, who reject the labelling of their differences as 'impairments', regarding themselves as a linguistic and cultural minority (Barnes & Mercer 2003, Davis 2002a). Describing themselves as a distinct cultural group with a unique language and history, they claim to be Deaf (capitalized like 'Italian'), rather than people with an impairment (Corker 1998b).

Recognition that the labelling of impairments is an ideological, culturally specific and unstable endeavour is not the same as pretending that impairments do not exist or imagining that they are the products of discourse (see Chapter 6). Nor does it seek to minimize the profound difficulties that people with some forms of impairment experience with problems such as pain, fatigue, incontinence, paralysis, spasticity, emotional anguish or reduced life expectancy. Indeed, impairments can impose their own forms of oppression. But if impairments are, indeed, variations from culturally specific "norms" rather than consistent "facts", then the classification of impairments must become a contested practice and the outcome of classification must be subjected to critical interrogation.

CLASSIFICATORY PRACTICES

Critics contend that societal practices that divide certain categories of people from others – e.g. by ability, religion or ethnicity – contribute to marginalization by establishing value: superiority and inferiority (Foucault 1977). They argue that marginalization results from classificatory systems whereby certain sorts of people are not only compared and categorized, but hierarchized, separated, excluded and institutionalized (Foucault 1977, Said 1979, 1993). Foucault (1977) identified *classificatory practices* as those techniques that enable the separation of the normal from the deviant. Classification is seen as integral to the practice of marginalizing those believed to deviate from the "norm".

Systems of classification that are based on bodily traits – ability, colour, gender – are perceived to promote and support the exclusion of certain people from 'the continuum of acceptable human variations' (Mitchell & Snyder 2003 p 861). Indeed, it has been argued that 'the real function of classification systems' is to 'oppress the people they define . . . First, they imply we are inferior. Second, they allow the dominant culture to institutionalize those of us they consider outcasts and misfits' (Charlton 1998 p 163). Critics contend that such taxonomies have always been oppressive tools of power, used to justify abhorrent social practices such as apartheid, slavery and the institutionalization of disabled people (Charlton 1998, hooks 1995, Mitchell & Snyder 2000). In apartheid South Africa, for example, the ways in which people were classified determined the 'rights' to which they were entitled (Bozalek 2000). Rather than insisting on the rights of all disabled people, South African therapists '(silently) accepted, and thus maintained, the status quo' (Cornielje & Ferrinho 1999 p 220). It was only at the Truth and Reconciliation hearings that the privileged, White health and social care professionals were forced to review their own complicity in the marginalization of the Black majority (Bozalek 2000). Healthcare professionals are not neutral players but active participants in enforcing specific political practices, for example through classificatory practices that are used to enable and justify the separation of the "normal" from the deviant.

DECONSTRUCTING DUALISM

The practice of dividing the world into binary opposites – normal and abnormal, 'us' and 'them' – has characterized Western thought since at least the time of Plato. Plato (1993) proposed, for example, the dualistic concepts of heaven and earth, body and soul, permanence and change. The dualistic concepts of mind and body that were further developed by Descartes became central to the ideology underpinning Western medicine (Cottingham 1988).

Dualistic thinking is specific to Western philosophy and does not represent a universal "truth". Eastern philosophies such as Buddhism and Taoism have long and intellectually rigorous histories centred not on compartmentalism but on the interconnectedness and 'oneness' of all life (Chuang Tzu 1964, Kupperman 2001). The Tai Chi T'u – the familiar black and white double 'fish' symbol – that represents yin and yang, for example, contains an 'eye' or seed of its other, indicating the interplay and fluidity of apparent opposites. Recent work by Western 'queer' theorists seeks to deconstruct dualistic 'thinking as usual', contesting the tendency to divide people into either/or categories such as straight/gay, white/black, man/woman, able/disabled. Shakespeare (1999 p 57), for example, observed that 'binary oppositions between straight and gay, disabled and non-disabled are inaccurate and oppressive ideologies, which obscure the continuities of disability and sexuality'.

Queer theory explores the ideological construction and presumed naturalness of "the norm" (McRuer 2003), the processes by which certain people become labelled as deviant (Epstein 1994) and demonstrates the instability of binary oppositions, such as homosexual/heterosexual or male/female (Stein & Plummer 1994). These issues are also central to the intellectual interrogation of disability. Formerly a term of homophobic abuse, 'queer' has been redeployed as an umbrella term for a spectrum of culturally marginal sexual self-identifications (Jagose 1996). Queer theory is an interdisciplinary school of thought that interrogates the kaleidoscope of human sex, gender and desire and critiques and destabilizes heteronormativity (Sherry 2004).

Transvestites, bisexuals and other sex rebels illustrate the diverse spectrum of identity and desire that precludes dualistic divisions of the global population into simple categories of straight/gay. Further, transsexuals, transgendered people, intersexuals (formerly termed 'hermaphrodites') and other gender benders demonstrate that the categories 'male' and 'female' lack rigid boundaries, thereby challenging the belief that the world can be neatly divided into two sexes (Davis 2002a, Marks 1999). Indeed, while the Hirja in India are clearly defined and accepted by the culture as a third gender, some scientists contend that the interplay of genes, hormones and anatomy can produce at least five distinguishable genders (Barnartt 2001, Roughgarden 2004).

Queer theorists problematize any theoretical stance that is based on a simplistic dichotomy of genders, observing that this essentializes the categories 'man' and 'woman' and falsely partitions the population into two homogeneous groups (Ingraham 1994, Seidman 1994). This has relevance for those rehabilitation researchers who elect to study just women, or just men, as if these simplistic, opposing categories somehow encompass people with uniform perspectives and experiences, irrespective of "race", ethnicity, class, caste, religion or sexual identity (Lugones & Spelman 1983). In reality, researchers have found more similarities than differences between men's and women's experiences of disability, suggesting that the master status of masculinity is almost wholly eroded by the stigmatized status of disability (Shackelford et al 1998, Shakespeare 1999). Indeed, it is only by studying the experiences of both men and women that any differences that are specific to gender identification can be illuminated and explored (Hammell 1998a).

To further complicate simplistic, dualistic thinking, feminist theorists like to claim that power is associated with gender, with the male and masculinity (Hartsock 1990), yet disabled men and women speak of relations of power within hospitals and residential institutions where they experience powerlessness relative to the more powerful, predominantly female staff. 'For disabled women [and men], the oppressor may at times be other women acting as colonizer, regulator or controller' (Meekosha 1998 p 170). Women who are confined within institutions are not subordinate to men, do not serve men, or labour for men. On the contrary, they are usually subordinate to women. Although power is unarguably distributed unequally in society, its distribution depends on more complex equations than a simplistic male/female dualism (Vernon 1999).

Queer theorists' deconstruction of binary opposites extends to the distinctions between 'mental' and 'physical' illnesses. Tremain (1996 p 23), for example, argued that this distinction 'relies upon a philosophically indefensible mind/body dichotomy' that is prevalent within Western thought and construes the mind and body as separate entities. It is intriguing that although the rehabilitation professions generally espouse a holistic orientation, their professional discourses tend to perpetuate dualism, rarely resisting the tendency to speak of physical *or* mental illnesses (Hammell 2001a).

FAILURE TO BE NORMAL

It is claimed that there are more points of overlap between disability and sexuality than between disability and either "race" or gender, thus highlighting the potential contribution that queer theory can make to understanding the experience of disability (Scheer 1994). 'Theorists and activists in both queer studies and disability studies advocate a scholarly and political confrontation with normative ideas and institutions that exclude individuals according to their physical, sexual, or ideological expressions of selfhood' (Serlin 2003 p 154). Queer theory and disability theory both critique the constructed ideal of "normality" and its inherent implication that those outside the normal range are, by definition, deviant and abnormal (McRuer 2002) and are therefore to be 'pitied, medicalised, ostracised or criminalised' (Rose 2004 p 29).

Danaher et al (2000 p 61) claim that we are all 'continually being judged in terms of the normality or otherwise of our mental attributes, our physical capacities, our feelings and attitudes, and our sexual preferences'. These judgements are neither apolitical nor benign. Disabled people and sexual non-conformists share histories of abuse, harassment, discrimination, persecution, violence and assault (Sherry 2004), having been 'variously exorcized, burned, incarcerated and experimented upon in attempts to purge their differentness from the accepted normative standards, or to eradicate them altogether' (Appleby 1994 p 19, Corbett 1994). Queer and disabled people have been subjected to various disciplinary mechanisms of 'treatment' and 'cure' in attempts to induce conformity with social norms (Sherry 2004). Sexual minorities thus share with disabled people 'a history of injustice: both have been pathologized by medicine; demonized by religion; discriminated against in housing, employment, and education; stereotyped in representation; victimized by hate groups; and isolated socially, often in their families of origin' (Sandahl 2003 p 26). It is hardly surprising that both disability and queer theorists have elected to focus critical attention upon the oppressive ideology of normality (explored in Chapter 2).

The ideas of "ability" and "disability" rely on deeply entrenched *'ideals of normality'* (Tremain 1996 p 23). Theorists have demonstrated that social power accompanies the possession of certain physical and sexual 'norms' such that physical, political, legal, economic and social environments are designed to exclude those who do not conform to this template (McRuer 2003). For example, certain policies of governments, insurance companies and housing agencies, and specific workplace practices, are designed solely for able-bodied, heterosexual people (Butler R 1999, Valentine 1993). Twigg (2002) explained that social policies are designed to assert and support the "norm" in such diverse issues as pensions, entitlement to financial benefits, access to fertility treatments, adoption regulations and sexual health services.

PRESUMING NORMALITY

Butler (1997 p 2) claimed that the apparent 'normativity' of the man/woman binary is supported by implicit presumptions of heterosexuality. The assumption that everyone's sexuality conforms to specific "norms" is termed 'compulsory heterosexuality' or *heterosexism* by queer theorists, who contest the tendency to portray a certain set of perspectives and experiences as universal (Butler J 1999). They claim, for example, that feminist research claiming to explore the situation of 'women' is premised on a false universalism and demonstrate that the experiences of lesbian women might have more in common with those of gay men than of other women (Fraser & Nicholson 1990, Stein & Plummer 1994).

The norm within rehabilitation is to assume that everyone is straight; a reflection of both homophobia and heterosexism (Crepeau 1998, King & McKeown 2004). This assumption – that heterosexuality can be both presumed and expected – has led to rehabilitation that is perceived to be inadequate, irrelevant and 'beyond ludicrous' by those who deviate from this presumed norm (Killacky 2004 p 59).

CLASSIFIED AS DEVIANT

Homosexuals have shared with disabled people the experience of being judged against a valued norm by those with more social power, and found wanting (Breckenridge & Vogler 2001). A Catholic bishop, for example, claimed that people who are blind, deaf or homosexual have 'a manufacturing defect' (Le Monde 5 February 2002); they are not just 'deviant' (different), but 'defective' (substandard). Like homosexuals, disabled people are perceived as failing to contribute to society, as posing a threat to public health or safety and as transgressing societal norms and values. Both groups tend to provoke negative responses such as unease and discomfort (Leary & Schreindorfer 1998). Both groups have been denigrated as 'deviant'.

The practice by which "normals" apply the label of 'deviance' to homosexuals and disabled people justifies prejudice and validates stereotyping. Although disability might no longer be viewed as a mark of sinfulness (see Chapter 4) 'it is still a stigma of inferiority' (Bickenbach 1993 p 143).

Queer theorists, like anthropologists, have demonstrated the ways in which human characteristics and behaviours are interpreted differently at different times and in different contexts (Foucault 1978). At times viewed as a probable cause of physical impairments (Martin 1997), homosexuality was admired by the ancient Greeks and was central to the code of honour of the samurai in medieval Japan (Crompton 2003). It has since been viewed as a sin, a crime, a psychiatric pathology and (most recently) one among many dimensions of the kaleidoscope of human sexuality (Swain et al 2003). It can therefore be seen that what counts as 'deviant from the norm' and what is included within the spectrum of 'acceptable human variations' is historically and culturally specific. Homosexuality is currently 'in'; impairment is still 'out'.

DIVIDING PRACTICES

The normal/abnormal ideology is not politically neutral. It reflects value judgements that equate "normality" with virtue (Barnes et al 1999). Fawcett (2000a) contends that the process of classifying some people as "abnormal" affirms the "normality" and superiority of others. The normal/abnormal dichotomy 'has been used as justification of oppression, discrimination, and marginalisation of disabled people' (Gillman et al 2000 p 395). Thus, critics contend that dualistic judgements of normality/abnormality, straight/gay, male/female, white/black are not mere binary labels, but expressions of power (Davis 1995). 'Dominant/subordinate relations are unequal relations between population groups in the society, based on group-level inequalities in political (decision-making) power, economic power (resources) and social power (prestige) or esteem' (Kallen 2004 p 33).

The process of distinguishing people on the basis of their proximity to normality is an example of what Foucault termed 'dividing practices': techniques by which different categories of people are created by separating, normalizing and institutionalizing certain populations (Twigg 2000). 'Dividing practices work to qualify or disqualify people as fit and proper members of the social order' (Danaher et al 2000 p 61). Marginalizing practices follow dividing practices.

OPPRESSION: MARGINALIZATION

Many disability theorists refer to the 'oppression' of disabled people: a result of domination and of ideologies of superiority and inferiority (e.g. Charlton 1998, Oliver 1990). *Oppression* describes the disadvantage and injustice experienced by some social groups (Northway 1999). Young (1990) identified five 'faces' of oppression that have provided theorists with a conceptual framework with which to examine the situation of disabled people: marginalization, exploitation, powerlessness, cultural imperialism and violence. These dimensions of oppression are raised by theorists throughout this book and will each be explored in more depth as they arise.

Marginalization has been shown to be the product of ideologies that create deviancy, abnormality and inferiority. More than just ideas, ideologies have direct consequences: marginalization, for example, results from material and social deprivation and powerlessness due to a lack of access to employment and other rights of citizenship (Young 1990). A further dimension of marginalization is segregation and confinement (Said 1993). Disabled people have a history of being confined within residential institutions and are frequently denied access to public spaces (Gleeson 1999a, Imrie 1996).

Bickenbach (1993 p 143) argued that disabled people share with members of 'discredited "races"' the experience of having 'an identifiable difference that sets them apart from the "normals"'. From his own experience of acquired impairment, Murphy (1990 p 5, 127) observed that disabled people are 'outsiders': 'marginal' people, occupying a 'tenuous position at the edge of society'. Ideologies provide the justification for marginalizing certain groups; specific social practices produce marginality.

MARGINALIZING DIFFERENCE

Seidman (1995) argued that the power of the ideology of "normality" lies in its capacity to justify the denial of basic rights and to enforce social marginalization. Feminist theorists observe that a hierarchy of physical traits – "race", gender, ability –'determines the distribution of privilege, status, and power' in society (Thomson 1997a p 6). Further, classification of certain people as inferior on the basis of sexual behaviour, religion, opinion or ability has historically enabled the dominant culture to institutionalize many considered to be deviant. This has included – among others – unmarried mothers, religious and political non-conformists and disabled people (Barnes & Mercer 2003, Fawcett 2000a).

The labelling of disabled people as 'deviant' (inferior), and the consequent provision of 'special' (inferior) segregated forms of housing, education, transportation, employment, cultural and leisure opportunities is understood by many disabled people to be a form of 'apartheid' (Rioux 2001, Shapiro 1994); a product of the colonial tendencies of the dominant population.

Arising from anticolonial ideals of freedom, human rights, equality and social inclusion (Namsoo & Armstrong 1999), *postcolonial* theories explore the ways in which the dominant, powerful social group privileges its own values and norms, defining, marginalizing and excluding others deemed inferior (Said 1979). Although any human trait could be selected for stigma, the dominant group has the authority and ability to determine which differences will be inferior (Coleman 1997, Thomson 1997a). Theorists have demonstrated that colonial powers reinforced and justified inequalities in power by privileging White, European, Christian "norms", thereby marginalizing others deemed to be abnormal, inferior, incapable of looking after themselves and requiring the paternal rule of others for their own 'best interests' (Said 1979, Young 2003). Indeed, the social organization of colonial societies was dependent on the inequality of its citizens (Namsoo & Armstrong 1999). The justification for marginalizing colonized people precisely replicates the justifications given for marginalizing disabled people who have been deemed to be abnormal, inferior, incapable of looking after themselves and requiring the p/maternal rule of others for their own 'best interests'. Disabled people have a history of institutional confinement based on this very premise.

Unlike much contemporary social theory, postcolonialism has a political dimension, being focused on those at the margins of society and dedicated to the elimination of inequality and other social hierarchies (Young 2003). It is valuable for its exploration of the value-judgements that underpin contemporary ideas of "normality", the effects of such judgements upon the opportunities afforded to those who are judged to be inferior, and the apparent justification these judgements provide for social inequities. Thus postcolonialism provides a way to talk about living in a world that seems to exist for others (Young 2003).

The division of people into binary categories was central to the colonial enterprise. These divisions were used to control and regulate the movement of people, such that colonized people were restricted from entering the space of the colonial power. Indeed, the power to regulate movement was an integral component of the practice of colonialism, of which apartheid was an extreme example (Danaher et al 2000). Those therapists who have worked with disabled people to attain physical access to social spaces such as public buildings and to systems of transportation will doubtless have experience of the social practices that prohibit the marginalized from entering the spaces of the powerful.

Said (1979, p 207) observed that 'colonized people' are those who are 'analyzed not as citizens or even people but as problems to be solved or confined'. Given the history of institutional confinement of disabled people

(Barnes 1991, Charlton 1998) and the problem-oriented modes of practice that proliferate among the nursing and rehabilitation professions (Johnson 1993), it is not difficult to translate the ideas of postcolonialists into an analysis of disability.

Said (1979, 1989) claimed that 'marginalized minorities' include all people who are designated as backward, inferior or 'lesser beings' when viewed in a framework constructed out of biological determinism. *Biological determinism* implies that one's life possibilities are wholly dictated by one's biology. In the past, for example, girls and women were considered unsuitable to undertake such activities as university education or to vote because of their biological 'inferiority'. Indeed, in many countries they were not legally deemed to be 'people'. 'These attitudes extended into the whole of the culture: social relations, politics, law, medicine, the arts, popular and academic knowledges' (Young 2003 p 5). The belief that 'biology is not destiny' later became a slogan for feminists who sought to demonstrate that their life possibilities were restricted due to social – not biological – factors.

Discrimination based on physical difference is not limited to gender but extends to a hierarchy of differences, in which gender often 'trumps' "race". For example, physical differences *between* women were used as justification for denying black women and men the right to vote in South Africa until 63 years after white women acquired this right for themselves (Guardian Weekly 9–15 October 2003). Thus, the rights of citizenship were traditionally allocated according to physique, with physical differences used to divide the powerful from the powerless. They still are. In many countries, for example, disabled people are prevented from voting due to the inaccessibility of polling centres (Hammell 2004d).

Postcolonial theorists contend that on the basis of biological determinism colonized people become fixed in 'zones of dependency and peripherality' (Said 1989 p 207), an apt description for the position of disabled people throughout the world. The practice of segregating disabled people in education, housing, employment, transportation, etc., echoes practices central to the colonial endeavour (Hurst 1995).

The postcolonial feminist theorist bell hooks (1995) explained that the achievement of colonialism does not require the assumption of power in someone else's country but can be achieved by dominant groups through *social apartheid* – a philosophy that determines 'inherent' inferiority and informs social priorities – and economic disenfranchisement in one's own country. Indeed, the most pervasive form of marginalization is economic. Even in resource-rich countries such as Canada, the UK and USA, the majority of disabled people are unemployed and poor (Barnes & Mercer 2003, Charlton 1998, Crichton & Jongbloed 1998). The history of disability has been central to the history of begging (Thomson 1997a); indeed begging remains the primary occupation for the majority of the world's disabled people (Groce 1999a).

Privilege and marginalization

Unequal opportunities of access to wealth, privilege and the production and consumption of resources result from being defined as a member of an undesirable social category. Conversely, class privilege can dilute the marginal experience of disability (Vernon & Swain 2002). Queer theorists share with black feminists the understanding that different identities intersect and are subject to different oppressions, such that disability and sexuality are entwined with class, "race", age and gender (hooks 1981, Stein & Plummer 1994, Vernon 1999). Thus, 'whilst disability may be the only aspect of disabled White heterosexual men's experience of oppression, the same cannot be said of disabled Black people, women, gay men and lesbians, older people and those from the working class', all of whom deviate from the established "norm" in several ways (Vernon 1998 p 208).

However, although many theorists contend that disabled people as a population are marginalized, few would argue that all disabled people are marginalized. Various dimensions of social stratification can mediate the effects of having an impairment (Vernon 1999). Thus, although many people experience the onset of impairment as a 'fall from privilege' (Rockhill 1996 p 184), material wealth, education, professional and employment statuses, gender, age, "race", ethnicity, citizenship status, class, caste, sexual orientation, marital status, religion, language and other dimensions of differentiation associated with distributions of power can combine and intersect to maintain social privilege for individual disabled people.

Accordingly, some disabled people are annoyed at the apparent disrespect of theories that seem to portray them as helpless victims of social oppression, when they view themselves as people who have worked hard to attain a high degree of personal achievement (Hockenberry 1995, Roberts 1996, Simpson 1996). Postcolonial critics have also challenged the patronizing élitism that underlies the assumed privilege to define others as 'oppressed' when this is not how they view themselves (e.g. Mohanty 1994, Prakash 1994). Mann (1995) invoked the term *theoretical imperialism* to describe the exercise of power through which academics authorize and privilege their own understanding and interpretations over those of the theorized.

Roberts (1996 p 15) suggested that while the disability movement's academic élites have been contemplating oppression, discrimination and injustice 'some of us disabled have been having a ball – we've done it all'. Sadly, not all people who have impairments are afforded the opportunity to 'do it all'. It is difficult, for example, to 'do it all' if confined within an institution or if unable to access affordable transportation.

Marginalization, depression and suicide

One of the assumptions of the rehabilitation professions that has enjoyed considerable longevity is the belief that depression is an inevitable consequence of a serious injury such as spinal cord injury (see Hammell 1992). Reflecting prevailing cultural beliefs that life with a spinal cord injury would not be worth living, early theorists guessed that depression would be both a natural and necessary reaction to injury; therefore the absence of depression signalled a failure to recognize the reality of loss (Burke & Murray 1975, Krueger 1984). Client behaviours tend to be interpreted according to prevailing ideologies, even when these lack an evidence-based foundation (Hale 1991, Wortman & Silver 1989). Accordingly, research has demonstrated that experienced healthcare professionals consistently overestimate the degree of distress or depression experienced by their spinal cord-injured clients (Bach et al 1991, Cushman & Dijkers 1990).

Most of the research investigating depression among people with physical impairments has significant methodological limitations (Jacob et al 1995, Widerström-Noga et al 1999). However, although studies suggest that clinical depression is exceptional rather than usual, researchers have reported that a significant minority of people with spinal cord injuries exhibit clinically elevated levels of depression and distress many years after injury (Fuhrer et al 1993, Hammell 1994a). High rates of substance abuse are also reported (Radnitz & Tirch 1995).

It is apparent that levels of anxiety and depression correlate with neither the level of spinal cord injury nor the degree of physical function, indicating that the severity of an impairment does not dictate the severity of psychological distress (Elfström et al 2002, Hancock et al 1993). Although data from mortality studies suggest that suicide rates following spinal cord injury are significantly higher than among the general population, this finding cannot be correlated with lesion level either (Soden et al 2000).

Researchers challenge the cultural assumption that disability is a prime predictor of suicide (Hartkopp et al 1998) and observe that the suicide rate among disabled people would be much higher if it reflected the frequency with which non-disabled people claim a preference for death over disability (Silvers 1994). Following her T12 spinal cord injury, Monica Bascio felt neither depression nor grief but a desire to get on with her life. When she was denied an occupational therapy clinical placement on the basis of discriminatory attitudes she explained 'for the first time disability was slammed in my face. It caused me to question my whole existence' (cited in Vogel 2004 p 30).

Research has found that gay men, lesbians and transgendered people are also highly susceptible to depression, substance abuse and suicide (King & McKeown 2004, McRuer & Wilkerson 2003). Solomon (2001) claims that this is due to their marginalized situation: a reflection of diminished social status and a life history of being demeaned and humiliated. As Sherry (2004 p 772) observed: 'living in a homophobic culture is incredibly traumatic'. Guter (2004 p 224) alludes to the efforts expended by gay men to reclaim their humanity and 'ameliorate the depression that results from being despised and rejected', noting that 'society is no help in this endeavour'. Perhaps depression among marginalized disabled people might have a similar, social, origin? In addition, research demonstrates that rates of mental illness and suicide are highest among people who have low socioeconomic status, those in boring, monotonous occupations and who have little opportunity for control and creativity in their lives (Swain & French 2004). Clearly, this encapsulates the plight of a majority of disabled people.

Byzek (2004) claims that it is absurd to suggest that an impairment is the sole determinant of depression but observes that 'being isolated, discriminated against, prejudged, and the target of ignorant comments will bring anyone down' (p 37). Following his spinal cord injury, Basnett (2001 p 459) explained that he became depressed when confronted with the reality that

'I could not live where and with whom I chose [or] make decisions about when to get up and go to bed'.

Craig et al (1994 p 228) suggest that frustrations encountered on a daily basis might contribute to depression in living with an impairment in the long term; for example 'the stresses of coping with architectural barriers, economic costs, vocational limitations, strains on family roles and relationships, and demands of others who lack an understanding'. This suggestion is supported by the findings of other researchers who claim that daily hassles and frustrations are more predictive of depression than major life events such as sustaining a spinal cord injury (Rintala et al 1996).

When a disabled person commits suicide this is inevitably viewed as a consequence of their impairment, yet when a depressed mother or a jilted teen commits suicide there is no equivalent judgement that suicide is an inevitable consequence of being a teenager or a mother. This is a cultural discourse reserved for disability (Gerhart & Corbet 1995). The belief that having a serious impairment leads inevitably to depression and a low quality of life underpins medical, legal and ethical support for euthanasia and eugenics. This belief is challenged by disability theorists who argue that political, economic and cultural forces contribute to the experience of marginalization and poverty, not biological ones (Morris 1991). Goble (2003 p 49) argued: 'disabled people may well be driven to a despair that makes them wish to end their own lives, not as a result of anything inherent in their biological or genetic make-up, but as a result of social discrimination, prejudice and inadequate, inappropriate and oppressive service systems'.

OUTCOMES OF CLASSIFICATION: ELIMINATING DEVIANCE

Although the intent of classifying, measuring and statistically analysing divergence from assumed norms (using tools such as the ICF) might, in some societies, be benign, the consequences for those classified as less than normal can be devastating (Hammell 2003a). On the basis of such classification, disabled people have been denied medical interventions, confined within institutions and used as 'guinea pigs' for medical research (Anand & Hanson 1997, Hayashi & Okuhira 2001, Rock 2000, Singer et al 1995). They have also been killed (Shapiro 1994, Pfeiffer 2000). Davis (2002a p 157) observed: 'Let us never forget that the deaf, the feeble-minded [sic], and other "defectives" were the first to be rounded up by the Nazis and sent to the death camps. Only when the camps had consumed people with disabilities did the Nazis begin to bring in the racial undesirables'.

It is thought that more than 250,000 disabled people were exterminated by the Nazis (Barnes & Mercer 2003, Priestley 2003), yet, as Parks (2001 p 55) observed, the targeting of disabled people 'has been largely overlooked in historical research and the collective remembrance of the Holocaust', perhaps because 'this persecution has often been viewed as less objectionable than that of other groups' (Parks 2001 p 56). It would be comforting to assume that what happened in Nazi Germany could not happen again. Human rights atrocities committed within our lifetime suggest otherwise. Further, Ghai (2002 p 91) claims that in a culture such as is found in India, 'in which there is widespread female infanticide, killing imperfect children will not even count as a crime'. As Hubbard (1997 p 195) suggests, 'we cannot afford to be complacent'.

It would also be comforting to believe that healthcare professionals – by definition – would actively resist any attempt to eliminate people based upon their impairments. In reality, it was medical professionals who invented, developed and carried out the euthanasia project in Nazi Germany (Goble 2003, Mitchell & Snyder 2003). 'Although participation was voluntary, there was no shortage of volunteers' (Priestley 2003 p 181). Indeed, 'racial hygiene' formed part of the curriculum in many German medical schools (Hubbard 1997). Further, by *classifying* the different and the abnormal, healthcare professionals singled out who would be killed (Gallagher 1990).

Pfeiffer (1998 p 520) noted that: 'One of the first things that an oppressive government does before it begins to eliminate a group of people is to classify them. Once classified it is easy to select subgroups for elimination as did Nazi Germany in the 1930s and 1940s'. However, because the public chooses to imagine that disabled people are treated with kindness (Davis 2002a), there is a cultural ambivalence about recognizing the disastrous legacies of defining, classifying, measuring and managing disabled people as 'deviant to the norm' (Mitchell & Snyder 2003). Healthcare professionals tend to share this ambivalence, yet to ignore history might be to repeat it.

OUTCOMES OF CLASSIFICATION: EXCLUDING DEVIANCE

Even today, people commonly state that they would rather be dead than endure life with a severe physical impairment, and healthcare professionals demonstrate attitudes that are little different from the society that spawns them (Dijkers 1996, Gerhart 1997). However, 'the notion that one is better off dead than disabled is nothing less than the ultimate aspersion against the physically impaired, for it questions the value of their lives and their very right to exist' (Murphy 1990 p 230).

When 'atypicalities' are deemed undesirable, genetic medicine is embraced as a way to '"select" those characteristics we value, and "select out" those characteristics we do not' (Goble 2003 p 46). In the UK, for instance, approval has been granted to abort a fetus because it had a cleft lip and palate (Guardian Weekly 4–10 December 2003): an impairment that is readily amenable to surgical remediation. Disability activists do not argue against a woman's right to abortion (Sharp & Earle 2002) but they do challenge that decision if it is based solely on the desire to avoid the birth of a certain sort of baby, arguing that this is the ultimate in aesthetic consumerism (Hughes 2000).

The cultural imperative to reduce the incidence of 'defectives' can place tremendous pressures upon women (Barnes & Mercer 2003). A leading embryologist claimed that prenatal screening will soon make it a 'sin' for parents to have a disabled child (Sunday Times 1999). Thus Shakespeare (2003 p 205) observed that the birth of a baby with Down syndrome 'has moved from being an unfortunate piece of bad luck, to being a blameworthy failure of surveillance and control'. Wolbring (2001 p 45) claimed that through new methods of prenatal screening for genetic 'defects': 'women lose their right to autonomy and reproductive freedom, becoming instead the quality control gatekeepers of human perfection'. Such practices devalue the lives of disabled people (Morris 1991) and send a message: '"We do not want any more like you"' (Wendell 1996 p 153). The public's perception that life with an impairment, by definition, is not a life worth living is grounded in the perception that an impairment is the defining feature of an individual's life and of their identity.

THE COMPLEXITY OF IDENTITY

Thomson (1997a p 12) observes the tendency of 'normates' to assume that 'disability cancels out all other qualities, reducing the complex person to a single attribute'. Negative cultural stereotypes turn a stigmatized difference into a 'master status [sic], the attribute that colours the perception of the entire person' (Coleman 1997 p 222). Indeed, disability is taken to be not merely a "master" status but an exclusive status (Asch & Fine 1988 p 3). For example, the apparent inability to imagine that someone might have an impairment and also be employed – even wealthy – is evidenced by the common experience among disabled people: of having a stranger drop coins into their empty coffee cups – 'and in one memorable incident, a full cup' (Hewitt 2004 p 15).

Professor Robert Murphy noticed that, in society's eyes, his severe physical impairment eclipsed all the achievements of his life, becoming his defining identity. 'I had moved subtly from the center of my society to its perimeter. I had acquired a new identity that was contingent on my defects' (Murphy 1990 p 110). In his classic study of 'stigma', Goffman (1963a) noted that because society views physical impairment as a 'spoiled' identity, stigma becomes a defining, "master" identity characterized by generalized incapacity. All the attributes of the individual are ignored except those that fit the stereotype associated with the stigma (Coleman 1997).

Supporting Murphy's and Goffman's observations, a young man with a high spinal cord injury noted the tendency for rehabilitation professionals to view him solely as a 'disabled person' rather than seeing him as a multifaceted person like themselves. He explained: 'the only thing I have in common with other disabled people is my disability! And, OK, so that's pretty big, but on the other hand, it's not who I am. This wheelchair isn't who I am' (Hammell 1998a).

Queer theorists contend that identities 'are always multiple or at best composites, with an infinite number of ways in which "identity components" (e.g., sexual orientation, race, class, nationality, gender, age, ableness) can intersect or combine' (Seidman 1994 p 173). Although society might attribute one, totalizing identity to those deemed deviant – 'gay', 'lesbian', 'disabled' – queer theorists demonstrate that all people have multiple threads to their identities –e.g. mother, nurse, daughter, lesbian, volunteer, golfer, white – such that their 'deviant' characteristic constitutes just one of many dimensions of who they are (Stein & Plummer 1994).

However, it is difficult to create and maintain a social movement in the absence of a collective sense of one-dimensional identity. Those disability theorists who are influenced by Marxism and who believe that necessary social changes can only be achieved through collective action claim the existence of a 'disability identity': a stable, distinctive group identity (Campbell & Oliver 1996, Finkelstein 1993). They espouse a unified disability culture, expressing a collective identity in which impairment is a source of pride and strength (Swain & French 2000). Through focusing on their difference they elect to turn a 'label into a badge' (Shakespeare & Watson 2001a p 20).

However, a minority of disabled people are involved in the disability arts movement, with the disability rights movement and with asserting pride in impairment as a defining identity, and it would seem that many disabled people, instead, are involved in a process of 'restructuring' what is considered to be 'normal'; 'trying to make difference *not* matter' (Watson 2002 p 522). By negating 'impairment' as a "master" status, they refuse to be classified on the basis of bodily difference, electing to identify with other dimensions of their experience, such as ethnicity, sexuality, marital status or parenthood (Shakespeare & Watson 2001a). Through focusing on their abilities and the 'ordinariness' of their lives, they redefine for themselves the meaning of 'disability' (Hammell 2004h, Watson 2002). Indeed, it might be more radical to reject disability as a "master" status than to embrace it as the basis for a common identity (Watson 2002).

IMPLICATIONS FOR REHABILITATION: RESTRUCTURING NORMALITY

To find oneself the only person of one's own colour in a large gathering is to discover what it is 'to be from a minority, to live as the only person who is always in the margins, to be the person who never qualifies as the norm' (Young 2003 p 1). Because this is also the experience of physical impairment (Murphy 1990), surely the rehabilitation process should be engaged in preparing people to resist enforced marginality and to challenge the distribution of opportunities that are justified by normative, dualistic thinking?

Rehabilitation is often said to be a process in which clients are assisted to 'accept', 'adapt to', or 'adjust to' living with an impairment; but what does this really mean? Safilios-Rothschild (1981 p 7) found that 'rehabilitation entails a highly stressful resocialization process into an "inferior" status' and that the process of 'acceptance' of disability necessitates 'the relinquishing of majority status rights'. 'Adjustment' to disability, it is argued, is not so much a psychological process as one of adjusting to changes in others' perceptions, in social positioning and in access to educational, economic and social opportunities (Linton 1998). If these claims are accurate, then rehabilitation professionals are doing a great disservice to their clients by acclimatizing them to inferior social status and low life expectations. The adequacy of rehabilitation services should, instead, be measured by the degree to which they enable people with impairments to transgress a minority status.

There is growing evidence that many people who have lived with physical impairments for some time undergo a conceptual transformation, such that they change the way they think about disability. Through choosing to minimize losses and focus instead on abilities and accomplishments, they perceive themselves to be competent and capable (Carpenter 1994, Duggan & Dijkers 1999, Gill 2001, Hammell 2004b); indeed many no longer view themselves as *dis*abled. A young man with a high spinal cord injury explained: 'I don't look at you as able-bodied and me as disabled ... We're [all] doing the best we can with what we have' (Hammell 2004f).

By redefining "normality", people who are defined by others as 'deviant' realize it is acceptable to be who they are (Coleman 1997). Rehabilitation therapists are ideally positioned to assist their disabled clients to begin the process of redefining normality by challenging ideologies that posit 'disability' as both 'inability' and 'ineligibility' and through encouraging them to refuse to accept a marginal, minority status.

Steve Biko (1978) claimed that the only vehicle for changing the circumstances of oppressed people is through infusing people with pride and dignity and by reminding them to resist complicity in allowing themselves to be oppressed. And there we have it. Rather than training disabled people to aspire to be marginal (see Chapter 5), rehabilitation professionals could engage in a process of infusing people with pride and dignity, encouraging them to see themselves as equal to other people; not denying their differences, but making 'difference *not* matter' (Watson 2002 p 522). This entails focusing upon abilities and upon what people can *do* (see Chapter 11), contesting social barriers that restrict opportunities to those whose abilities conform to certain ideological norms and refusing classificatory practices that divide people, one from another.

IDEOLOGY AND POWER

This chapter, and the one that preceded it, have sought to deconstruct the ideologies of normality and deviance that underpin current rehabilitation theories and practice, demonstrating that ideologies are neither politically neutral nor devoid of consequences. Ideologies inform classifying practices, which enable dividing practices and justify the marginalization of specific groups. These, in turn, have been the precursors of the exclusion and elimination of disabled people. Although seemingly benign, ideologies cannot be divorced from power.

Anthropologists confirm that impairments are normal and have been experienced throughout history, in every culture, by people of all ages, religions and "races" and in all social classes and castes (Luborsky 1993). They will continue to be so. Impairment is not something abnormal or peculiar, but is 'fundamental to the human experience' (Barnes 1996b p xii); *a dimension of normality*. Impairment is also the one dimension of devalued human status to which we are all vulnerable (Hammell 2004d).

Far from reflecting deviations from *the* "norm", impairments are a normal component of human diversity; a normal part of everyday life, not just for people who have impairments at the current time, but for humanity as a whole. Attempts to establish parameters of an ideological norm and to classify deviations from this assumed norm are thus not just futile endeavours but an attempt to deny the normality of human diversity. Worse, they are endeavours that have led to profound abuses of human rights.

This chapter explored ideologies of abnormality – of deviance from an assumed and privileged norm – and the issues of power/powerlessness that these ideologies reflect and promote. The following chapter examines theoretical models of disability, demonstrating that the ways in which theories are constructed determines the response to disability: by disabled people, by rehabilitation professionals and by societies.

Chapter 4

Theoretical models of disability

Our exclusion from society is a human rights issue.
(Campbell & Oliver 1996 p 62)

INTRODUCTION: THEORETICAL MODELS OF DISABILITY

So far, this book has sought to demonstrate that ideas are not merely events within our minds devoid of consequences. Ideas inform and shape behaviour, and ideas about impairments shape the responses of individuals and societies to people who have various forms of impairment. Pursuing the contention that specific ways of thinking about disability have consequences for the lives of disabled people, Chapter 4 explores three influential models of disability.

A *model* is a framework that is used to make sense of information (Coleridge 1993); it encapsulates specific knowledge and perspectives and posits links between data. A model is both shaped by ideas and serves to shape ideas. Indeed, a model may shape ideas so successfully that it is eventually regarded as the natural or "right" way of thinking about an issue. At its best, a model helps to organize theories and ideas; at its worst, a model may limit the possibilities for alternative ways of thinking. Engel (1977 p 130) observed that 'in science, a model is revised or abandoned when it fails to fit all the data. A dogma, on the other hand, requires that discrepant data be forced to fit the model or be excluded'. It is because ideas about disability have consequences for disabled people that theoretical models need to be constantly challenged.

This chapter describes and explores three models of disability: the moral/religious, the individual/medical and the social/political. Although these models originated at very different times, they are all evident in contemporary societies, demonstrating the persistence of certain patterns of thought – models – in shaping ideas about disability. The chapter outlines the assumptions of the models and examines the consequences of these modes of thought for disabled people and for the rehabilitation professions.

THE MORAL/RELIGIOUS MODEL OF DISABILITY

The moral/religious model probably represents the oldest and also the most pervasive framework for understanding disability. Shared by most cultures throughout the world, this model is also evident in all the major religions (Hughes 1998, Mackelprang & Salsgiver 2000). The moral/religious model is primarily concerned with ascribing a cause for impairments, perhaps responding to a human need to explain why 'bad' things happen. Further, by promulgating the belief that impairments are the result of sin, witchcraft, the evil eye, the wrath of God/gods or an ancestor's anger, for example, religions have sought to regulate and control the behaviour of their adherents through fear and the threat of supernatural punishment.

The moral/religious model attributes impairment to the consequence of possession by evil spirits, as punishment for wrong-doing (such as breaking taboos) or of sin committed by either the individual (in this or a previous incarnation) or the parents (particularly the mother). Within the Christian New Testament, for example, Jesus is reported to have healed a paralyzed man by telling him 'Your sins are forgiven' (Matthew 9:2). Thomson (2002) notes that, from the New Testament to modern 'healing miracles', the theme of bodily restoration as spiritual redemption is essential to Christianity.

Indeed, it has been argued that the Christian rhetorical tradition demonizes disabled people (Wilson & Lewiecki-Wilson 2002). In the Old Testament, disabled people were regarded as 'unclean', like prostitutes and, within certain Jewish sects, disabled people were prevented from eating with other members of their communities (Stiker 1999). Hindu mythology portrays impairments in extremely negative terms: as flaws or deficiencies that must be endured to repay past sin; associating impairment with deceit, mischief and evil (Ghai 2001). Buddhism teaches that impairments constitute a form of 'educational rebirth' for wrong conduct in previous incarnations (Miles 2000). The ways in which religions have passed moral judgements on impairments has virtually guaranteed that disability is generally equated not with difference, but with deviance (Hughes 1998).

Because an impairment is viewed as evidence of an inherently sinful person or one who is fundamentally flawed, disabled people are commonly prohibited from assuming leadership roles within their faith communities and may be limited in their worship (Hughes 1998, Mackelprang & Salsgiver 2000). Some sects, such as Roman Catholicism, have prevented disabled people from marrying. Hinduism, Buddhism, Jainism, Zoroastrianism and Judaism all have laws that have excluded disabled people from their right of inheritance and from becoming priests, kings, monks or doctors (Miles 1995). Social inequities are therefore sanctioned and legitimated within this model.

When Aids initially appeared to be centred within the gay community in North America, the fundamentalist churches claimed this was divine punishment for sinful, homosexual practices. Conveniently overlooking the reality that lesbians have the lowest incidence of HIV and Aids throughout the world, this perpetuated the notion that impairment demonstrates divine displeasure and retribution.

Disabled people serve as a reminder that we cannot control our own destiny – or that of our children – and that we are always vulnerable to illness or injury (Marks 1999); often irrespective of our behaviour or lifestyle. Although many people would denounce the suggestion that impairment constitutes some form of punishment for sin – that 'bad' things justifiably happen to 'bad' people – the commonly cited belief that 'everything happens for a reason' would seem to reflect a need to attribute a divine agenda to the 'bad' things that happen, and a belief that we are all helpless pawns in a bizarre supernatural chess game.

Thomson (1997a p 36) suggests that 'the human need for predictability gives rise to a belief that people get what they deserve . . . if something "bad" – like having a disability [sic] – happens to someone, then there must be a "good" reason – like divine or moral justice – for its occurrence'. She proposes that this is 'a psychological safeguard against the intolerable randomness of experience' (Thomson 1997a p 36). Qualitative research undertaken by McColl and colleagues (McColl 2000, McColl et al 2000) among people who had sustained a neurological injury found that some people believed their injuries 'happened for a reason', although they tended to be unclear about what this reason might be. Some viewed their impairments as a mission, demonstrated by comments such as: 'I just believe I was saved for a purpose' (McColl 2000 p 222). Although there tended to be a vagueness about what this purpose was, there was a belief that it would be revealed in time (McColl et al 2000). Others believed their injury was a test or a form of punishment: 'I take it as a punishment . . . I look at it as the way God has of repaying'; or a divine warning: 'if you start to get off the track, that's when He steps in and makes a correction' (McColl et al 2000 p 821). These ways of explaining impairments reflect a moral/religious interpretation or model.

Researchers have found that many people re-evaluate their life priorities following the onset of serious illness or impairment, although the majority do not subscribe to the belief that this was the 'reason' they became ill or impaired (Hammell 2004h). The actor, Christopher Reeve, for example, commented: 'I wasn't injured for a reason. It was an accident, it just happened. But now I have the opportunity to make sense out of it. I believe it's what you do *after* a disaster that gives it meaning' (Time 1996 p 44). To suggest that illnesses, injuries or impairments 'happen' for a purpose, to teach patience, to strengthen relationships, to punish, or to prompt a life review, for example, is to subscribe to the moral/religious model and its belief that impairments are a deliberate part of a grand supernatural scheme.

Consequences of the moral/religious model

The idea that impairments are deserved leads easily to derision, ostracism, abuse, ridicule and pity. The belief that disabled people are 'pitiful' (a word that implies both compassion and contempt) underpins the concept of charity or alms-giving. Notably, the 'moral obligation' to donate to charities that claim to help those 'less fortunate than ourselves' is action directed towards individuals (Richardson 1997). This is not effort directed towards changing the circumstances of disabled people as a population or of striving to equalize opportunities so that others might, instead, become *as* 'fortunate as ourselves'. Ghai (2002) notes that many charitable gestures are made not from a sense of solidarity but from a cultural obligation to do one's religious or dharmic duty. Because charitable donations are, by definition, of a voluntary nature, the amount of assistance available to disabled people fluctuates, with no relationship to the actual need for support (McColl & Bickenbach 1998a). Rather than seeking to promote social justice, acts of charity reinforce relationships of superiority and inferiority, perpetuating the status quo of inequality (Coleridge 1999). In reality, charitable giving is often viewed as a way to attain 'riches in heaven' for oneself.

By explaining disabled people's oppression as a form of punishment, the religious model provides moral and ideological justification for violating disabled people's rights (Vasey 2004). The traditional belief that impairments constitute a form of divine punishment often leads to guilt and shame, such that the presence of a disabled family member is perceived as a blight on the honour and reputation of an entire family (Abu-Habib 1997, Turmusani 1999). To preserve a façade of "normality", disabled people may be hidden from view, often in appalling conditions of confinement and deprivation (Camilleri & Callus 2001); a lifetime of 'house arrest' for the 'crime' of impairment. By virtue of its global dominance, the moral/religious model has been particularly influential in informing and justifying widespread discrimination against disabled people.

THE INDIVIDUAL/MEDICAL MODEL OF DISABILITY

Commonly labelled either the medical model or the individual model of disability, this is the model that has traditionally underpinned the rehabilitation professions. Arising during the Enlightenment period in Western history with the belief that science could solve any problem, the medical model sees disability as an individual deficit amenable to "expert" solutions (Mackelprang & Salsgiver 2000). The model works like this: an individual whose body structure or function is perceived to deviate from socially recognized norms comes to the attention of healthcare professionals who assess, diagnose and legitimate the person's impairment. Any restriction of activity or social disadvantage that the individual confronts in his or her everyday life is deemed to be the inevitable and tragic consequence of this impairment (Thomas 2002). This implies that there is no hope for social inclusion in the absence of a cure for the impairment.

'The medical model assumes that there is an optimal level of human functioning to which all human beings should aspire' (Leplége & Hunt 1997 p 48) and this assumption has been largely unchallenged by the rehabilitation professions. Thus, medical and rehabilitation services are directed towards the application of treatments that might enable individuals to overcome their functional deficits and appear in a manner that is as near to normal as possible. In addition, a process of psychological adjustment is deemed necessary to enable the person to come to terms with their deficits.

Oliver (1983) suggested that because theorists imagined that it would be a tragedy to have an impairment, they decided that a process of psychological adjustment would be required to enable individuals to adjust to their situation. Indeed, this process was reified in a stage theory of adaptation, which required the individual to pass through recognizable phases of shock, grief, denial, anger and depression (Oliver 1981). Lack of supportive evidence – and indeed, plenty of disconfirming evidence – has not completely dampened therapists' enthusiasm for this dogma (Hammell 1995). It is suggested that this ideology has served professional interests: if disabled people fail to achieve the rehabilitation goals established by their therapists, 'blame' can be laid on the clients' difficulties in adjusting to impairment, leaving the rehabilitation process unchallenged (Oliver 1981).

The individual/medical model was clearly reflected in the United Nations' International Year of Disabled Persons, which declared its primary aim as being to 'help disabled people in their physical and psychological adjustment to society' (Barnes & Mercer 2003 p 145). The onus within this model is on disabled people to adapt themselves to a society designed to meet the needs of the dominant population; there is no obligation for society to change to accommodate all its members. Indeed, there is no room within this model to identify societal, rather than individual, problems.

The original WHO (1980) ICIDH system for classifying impairments, disabilities and handicaps neatly encapsulated the individual/medical model from which it arose, proposing that any difficulty encountered in everyday living was caused by an individual's difference. Although the more recent incarnation of the ICIDH – the ICF – has attempted to adopt a broader perspective (see Chapter 2), the focus of the classification remains those individuals deemed deviant from the norm and the problems that they face, as individuals, in their daily lives as a result of their deviant characteristic.

Consequences of the individual/medical model

The individual/medical model has dominated the rehabilitation professions in such a way as to make this model appear to be the "right" way of thinking about disability. Indeed, the existence of a competing model (see below) has rarely been acknowledged. Hunt (1996 p 243) observed: 'I think it is reasonable to say that occupational therapists, like most of their professional colleagues, have held the view that . . . rehabilitation can be used to reduce disability by helping people to relearn skills and adapt themselves to a world in which able-bodiedness is the norm'. By defining disability as a medical problem the rehabilitation professions have delimited their mandate to 'the cure or restoration of the disabled individual to as nearly a normal existence as possible' (Groce & Scheer 1990 p v); somehow viewing this as an adequate, useful and benevolent response to disability. Critical disability theorists reject the premise that the intent of the individual/medical model is benevolent. Rather, they view attempts to normalize individuals as inherently repressive and they challenge models of practice within which powerful "experts" determine treatment plans for powerless 'patients' (see Chapter 2). Reynolds (2004a) notes that because the medical model privileges "expert" biomedical knowledge there is no role for clients in making treatment decisions. 'If disease, disability and diagnosis are framed squarely in terms of body pathology, then individual experience, values and goals seem quite irrelevant to decisions about treatment, care and support' (Reynolds 2004a p 19).

There are occasions when the individual/medical model is highly appropriate; for example, in the instance of someone who has a torn cruciate ligament and a realistic hope for full restoration. However, although intervention in such an instance might reasonably be labelled as 'treatment', it cannot be labelled as 'rehabilitation'. By definition, treatment that aims to cure or restore is not rehabilitation, i.e. the process of enabling individuals to live well with an impairment in the context of their environment. Indeed, although the term 'treatment' is appropriate to the individual/medical model, 'intervention' is more appropriate within the social/political model (see below). This is not solely because 'treatment' implies client passivity but also because 'intervention' reflects a mode of practice that might focus on environmental changes – such as workplace modifications – rather than attempts to modify the individual (Hammell 2004a). Engel (1977) argued that the medical model is inadequate for either the scientific or social responsibilities of medicine and that it embraces mind–body dualism, ignores human experience and reflects a culturally specific perspective. Nonetheless, he claimed that the model 'has acquired the status of *dogma*' (Engel 1977 p 130).

Illness and impairment

Congruent with the medical model, many social policy experts, therapists and researchers equate chronic illness with disability (Rock 2000, Stalker & Jones 1998) as if these terms are interchangeable and insights from the study of chronic illness may be universalized to the experience of disability (e.g. Wendell 1996).

The term 'illness' is commonly used to describe the 'subjective feeling of being unwell and may include symptoms of pain, breathlessness, tiredness, nausea and vertigo' (Finkelstein & French 1993 p 29): problems that are experienced by most people at some time but that occur much or all of the time among people with chronic illnesses. Although some people with impairments can experience physiological consequences that require medical treatment (e.g. people with multiple sclerosis) others with impairments such as learning difficulties, short stature and amputations might not (Barnes 1998a, Frank 1986). In addition, Mitchell & Snyder (1997 p 3) observe that 'disabled people, by definition, do not enjoy the biological luxury of recovery' that may accompany the experiences of illness or disease.

Disability is not an issue of health. Many disabled people regard their health as 'excellent' (Wilcock 1998) and have no need for extensive medical services (Amundson 1992). Despite profound impairments, people with congenital amputations or who are blind, for example, are not ill and cannot be made to 'fit' within the medical model of disability. Illness involves varying degrees of suffering and of bodily dis-ease, whereas impairments are not necessarily equated with any degree of suffering. However, mental illnesses can entail profound suffering and might also *impair* functioning at the level of feeling, cognition and behaviour (Ferguson 2003). Although Michalko (2002) argues that disability and suffering have always been paired, this equation perpetuates the myth that any and all disadvantages experienced by disabled people can be attributed to their 'affliction', provokes pity and enables social exclusion to remain unchallenged. Kasnitz & Shuttleworth (2001 p 20) observe that 'disability exists when people experience discrimination on the basis of perceived functional limitations'. Thus, Amundson (1992 p 114) observed that 'unlike ill people, disabled people are not (typically) globally incapacitated *except insofar as an environment helps to make them so*' [emphasis in original].

THE SOCIAL/POLITICAL MODEL OF DISABILITY

The social/political, or 'social' model arose from the declaration by the British Union of Physically Impaired Against Segregation (UPIAS 1976 p 3–4) that 'In our view it is society which disables physically impaired people. Disability is something imposed on top of our impairments by the way we are unnecessarily isolated and excluded from full participation in society ... disability is therefore a particular form of social oppression'. This model was subsequently adopted by Disabled People's International (Siminski 2003). Just as feminist theorists have made a distinction between sex (being male or female) and gender (the social experience of being a man or woman), so disability theorists distinguish impairments (perceived bodily differences) and disability (the social experience of having an impairment) (Shakespeare 2003).

In the social model, *impairment* refers to 'perceived abnormalities of the body and/or the mind, whether real or ascribed' (Barnes 2003 p 829) and *disability* refers to 'the loss or limitation of opportunities to take part in the normal life of the community on an equal level with others due to physical and social barriers' (Barnes 1991 p 2). Thus, 'disability' refers not to something wrong with an individual (as the individual/medical model would contend); rather, 'disability is something wrong with society' (Oliver 1996a p 129). It has therefore been suggested that disability should fall under the remit of government departments of the environment, rather than of health (Finkelstein 1991).

'The social model of disability is an analysis of a process of marginalization, oppression, discrimination, exclusion, or in other words disablement, that affects people with impairments' (Sapey 2004 p 273). According to the social/political model, 'disability' 'is all the things that impose restrictions on disabled people: ranging from individual prejudice to institutional discrimination, from inaccessible public buildings to unusable transport systems, from segregated education to excluding work arrangements, and so on' (Oliver 1996a p 33). Richardson (1997 p 1269) explains that someone who has a physical impairment due, for example, to cerebral palsy 'may not be disabled from living a full life if social prejudices in the home, work place, public facilities, public buildings and public transport are absent and wheelchair access is present'.

Chapter 1 explored the contentious issues surrounding the terms 'disabled people' and 'people with disabilities' and cited Neufeldt's (1999 p 32) explanation that 'disability results when a person with an impairment encounters an inaccessible environment. It is therefore the environment which disables the person and so the term "person with a disability" is incorrect'. It can be seen that using the term 'disabled people' reflects an acknowledgment of the social model and the theoretical perspectives of disabled people. As Priestley (1999 p 7) observed, 'the choice of appropriate terminology is not just a semantic decision. It is also a political one'.

Disability as oppression: exploring the social/political model

Critical disability theorists claim that disabled people are oppressed, citing evidence of the 'highly unequal distribution of material resources and uneven power relations and opportunities to participate in everyday life, compared to those available to non-disabled people' (Barnes & Mercer 2003 p 19). The recent turn to qualitative research methods by the rehabilitation professions has enabled the perspectives of disabled people to emerge in ways that are prohibited by those forms of data collection that are limited by the hypotheses of researchers (Hammell & Carpenter 2000). Such research enables clients' perspectives to test the validity of various models. For example, Mary Law (2004) described research undertaken to identify factors that affect the daily life patterns of children who have physical impairments. The main research findings centred not on the inherent problems of impairments but on the role that social and physical environments play in supporting or hindering the everyday activities of disabled children. These were primarily negative social attitudes, significant physical barriers and inappropriate social policies. Thus, through an exploratory, qualitative and participatory approach to research, findings emerged that provided clear support for the social model of disability and its contention that 'disability is created in interactions with a physical and social world designed for non-disabled living' (Swain et al 1993 p 2).

In an attempt to identify those factors that have been found to influence perceptions of quality of life following spinal cord injury, a review of approximately 70 peer-reviewed, published research reports was undertaken. These studies demonstrated that dissatisfaction with life after spinal cord injury primarily arises not from the injury itself but from social disadvantages such as confinement to a residential institution, unemployment and reduced community access (Hammell 2004i). Quality of life appeared closely linked to equality of life. Clearly, such findings provide evidence-based support for the social model of disability. They also suggest that efforts by rehabilitation practitioners to enhance the quality of their clients' lives through enhancing physical function may be aiming at the wrong target.

Importantly, the environment is not solely a physical entity. Recent attempts by geographers (e.g. Butler & Parr 1999, Gleeson 1999a) to explore the experience of impairment from within their narrow field of expertise – place and space – demonstrate the futility of this task in isolation from those economic, social, legal, cultural and political structures that inform specific configurations of place and space and that shape individual lives.

Critiques of the social/political model

Although some critical disability theorists argue for an adherence to the social model (Shakespeare 1997b, Ward 1997), a theoretical model should act as a lens to sharpen one's thinking, not as a set of blinkers to restrict ideas and enforce conformity. Clinicians, researchers and theorists should not be slaves to theory but open to different explanations and interpretations that might serve to expand, revise or renew current theories. Stone (2001 p 51) suggested that 'using the social model of disability as an analytical framework is not the same as using it as a blueprint'. In reality, the social model has been subjected to considerable debate and critical analysis and these perspectives will be outlined in turn.

Does the social/political model ignore impairment?

One contention reflects a belief that the embodied experience of disability (Toombs 1995) and the frustrating and 'oppressive' aspects of impairment (Barnes & Mercer 2003, Clare 1999, Mulvany 2000) have been ignored by the social model. This contention has been raised primarily by disabled feminists who, while acknowledging the disabling impact of physical and social barriers, reject the idea that their problems are wholly social, believing that this ignores such experiences as pain, fatigue, paralysis and reduced life-expectancy (Clare 1999, Crow 1996, French 1993a, Morris 1991, 1994, Pinder 1995). However, the contention among social model theorists that 'disablement is nothing to do with the body. It is a consequence of social oppression' (Oliver 1996a p 35) does not contradict the assertion that bodies can exert their own forms of oppression (e.g. pain, incontinence, spasticity); rather, it emphasizes that disablement is a form of social oppression that is superimposed on those with impairments. As Thomas (2004 p 25) explained: 'while impairment is not the cause of disability, it is the raw material upon which disability works'.

Critical disability theorists do not argue naïvely that the problems they face in their everyday lives are 'nothing more than social oppression' (Oliver et al 1988 p 12). 'Clearly, this view is inadequate, for having a spinal cord injury [for example] imposes a number of personal problems, such as . . . urinary infections, risk of pressure sores, and so on, which cannot be explained in terms of social oppression' (Oliver et al 1988 p 12). However, there is an analytical division between the problems associated with the body – impairment – and those imposed by society – disability. As Thomas (2002 p 43) explained, 'the potential for impairment to limit activities is not denied, but such limitations do not constitute *disability*'.

Removing the body/mind from the social model's definition of disability makes it possible to identify the range, form and types of discrimination that make the world a difficult place for disabled people (Barnes 1991), to differentiate these from impairment issues and to explore the intersection and interaction of impairment and disability (Thomas 2001). Stone (2001) explained that there is an important difference between the ways in which one's life chances are diminished because of an impairment and the ways in which one's life chances are diminished as a consequence of disabling responses to that impairment. The social model facilitates exploration of these differences.

The struggle for social inclusion does not constitute a rejection of the healthcare interventions that alleviate impairments (Ahmad 2000). On the contrary, disability researchers advocate for appropriate, specialized medical services to be available from 'cradle to grave', or 'accident to grave' (Oliver et al 1988 p 33). In a just world, disability would be eliminated but pain, spasticity, tremor and other problems related to impairments might persist. As Morris (1991 p 70–1) observed: 'While the negative parts to the experience of being Black or gay in a white, heterosexist society can be identified as wholly socially created, there are negative aspects of being disabled which would persist regardless of the society in which we live'.

Research among people with high spinal cord injuries found that the physical manifestations of their impairments were of central concern and that these presented barriers to employment: 'because sometimes you just can't get out of bed: you may have a pressure sore or not be feeling well . . . it's not as easy as an able-bodied person' (Hammell 1998a). This lends support to the argument that 'although the medical model has ignored sociocultural issues, it cannot simply be replaced by a socio-cultural model which ignores medicine' (Groce & Scheer 1990 p 1443).

Is the social/political model inescapably dualistic?

Some theorists protest that the social model reproduces an outmoded and discredited form of dualistic thinking, with artificial boundaries dividing the bodily experience of impairment from the social experience of disability

(Corker & French 1999). This overlooks the relationship between these two dimensions of experience. It is possible to examine the problems that may accompany an impairment – for example pain or spasticity – from both a physical and a social perspective. Fatigue may only become a barrier to shopping, for example, if shops do not provide any seating on which one might rest.

The argument that impairment and disability are two different, but related, dimensions of experience would seem to be no more dualistic than the premise that gender (cultural) and sex (biological) are related but different concepts. Being biologically female, for example, can be accompanied by negative physical experiences, such as dysmenorrhoea or menorrhagia. Not only does social taboo forbid mention of these issues but the limited number of toilets provided in public spaces may serve to restrict the mobility of women at certain times. Thus the (sometimes negative) physical experience of being female can have social dimensions. Further, being gendered as female may also be a cultural experience of diminished opportunities, with restricted access to social spaces and negative and demeaning social attitudes: disadvantages that are not attributable to female biology but to gender discrimination.

Some critics have argued, however, that the sex–gender system reflects the imperialistic tendencies of feminists who have simplistically seized on gender as culturally constructed yet failed to question the ways in which cultures can construct anatomical or biological sex (Tremain 2002). Research has found that the birth of an intersexual baby, who does not conform to clear male or female "norms", is regarded as an 'emergency' because it threatens social and cultural normativity (Fausto-Sterling 2000). Immediate 'correction' occurs by means of surgical intervention or chemical control (Tremain 2002): 'technologies of normalization' (Fausto-Sterling 2000 p 275) that serve to uphold binary sex categories (Tremain 2002). Human biology is a product not just of science but of cultural and social pressures (Rose 2004).

Wolbring (2001 p 43) notes that 'in the West, the positions of women, gay men and lesbians are now widely viewed within a social model, suggesting that the disadvantage they experience is caused not by an intrinsic characteristic of being female or gay but by the behaviour of male/heterosexual-dominated societies towards them'.

Rather than reinforcing dualistic thinking, a social model compels consideration of both the physical and the sociocultural sequelae of both impairment and disability. Indeed, Ahmad (2000) argued that it is necessary to reconceptualize disability as a social issue to ensure that the marginalization and discrimination experienced by disabled people is seen in similar terms to racist, homophobic and sexist discrimination.

Is the social/political model relevant in the majority world?

Some critics have suggested that the social model is inappropriate for people beyond the minority ("developed") world (e.g. M. Miles 1996, Stone 1997). In response, Stone (1999 p 3) argued that 'the evidence from many disabled people who live in the majority world is that the social model makes sense across cultures and countries'. Comparing the situation of disabled people in the minority and majority ("third") worlds, Turmusani (1999) notes shared experiences of disadvantage in every area of life, with reduced access to educational, training and employment opportunities, to health care, transportation and religious and public buildings. The overall picture for both is of 'inadequate services, socioeconomic structures that exclude disabled people, and a lack of access and equal opportunity. It is also one of negative social attitudes' (p 195–6). Turmusani claims that the situation for disabled people will only improve if the social model of disability is promoted.

Miles & Hossain (1999) contend that social model rhetoric is incomprehensible to those people for whom losing one's eyesight, for example, is an 'unmitigated personal disaster' (p 80). They also argue that although such models might be relevant in countries wealthy enough to adapt their environments to meet the needs of their citizens, they are neither relevant nor appropriate for impoverished countries; and that 'foisting' these ideas onto countries of the majority world 'displays some arrogance about the practical realities of development' (p 80). This completely misses the point of the social model, which does not argue that impairments are of no consequence, nor that they might not be personal disasters, but insists that the inherent difficulties faced by people with impairments are compounded by oppressive social circumstances. Clearly, poverty is *the* oppressive circumstance, *par excellence*. Indeed, given the strong relationship between poverty and impairment (Reviere & Hylton 1999, Stone 1999) and the reality that neither governments nor most non-governmental organizations have auspicious records for including disabled children and adults in their education, employment or development programmes (Frost 1999, Turmusani 1999), the social/political model appears to be especially relevant to the majority world. In the majority world, disabled people are disadvantaged by social and political inequality, negative cultural stereotypes and inequitable access to education, employment, health care, economic assistance and to the everyday life of their communities. This does not negate the oppressive dimensions of many impairments, but it does support the social model.

After exploring the situation of disabled people in Bangladesh, Waldie (2002) reported that the primary problem facing disabled people was that of negative social attitudes – stigma and prejudice – and that these attitudes led directly to their secondary problems, of inequality of opportunity and of the inability to participate in society due to social and physical barriers. Clearly, this supports the social model, indicating global discrimination towards those with attributed impairments. Indeed, Swain (2004a p 57) noted that an international, human rights approach to social change has emanated 'from the social model of disability and the global challenge to the oppression of disabled people'.

Problems of identity and universalism

It can reasonably be argued that the social model reproduces the medical model's problem with respect to identity. The individual/medical model focuses on the physical and psychological aspects of impairments. The social model turns its attention to the social constraints upon those who are 'different'. However, both models focus on disability as the most salient and important dimension of the individual's life, reducing disability to a defining identity. This ignores other dimensions that contribute to identity, such as professional status, age, "race," class, gender or sexual identity, and that intersect and influence the ways in which the world is experienced (e.g. Vernon 1996). (Issues of identity were explored in Chapter 3).

Further, because of its emphasis on oppression, the social model tends to portray disabled people as universally poor, unemployed and socially marginalized (e.g. Oliver 1996a). Although it is undoubtedly true that a disproportionately high percentage of disabled people do, indeed, fit this description (Charlton 1998, Crichton & Jongbloed 1998), impairments pervade all strata of society and can occur at any time and in any family. For example, among the fifteen men who participated in a study into severe head injury there were an architect, an air traffic controller and two university professors (Hammell 1994b). Although this was undoubtedly an unusual sample, it was one that demonstrated our universal vulnerability to impairment, irrespective of wealth or class.

The reality that many people with a specific impairment are fully integrated into the social and economic lives of their communities, whereas others with similar impairments are not, lends credence to the argument that disability is a social and not a biological phenomenon. Nonetheless, although the experience of disability is impacted by its intersections with "race," gender, class, age and sexual orientation, Vernon (1998) contends that the stigma of impairment over-rides all other boundaries, leading to a critical similarity in the experience of all disabled people.

Is the social/political model an urban model of disability?

The social/political model insists that all problems associated with disability could be solved in a just society. So now I must add my own criticism: that the social model is an urban model of disability. The reality of the experience of disability in rural areas and in countries of the majority world is centrally concerned with mud and sand, snow and cold, trees and vegetation, rough ground, unpaved roads, mountains and hills: problems that will present insurmountable barriers in even the most just society. In winter in northern Saskatchewan, for example, 'seeing eye' dogs are unable to function because they cannot distinguish kerbs from the packed snow in which these kerbs are encased (Hammell 1998a). Thus a disabled feminist observed: 'I believe that some of the most profound problems experienced by people with certain impairments are difficult, if not impossible to solve by social manipulation' (French 1993a p 17). This problem with the social model is not surprising when one considers that most disability theorists live in urban areas in the minority world. However, 80% of disabled people live in the majority ("developing") world and 90% of these people live in rural areas (Marks 1999). Nonetheless, as a deliberate political strategy, social model theorists have chosen to focus on those physical, economic, legal, political, cultural and social barriers that are the products of discrimination and thus amenable to change.

Consequences of the social/political model

The social/political model arose out of the experiences of disabled people, was originally articulated by disabled activists and has been embraced, debated and promoted by disabled and disability theorists. In the terms of Antonio Gramsci (1971), the social model represents an *organic* model: arising from the very people whose experiences it aims to encapsulate. It is also a postcolonial model in that it describes the experiences and perspectives of the dispossessed in their own terms and counters the imperialistic definitions imposed by those wielding more power (Young 2003). By articulating the social model, disabled activists and academics contested the assumption that the problems faced by disabled people are a direct consequence of their impairments. When disabled people first encounter the ideas that inform this model it is often an experience of both revelation and liberation; a recognition that their impoverished social circumstances are not their 'fault' (Campbell & Oliver 1996, Crow 1996, Thomas 2002). Indeed, Hevey (1992) likened his discovery of the social model to a religious conversion, or 'road to Damascus' encounter.

Beyond being an organic theory arising *from* a social movement, the social model of disability has played a significant role in influencing the social movement from which it originated (Campbell & Oliver 1996): the model is thus both social and political. Disability theorist and activist, Liz Crow (1996 p 207) observed that it has 'enabled a vision of ourselves free from the constraints of disability (oppression) and provided a direction for our commitment to social change. It has played a central role in promoting disabled people's individual self-worth, collective identity and political organization'.

The social/political model has had a major global impact. Gabel and Peters (2004 p 585) note 'evidence for the influence of the social model abounds in international declarations and conventions, in national legislation, in global expansion of Community-Based Rehabilitation programmes, in the growing number of Disability Studies degrees in universities, in the push for inclusive education . . . and in the research literature'. Canada's Charter of Rights and Freedoms, for example, understands disability as a social status rather than a problem of individual deficits (Rioux 1999).

THE RESPONSE OF THE REHABILITATION PROFESSIONS TO THE SOCIAL/POLITICAL MODEL

Amundson (1992 p 111) observed that rehabilitation is an imperfect response to disability, noting that, as a society 'we design our environments to suit a range of biomedically normal personal abilities. Rehabilitation in itself does nothing to change these environments. It only changes the skills of disabled people so as to increase their ability to function in the pre-existing environment'. It is difficult to argue against this observation and it must surely prompt the rehabilitation professions to reflect on whether an individualized response to disability is in any way adequate.

Physiotherapists and occupational therapists have acknowledged the importance of physical, social, cultural, economic, political and legal environments in their theories of movement (Cott et al 1995) and of occupational performance (CAOT 1997). It makes little sense, therefore, to focus on modifying individuals' functional abilities while ignoring the environments within which these skills are required. Although the individual/medical model will always have some utility in informing interventions for acute medical problems, it is inadequate for identifying, examining or addressing the experience of disability. In addition to teaching mobility skills, for example, rehabilitation professionals must surely ensure that clients have somewhere they can go and something they can do?

The social model has influenced and shaped the ways in which some clinicians and researchers confront disability (Hahn 1988). As early as 1983, the social work profession began to engage with the social model and to learn from the perspectives of disability activists and theorists (Oliver 1983, Oliver & Sapey 1999), although Oliver (1996a) has questioned whether this has had much impact on practice.

In 1990, Jongbloed & Crichton observed, 'rehabilitation professionals still have a largely clinical or individualistic ideology and focus very little on improving the circumstances of disabled people through changes in laws or social policies' (1990a p 32). They challenged occupational therapists to embrace a sociopolitical model of disability and 'be less willing to accept individual explanations for problems that are essentially economic, social or political' (1990a p 32). However, the occupational therapy profession has been slow to respond to the social model (Craddock 1996a, 1996b). Although there are a few notable exceptions (e.g. CAOT 1997, Stalker & Jones 1998), many textbooks still conform to the individual/medical model. Indeed, the definition of disability employed throughout McColl & Bickenbach's book (1998b) is used by critical disability theorists as an exemplar of the individual/medical model (Swain et al 2003 p 28).

Acknowledging the social dimensions of disablement does not require that therapists neglect the individual physical or psychological issues of impairment. Of course not. Instead, it requires a more holistic focus – one that acknowledges that individuals do not live in vacuums but in complex physical and social environments – and this requires use of an appropriate model. The medical model has not been disproved. Rather, it has proved to be often appropriate to medicine and always inappropriate for rehabilitation.

Stone (1999 p 3) has argued that the rehabilitation professions should be 'allied to disabled people and the community, not allied to medicine or administration'. However, the rehabilitation professions – occupational therapy, physiotherapy, social work, speech and language pathology and nursing – are still more closely aligned with each other than with those of architects, lawyers, economists, politicians, social policy makers or with disability activists. They thus remain mired in the medical model and firmly focused upon individualized 'health care services' (Hammell 2003a).

Jongbloed & Crichton (1990a) observed that the rehabilitation professions have been largely indifferent to the social disadvantages experienced by their disabled clients and have an unauspicious record in the struggle to remove disabling barriers. This is the unsurprising consequence of an individual, medical approach to disability.

IMPLICATIONS OF THE SOCIAL/POLITICAL MODEL FOR REHABILITATION

Writing in the nursing literature, Richardson (1997 p 1270) claimed that: 'Once professionals working with disabled people accept the barriers [social] model it behooves them to form alliances with disabled people, assisting them with citizenship rights, with managing personal support, liaison with other services and advocacy in support of the removal of social and physical barriers in the local environment'.

Jongbloed & Crichton (1990b) outlined the difficulties in shifting from an individualistic to a sociopolitical approach to disability policy. It is apparent that it is equally difficult for the rehabilitation professions to shift from an individualistic, medical model of disability to a social/political model, perhaps because this will entail dismantling unequal power relationships with clients and will demand a commitment to social change rather than a preoccupation with changing individuals. Indeed, Schriner (2001) suggests that the term 'rehabilitation' ought to be used to describe practitioners' efforts to make social, attitudinal and physical environments more hospitable to disabled people; 'rehabilitating' the environment.

The social/political model requires therapists to expand the focus of their interventions from modifying individuals (for example, by teaching mobility skills) to also modifying environments (for example, by actively lobbying for accessible public transportation). It does not permit therapists to acquiesce to the status quo but demands a level of commitment and engagement that is alien to traditional stereotypes of professionalism. While some therapists have embraced the challenge of the social model in both research and practice (e.g. Hawkins & Stewart 2002), this model faces considerable resistance from those whose power is reinforced by the individual/medical model.

IDEOLOGY AND POWER

Barnes (1991 p 132) claimed that 'if the economic and social barriers which confront disabled people were removed the need for rehabilitation in its present form would be greatly reduced, if not eliminated altogether'. McKnight (1981) argued that the very existence of many healthcare professions depends on viewing disability from the perspective of the individual/medical model and that the forms of assessment and intervention the professions promote serve to define and individualize problems for which they hold 'solutions'. This suggests that the rehabilitation professions may have a personal investment in perpetuating the ideological dominance of the medical model that has little to do with client-centred practice and everything to do with maintaining power.

Some disability theorists view rehabilitation professionals as agents of the State, protecting the social status quo by 'pathologizing and individualizing problems that have been socially and economically created' (French & Swain 2001 p 736). Describing his awareness that the barriers he encountered in his life were a consequence of his environment rather than his impairment, Ian Basnett, a physician who sustained a spinal cord injury, has pondered who benefits from perpetuating the individual/medical model of disability: a model Basnett found to be woefully inadequate. Answering his own question, he suggests 'an individualistic model clearly suits the health professions . . . It emphasizes the importance of their skill and assists in their professional dominance' (Basnett 2001 p 452). He argues that health professionals are 'active promoters of a paradigm that strengthens their own role' (Basnett 2001 p 452).

Schriner (2001) notes that the individual model is politically conservative, avoiding confrontations with the structural and attitudinal barriers that discriminate against disabled people and attracting to the rehabilitation professions those people who are more interested in modifying individuals than achieving social change. The practice of changing people to closer approximations of "normality" and conformity is an implicitly political practice.

French & Swain (2001) contend that the emergence of the social model constitutes a fundamental challenge to professional ideologies and models. However, power has determined whose perspectives are accorded privilege and which model predominates. As French (1994b p 3) observed: 'the models put forward by powerful groups within society, such as the medical profession . . . tend to dominate the models of less powerful groups, such as disabled people themselves'. Consistent with the findings of the previous chapters – that ideologies are inseparable from power – it is apparent that the triumph of one model of disability over another reflects a collusion of ideology and power.

A considerable body of evidence demonstrates that disabled people are excluded from many dimensions of social life, such as education, employment, housing choices and transportation (Priestley 2003). Why and how does this happen? Is it part of a supernatural plan? Is it because of innate inabilities (and if so, why are people with tetraplegia, for example, able to attend university, work, travel and live in the community today when this was impossible for people with identical impairments in the recent past)? Is exclusion due to a society designed to meet the needs of the dominant population? Choice of an answer dictates the choice both of a model and of an approach to rehabilitation intervention.

'Disabled writers have argued that the most radical improvements in the lives of disabled people over the past decade have come not from the charities, health or social services professionals but via disabled people themselves becoming politically active' (Richardson 1997 p 1272). How might the rehabilitation professions and individual rehabilitation professionals contribute to the process of achieving a non-disabling society and equality of opportunity for disabled people? 'The social model message is simple and strong: if you want to make a difference to the lives of disabled people, you must change society and the way society treats people who have impairments' (Stone 1999 p 2–3). Embracing the social/political model of disability might be a useful place to start.

Building on the chapters that explored ideologies of normality and deviance, this chapter has interrogated various models of disability, outlining the need to employ theory that can capture the experience of oppression that circumscribes the lives of disabled people. The following chapter examines the cultural creation of disability to try to understand the origins and perpetuation of this oppression.

Chapter 5

The cultural perpetuation of disability

What disabled people have to "cope with" is not their impairment, but the hostility, prejudice, and discrimination that they meet every day of their lives. (Coleridge 1993 p 27–8)

INTRODUCTION: THE CULTURAL PERPETUATION OF DISABILITY

The previous chapter outlined the social/political model of disability and its contention that people with impairments are disabled by the ways in which they are 'unnecessarily isolated and excluded from full participation in society' (Union of the Physically Impaired Against Segregation (UPIAS) 1976). Through spotlighting the material dimensions of oppression – the physical, economic, political and legal aspects of disabling societies – social model theorists have sought to focus attention on the disabling barriers that prohibit equal participation and diminish opportunities for disabled citizens. However, this leaves unanswered some basic questions: *why* do disabling barriers exist and persist? *Why* does disability – disadvantage – appear to be an almost inevitable consequence of impairment? *Why* does the onset of impairment so frequently constitute a 'fall from privilege' (Rockhill 1996)?

Disability theorists contend that the relative powerlessness of disabled people and the social and economic inequalities they experience are due to social beliefs and values that perpetuate prejudice, discrimination and unequal life opportunities (Johnstone 1998). Prejudice is perceived to be an attitudinal response to impairment (abnormality) that *precedes* the creation of disabling environments (Shakespeare 1994). This chapter will draw on the work of cultural critics in an examination of the ways in which ideas of inferiority and deviance are perpetuated and used to justify the unequal distribution of life opportunities. These critiques are important for workers in the fields of health and social care, who are themselves products of particular cultural environments.

LIMITS TO THE SOCIAL/POLITICAL MODEL

When examining the social/political model (Chapter 4), it was clear that this model – like all theoretical models – has limitations. Although providing a useful framework within which to understand and interrogate the experience of living with an impairment, it was seen that the model is perceived, by some, to be unhelpfully narrow. The criticism of particular relevance to the present chapter is this: that the desire to redirect attention from the traditional preoccupation with assessing, classifying and modifying people to critiquing, challenging and changing environments has ignored or downplayed the role of culture in the oppression of disabled people (Thomas 1999).

Drawing from a very limited quantity of historical evidence, those disability theorists whose work is informed by Marxism infer that discrimination against disabled people arose as a consequence of capitalist industrialization and its inflexible work practices, which eliminated rural-based trades and introduced a separation of home and workplace (Finkelstein 1981, Gleeson 1999a, Oliver 1990). This overlooks the reality that white women's work remained focused in the home for considerably longer and that Black women in North America had been separated from their own homes since the 1600s and enslaved in those of white women (hooks 1981). Nor do these claims account for the ostracism of disabled people in rural areas of the majority world in the early twenty-first century (Kabzems & Chimedza 2002). Further, by limiting their analysis to 'work', these theorists ignore other important dimensions of people's lives, such as the opportunity to marry and form families and to participate in the cultural and spiritual lives of their communities. In these areas of life it appears that social rejection has been an enduring component of disabilism (Deutsch & Nussbaum 2000a). In the fifteenth century, for example, a Spanish nun wrote not only of the physical pain of impairment but of her social suffering as she was humiliated, despised and treated with contempt and scorn by her religious and social communities, who viewed bodily suffering as a punishment for sin (Juarez 2002).

Some observers contend that the primary problem facing disabled people is negative social attitudes – stigma and prejudice – and that these attitudes lead directly to their secondary problems of inequality of opportunity and of the inability to participate in society due to social and architectural barriers (Tomlinson & Abdi 2003, Waldie 2002). Shakespeare (1994) argued that prejudice precedes and justifies the oppression of disabled people, normalizing it and making exclusion appear to be 'common-sense'. Accordingly, it is claimed that aspects of social policy and the built environment that have an unequal or discriminatory effect on disabled people cannot be attributed to 'happenstance or coincidence' (Hahn 1993 p 741). Rather, they reflect a cultural fabric that created and perpetuates relationships of domination and inferiority. Gleeson (1999a) contends that improved building standards, for example, will not, on their own, solve the oppression faced by disabled people because disabling practices are a reflection of underlying patterns of social organization. The reality that people with facial disfigurements are unable to compete in the labour market on equal terms, for example, suggests that discriminatory barriers are the consequence of something other than market economics, poor architecture or the demands of a uniformly 'able' workforce (Arner 2004).

Said (1993) identified two processes through which colonized people resist the domination of a colonizing power: (1) fighting against intrusion and recovering geographical territory (or, in the instance of disabled people, fighting against *ex*clusion and *for* geographical access), and (2) changing the ideological and 'cultural territory' (p 209) that dominates their lives. Thus culture is centrally implicated in the perpetuation of power and powerlessness. It is also a potential site of resistance.

It is argued that disabled people are disempowered by cultural stereotypes and the social and political inequality these foster and promote (Groce 1999c). Poore (2002 p 261) suggests that a major task of a critical approach to cultural analysis is 'to expose and critique the omnipresent stereotypes and negative metaphors of disability in our cultural heritage'. Because societal practices are a reflection of societal attitudes – because prejudice precedes and justifies oppression – it is important to include the cultural environment in any examination of the interaction between disabled people and the world in which they live.

EXPLORING CULTURE

The concept of culture, most thoroughly explored by anthropologists, is used to define the knowledge, beliefs, attitudes, morals and customs that people acquire through membership of a particular society or group (Ferraro 1995, Peoples & Bailey 1994). *Culture* includes the ways in which people think about the world, their values, and their beliefs about how people ought to live. Anthropologists emphasize that culture is shared among groups and societies of people; and that culture is learned (Peoples & Bailey 1994). They identify two interlinked components of culture – mental and behavioral – demonstrating that learned attitudes, ideas, beliefs, values and perceptions inform particular actions and patterns of behaviour. Thus, cultural norms influence how people act and the unquestioned values that inform their actions. Through the transmission of cultural values, beliefs and attitudes, certain ideas acquire the status of 'common-sense', appearing both 'normal' and 'natural'.

Gayle Rubin (1997 p 101) claimed to have a 'quaint' attitude that 'statements about living populations should be based on some knowledge of such populations, not on speculative analysis, literary texts, cinematic representations, or preconceived assumptions'. However, these are precisely the ways in which cultures derive their beliefs and attitudes about 'other' groups, such as people who differ from themselves in terms of sexual orientation, "race" or disability. Cultural ideas are transmitted through such means as religious teachings, folklore, mythology, literature, art, film, news media and language. Stables & Smith (1999) observe that the mass media holds the power to transmit and reinforce those attitudes that operate in the interests of dominant groups. Indeed, dominant cultural ideas are produced and reproduced so successfully that they acquire the appearance of 'common-sense'.

Thomas (1993 p 3) claimed that 'our culture entraps us in common sense'. This cultural common sense informs each person's 'system of meanings, goals and values, *even* when the person is not explicitly aware of this system' (Charmé 1984 p 25). The French philosopher, Jean-Paul Sartre (1956) observed that one does not examine one's values or beliefs when engaged in the predictable routine of daily activities – when cultural values appear so natural and self-evident as to be indiscernible – but when crisis compels reflection. Disability researchers confirm that the crisis, or life disruption, occasioned by the onset of serious illness or impairment frequently compels people to question cultural norms and values (Becker 1997).

'Nicholas' was 46 when he sustained the high spinal cord injury that disrupted a life of significant material possessions, successful employment and social prestige. His injury, and subsequent abandonment by his wife of many years, prompted a confrontation with, and examination of, the values and priorities that had previously informed his life. Rejecting a lifestyle he now views as shallow and superficial, Nicholas is dedicated to spending time with his children, reading and studying philosophy. He enjoys looking at paintings, values time spent in quiet contemplation and the opportunity to 'sit in solitude – enjoy the fresh air' (Hammell 2004f). As Sartre suggested, crisis had brought formerly unchallenged values, beliefs and attitudes into sharp focus, providing the opportunity to discover new values and new priorities.

A similar sort of cultural disjuncture is often identified by people returning from prolonged periods in countries of the majority ("third") world who find that 'culture shock' is harder on return to a Western culture whose materialistic and self-oriented values they no longer share (Hammell 2004h). Leavitt (1999b) explained that 'culture shock' develops from having one's formerly taken-for-granted values questioned, one's beliefs challenged and one's ethnocentrism threatened. (*Ethnocentrism* is the belief that one's own culture is superior to others and is the standard by which all other people should be judged; Leavitt 1999b).

Social theorists have noted that within a particular culture the ideas and values of the dominant group pervade society in such a way as to appear 'natural', and have developed the concept of *hegemony* to describe how this occurs. Although the idea of hegemony is unfamiliar to many rehabilitation professionals, it is an important concept in seeking to understand how ideas about disability permeate cultures.

THE CONCEPT OF HEGEMONY

The concept of hegemony was developed by the Italian political theorist, Antonio Gramsci (1971). Gramsci's experiences of injustice, due, in part, to the discrimination he encountered as a disabled person, fuelled his analysis of social power (Dombroski 1989, Ransome 1992). Gramsci used the concept of hegemony to define the process through which power is exercised by a dominant group over a subordinate group. He recognized that the power of dominant groups need not be achieved or maintained through the use of force but can be accomplished through the diffusion of 'common-sense' ideas (Frankenberg 1988). Gramsci contended that the domination of certain ideas is achieved by engineering consensus, such that those ideas and beliefs that benefit the powerful appear 'natural', even to the powerless (Bocock 1986). These pervasive ideas serve to legitimate inequality, justify subordination and disguise exploitation and oppression (Frankenberg 1988).

Social theorists have demonstrated that prevailing cultural ideas are neither benign nor of equal benefit to everyone living in a particular society or group. Rather, dominant (or mainstream) cultural norms 'will always reflect the interests of those within particular social groups or societies who have the power to define situations and the resources with which to ensure that their own definitions are accepted as true' (Swain et al 2003 p 20). Thus ideologies and beliefs prevail, not due to their intrinsic superiority or inherent "truth", but as a consequence of power (Foucault 1980). As Priestley (1999 p 53) observed: 'the relative influence of opposing value systems is contingent upon the distribution of power within a given society', the result being that 'the dominant group's vision of reality [is] presented as universal and valid for all groups' (Abberley 2002 p 132). This is hegemony.

Some disability theorists have used the concept of hegemony to draw attention to the ways in which seemingly innocuous and apparently self-evident ideas serve to reinforce social superiority and inferiority, power and powerlessness, and to justify inequality (Charlton 1998, Oliver 1990). The 'hegemonic' ideology of disability equates impairment with helplessness, dependency, loss, tragedy, incompetence, inadequacy and deviancy: to be disabled is to have little value. For example, a common Chinese way of writing 'disability' combines two characters: 'broken' and 'useless' (Lewis 1999). To attempt to counter hegemony and to assert, for example, the value of disabled people's lives is to engage in revolutionary politics (Bickenbach 1993) and to strive to 'decolonize the mind' (Ngugi 1986).

Foucault showed that the process of achieving ideological domination can be quiet, systematic and hidden, all because certain ideas appear to be natural and inevitable (Said 1976). Ideological hegemony has been successfully achieved when certain viewpoints pervade the culture and are accepted as 'normal' and 'common sense', even by those demeaned by these points of view (Barnes & Mercer 2003). Several disability theorists have lamented the 'felt stigma' or 'internal oppression' experienced by those disabled people who have so thoroughly internalized the dominant hegemony that they see themselves as inadequate, useless and valueless (Barnes et al 1999, Coleridge 1999, Thomas 1999). This hegemony is not always resisted by those in the rehabilitation business.

Research shows that healthcare professionals often fail to challenge negative cultural stereotypes, encouraging disabled people to 'adjust' or 'adapt' to a life of diminished opportunities and 'accept' their reduced social status (Hammell 1998a, Oliver 1990). 'David', for example, described the dismal future his healthcare professionals predicted following his C1 spinal cord injury. He recalled receiving a consistent message (also recalled by other research participants): 'you will be dead within two years, you will never leave the hospital, you will never have a home, a job, a family and you will never travel: don't even think about it'. (Still alive, David has accomplished all this, and more). David's rehabilitation professionals encouraged him to envision a future in which he might be able to cross the street to a restaurant opposite the hospital and suggested: '"We'll teach you how to type on a typewriter so you can write letters" – to God knows who! And of course, everybody lived in town anyway; I didn't need to write! . . . but this was my rehab. and this was my future' (Hammell 1998a). The attitudes and beliefs of the therapists clearly reflected, rather than contested, prevailing cultural stereotypes and the assumption that diminished physical ability inevitably leads to a diminished life.

Perhaps therapists believe that by encouraging clients to 'aim low' they will protect them from disappointment and frustration? This p/maternalistic attitude reflects another prevalent cultural attitude that, unlike other ("normal") people, disabled people are unable to cope with the stressors in their lives. This is a disrespectful form of practice that lacks evidence-based support. Instead, research has demonstrated that those people whose expectations are higher than the judgements made by their clinicians do substantially better than people whose expectations accord with or are less than those of their 'treating clinicians' (Batterham et al 1996 p 1222). It is therefore ironic that researchers have found that physiotherapists and occupational therapists frequently strive to change clients' expectations and reduce their goals to match the therapists' own (Abberley 1995, Johnson 1993). This process is deemed by therapists to be 'educational' and is justified by their claims to superior knowledge (Abberley 1995). The evident impotence of such claims provokes a brief enquiry into what constitutes *knowledge*.

Knowledge and beliefs

Knowledge is a combination of factual information and belief. The instability of the boundary between these two dimensions is readily demonstrated by the shifting nature of knowledge. Within medicine, for example, ideas and facts once held to be "true" are now dismissed as erroneous or misguided beliefs. Nonetheless, there is a tendency within the healthcare professions to lay claim to the possession of factual knowledge (i.e. the knowledge they currently hold to be "true") while dismissing alternative perspectives (knowledge that conflicts with their own) as 'beliefs' (Gaines 1998, Good 1994). Foucault (1980) demonstrated that the dominance of one theory over another reflects, not the superiority of the theory, but an alignment of knowledge and power, enabling the perception that 'we' are rational and superior, 'they' are inferior; 'our' beliefs are 'scientific' and 'objective', 'theirs' are not (Said 1979).

Central to Foucault's work was the assertion that 'knowledge . . . authorizes and legitimates the exercising of power' (Danaher et al 2000 p 26). In turn, power legitimates knowledge, determining whose perspectives 'count'. Rather than official knowledge being the only or "true" explanation of things, Foucault's work demonstrated that 'it was really a case of some explanations winning out over others – often for political reasons' (Danaher et al 2000 p 3).

Researchers inevitably interpret research data (both qualitative and quantitative) according to their beliefs (Armstrong et al 1997, Holman 1993, Said 1979, Shakespeare 1996a), demonstrating that even the production of 'factual' and informational knowledge is inseparable from beliefs. Indeed, postmodern theorists have demonstrated that knowledge is never value free but replete with contradictions and cultural prejudices (Danaher et al 2000, Mitchell 1996). For example, many African paediatricians and psychiatrists believe that push-chairs ('prams' or 'baby-strollers') damage the relationship between a mother and child and lead to emotional instability; yet many paediatricians in Europe and North America – encultured with different values and beliefs – do not contest the use of these devices (Wax 2004).

Because beliefs permeate knowledge and inform both attitudes and actions it is important for the rehabilitation professions to evaluate their beliefs, recognize that their knowledge (like all knowledge) is saturated by culture and strive to understand the impact of culture in transmitting and promoting specific beliefs.

The knowledge and beliefs of disabled people, themselves, have been buried under the knowledge and beliefs of the dominant "normals". Indeed, when disabled people's knowledge contradicts or challenges dominant ideology – for example, when some claim to enjoy a more meaningful life after injury than they did prior to injury – they are labelled as suffering from 'false consciousness'. This élitist concept, originated by Marxists (Jary & Jary 1991), is deemed to encompass any idea or ideology that is held to be inappropriate in light of the "true" or "objective" situation as this is "correctly" perceived by those wielding greater power. Social scientists contend that use of the term 'false consciousness' implies that the truth of a given situation is understood correctly and with certitude by someone who is both more enlightened and in possession of a superior consciousness; that those deemed to be inferior are also deemed to be in error, and suggest that use of the term demonstrates contempt for those whose perceptions are being disparaged (Jary & Jary 1991, Somers & Gibson 1994, Wolf 1996). However, 'non-disabled people's greater access to the means of communication and representation effectively ensures the dominance of their world-view and values' (Barnes & Mercer 2003 p 88). This is the power of cultural imperialism.

OPPRESSION: CULTURAL IMPERIALISM

Oppression (disadvantage and injustice) is not solely the product of deliberate action but can result from social practices that are informed by specific values and norms. Importantly, 'oppression may arise not just because society actively seeks to disadvantage some groups of people but rather because of the effects of societal norms, laws and unchallenged assumptions' (Northway 1997 p 738). Oppression can result from both commission and omission.

Chapter 3 introduced Young's five 'faces' of oppression, which included cultural imperialism (Young 1990). *Cultural imperialism*, described by Northway (1997 p 738) as being 'the primary form of oppression experienced by disabled people', refers to the process by which a defined group is demeaned, devalued and stereotyped by those values of the dominant culture that are established as seemingly universal norms or common-sense (Lugones & Spelman 1983, Young 1990). Young (1990 p 123) claims that 'culturally imperialist groups project their own values, experience, and perspectives as normative and universal'. Thus, the cultural imperialism of colonial racism in apartheid South Africa, for example, informed specific interpretations of the Bible and of biology to justify the withholding of civil rights from those deemed 'inferior'. The function of this ideology was to preserve, protect and perpetuate minority white power; ideology and power, in combination, served a specific purpose. Indeed, ideology served to maintain power and dominance with such effectiveness that the white minority group wielded the majority of power and the statistical majority was accorded minority status.

Charlton (1998) observed that the dominant culture portrays certain beliefs concerning superiority and inferiority as natural and taken-for-granted, rather than as historically and culturally specific. Devalued groups are 'submerged in negative stereotypes' (Barnes & Mercer 2003 p 88). Central to cultural imperialism is the desire to assert the "normality" and "superiority" of the dominant group, hence critics contend that the purpose of displaying negative imagery of disabled people in literature, film and the media is to affirm how different 'they' are from 'us', and thus how admirably normal 'we' are (Thomson 1997a). Lorde (1984) claimed that the 'mythical norm' is always at the edge of consciousness.

Disability has been used to represent the deviance of difference from valued gender "norms". In the eighteenth century, for example, it was believed that 'what makes a *woman* elegant, makes a *man* deformed' (cited in Deutsch & Nussbaum 2000b p 12). The argument that deviance serves as a foil against which "normality" can be claimed was explored in Chapter 3.

Disability has also been used to represent the deviance of difference from valued racial "norms". The freak shows of the nineteenth century displayed people with evident physical/mental impairments and the native people of colonized countries under the single heading of "freaks" (Bogdan 1988). Davis (2001) notes that this practice expressed a form of nationalism, with disabled people viewed, not as citizens (with rights), but as aliens. The list of "inferior races" included all non-European people and those who were blind, deaf, hunchbacked, intellectually impaired and mentally ill (Scholnick 2002).

Postcolonial theorists have sought to expose the 'ideological nature of representation and the ways in which powerful representations become the "true" and accepted ones, despite their stereotypical and even caricatured nature' (Ashcroft & Ahluwalia 1999 p 63). From the perspective of postcolonial theory, cultural imperialism can be seen as one dimension of the process through which certain groups of people are marginalized. Moreover, it is because the ideas that benefit those wielding more social power enjoy such pervasive cultural circulation that they tend to be reproduced and perpetuated with little challenge. Thus, the idea that disabled people are both inferior and fundamentally deviant has been reinforced by the work of academics, authors, playwrights, artists, historians, film-makers and others.

Although people with different impairments and social positions do not share the same perspectives or experiences as other disabled people, 'there is a cultural gulf between the disabled and the non-disabled; to become disabled is to enter a different world' (Wendell 1996 p 65). Because disabled people do not regularly see themselves in dominant forms of representation, such as television, theirs is a largely unscripted world.

CULTURAL SCRIPTS

Cultures have been shown to transmit particular values and beliefs that serve to shape and govern behaviours among members of societies or groups. These values and ideas form 'cultural templates' that frame the ways in which it is believed that lives ought to be lived. A template, *cultural narrative* or *cultural script* constitutes a sort of story-line that frames the life possibilities for a member of that culture (Goffman 1959). The culture of a society provides the expected and accepted scripts for various social roles (Barnartt 2001), such that "normal" behaviour becomes desirable behaviour (Swain 2004b). For example, a Western, white, middle-class cultural narrative, or script, for young women might comprise university education, successful employment, marriage and children (supporting heterosexist "norms"). The cultural narrative for a young woman in many countries of the majority ("third") world will often omit the possibility of any education or employment, with marriage and children prescribed at a far younger age and with little opportunity for alternative scenarios. Cultural narratives thus shape one's expectations and visions of what sort of life might be possible.

Cultural scripts are reinscribed and reinforced by their apparent inevitability: one sees the lives of others, hears their stories (or narratives) and envisions a similar storyline for one's own life. Indeed, socialization within a particular culture is a process of 'learning the scripts' (Barnartt 2001 p 64). Journalist John Hockenberry (1995 p 24) observed that until the accident in which he sustained a spinal cord injury: 'I understood the world only as an evolving landscape of clockwork challenges and gradual change. I would grow up. I would graduate. I would have a career. I would be happy'. He referred to this sense of life's inevitability as 'the seductive predictability of day-to-day, so called "normal" life' (p 79). Hockenberry's observations demonstrate that he had so thoroughly internalized a particular cultural script, or life template, as to make his life course appear inevitable.

Although each individual is free to make their own life choices, these choices are made within the confines of a limited repertoire of available cultural scripts that are 'rarely of our own making' (Somers 1994 p 606). Notably, 'being oppressed means the *absence of choices*' (hooks 1984 p 5).

Until comparatively recently, people with severe physical impairments were caught in a cultural script that cast them in the role of helpless, dependent victims in need of constant care in residential institutions. However, once a few disabled people contested this 'script', attaining changes in social policy that enabled them to live autonomously in the community (with the help of assistants they employed through direct government funding), a new cultural script – or possible life course – became available to other disabled people. Once this new narrative, or script, was heard by others, discharge from rehabilitation to the community became the new norm for people with severe physical impairments in some countries (Hammell 2003a). However, Smith & Sparkes (2004) contend that rehabilitation institutions are not awash with counternarratives in which to frame possibilities following a life disruption, tending to reinforce dominant "norms".

Richardson (1990) suggested that individuals create new narratives to counteract or contest existing cultural narratives that serve to marginalize or oppress them and that these new cultural narratives can provide others with new life choices: 'hearing [about] them legitimates a replotting of one's own life. New narratives offer the patterns for new lives' (p 129). Richardson observed that new narratives become part of a cultural heritage thereby affecting future stories and future lives. She noted that the new cultural narrative can therefore galvanize other 'category members' (p 129), such as other disabled people.

'There is an inevitable connection between what people do and what they think they can do' (Saleeby 1994 p 356): the 'possible parameters' for lives of people 'like me' (Rogers & Swadener 2001 p 4). Through exposure to peers during rehabilitation, disabled people are enabled to glimpse possible life-courses that deviate from standard scripts (Smith & Sparkes 2004): what Rogers and Swadener (2001 p 4) refer to as 'narratives of imagined possibility'.

The absence of templates

Duggan et al (2002) observed that adjustment to an impairment such as a spinal cord injury can be difficult 'because there is no readily retrievable template upon which to anchor expectations for the future life course' (p 114). Research suggests that because there is no culturally accepted 'template', or script, for how one 'ought' to live with a severe impairment such as high spinal cord injury, each individual has the unusual opportunity to define his or her own priorities and possibilities (Hammell 1998a, 2004f). Daily life experiences therefore range between individuals who express great satisfaction in being employed full-time, running their own businesses or attending university (reflecting prevailing cultural values) and those whose primary occupation and source of profound satisfaction comprises watching their children, volunteering, spending time with special people or reading (contesting dominant values that dictate what adults of working age 'ought' to do; Hammell 1998a, 2004f).

Some researchers have reported, perhaps counterintuitively, that people with high spinal cord lesions have higher self-esteem and are more satisfied with their lives than people with incomplete or lower lesions (DeVivo et al 1991, DeVivo et al 1995, Gagnon 1990) and that suicide rates among those with minimal impairments following spinal cord injury are nearly twice as high as among those with more severe injuries (Hartkopp et al 1998) (although the latter finding is not consistent across studies; Soden et al 2000). Researchers have been at a loss to explain this paradox, but it is possible that people with paraplegia and low tetraplegia feel compelled to try to live up to cultural narratives that extol employment and celebrate physical independence. In a world designed to support the needs of the dominant, able-bodied population – in which discrimination and disabling barriers present sometimes insurmountable obstacles to the physically different – these expectations are prohibitively difficult for many disabled people to achieve (Hammell 2004f).

By contrast, people with high spinal cord injuries are not expected to participate in culturally valued activities (although they may *choose* to participate) and perhaps the reality that little is expected liberates them to choose what they will do and what values will inform their choices. Ville & Ravaud (1996) observed that although a failure to recognize the right of disabled people to work 'is a form of alienation, so is the imposition of work as an inevitable objective for all', and argued that work should not be 'an objective to be attained at any price' (p 250). Clearly, this has implications for client-centred goal-setting throughout the rehabilitation process and suggests the need to explore lifestyles that best reflect individuals' values and priorities (see Chapter 9). However, unlike those in the dominant population, disabled people cannot turn to literature, film or theatre for examples of possible life courses to which they might aspire (Kent 1988).

CULTURAL REPRESENTATIONS OF DISABILITY

While disability theorists in Britain have been primarily engaged in exploring the social, political, economic and legal dimensions of disability, their American counterparts have tended to focus, instead, on cultural issues, examining disability from the perspectives of the humanities: history, art and literary studies (Barnes & Mercer 2004, Shakespeare 1998a). Mitchell & Snyder (2000), Snyder (2002) and Thomson (1997a), for example, have examined the complicity of literature, art, photography and film in the devaluation of disabled people.

In an essay on classic American literature, Toni Morrison (1992) demonstrated that white writers historically managed to create a body of work that avoided direct mention of the significant population of black people on which white American life depended. She argued that the formation of this literature necessitated coded language and purposeful omissions. Readers shared the code, such that it was unnecessary to state that a character in an American novel was white. This was understood.

Morrison's insights suggest a parallel with the place of disabled people in art and literature: disabled people are often 'missing' in both literature and the media (Northway 1997). Further, readers do not need to be told that the characters in a book are able-bodied: we share the 'code' and readily understand that able-bodiedness is to be assumed unless we are specifically told otherwise. That we understand this, it might be argued, is because ableism is institutionalized in the very fabric of our culture.

Longmore (1987) observed that disability has long been used in literature as a melodramatic device such that deformity of body symbolizes deformity of soul. However, while embittered disabled villains frequently exhibit a pervasive malevolence towards society, Longmore notes that throughout history it is non-disabled people who have at times endeavoured to destroy disabled people.

Although some authors have seized on disability as a handy metaphor for the weakness and sickness of a nation (Scholnick 2002); for social inequities and the powerlessness experienced by colonized people (Kyeong-Hee 2001); as a way of embodying ill-will and provoking fear (e.g. Shakespeare's Richard III, Barry's Captain Hook); to engender pity (e.g. Dickens's Tiny Tim), or as a dramatic device to demonstrate perseverance and spiritual depth (Valentine 2001), disabled people are rarely permitted to occupy 'ordinary' roles, for example, as parents, lovers or workers (Barnes 1994).

Oliver (1990) sees cultural images of disabled people as portraying either superhumans or subhumans. He suggests, for example, that Sir Clifford in *Lady Chatterley's Lover* is portrayed as being pathetically less than human, while in *Reach for the Sky* Douglas Bader is portrayed as being more than human. Before sustaining a paralyzing injury, Nawaf Kabbara shared the prevailing cultural attitudes towards disabled people: pity for their impairment and admiration if they appeared to 'cope' well. His ideas changed after injury and prompted him to query: 'Why is it wrong to regard disabled people as heroes? Because we are not heroes' (in Coleridge 1993 p 39). He explains that although disabled people face challenges and accomplish things in a different way 'it is not heroism. It is just a life you have to carry out' (p 39).

Kent (1988) explored portrayals of disabled women in novels and plays, identifying recurring images of girls who could never aspire to be 'real women': those whose existence would eventually be validated by the love of a man. Instead, disabled women were portrayed as pitiful victims, helpless, useless and above all, undesirable. As a feminist, Kent lamented the reproduction of these stereotypes in the work of women writers, observing that although women have increasingly portrayed their female characters as vibrant, powerful, intelligent and passionate, they continue to exploit disabled womanhood to symbolically depict frailty, passivity and helplessness. These themes are not unique to Western writers. On Japanese television, for example, disabled women are used as role models of endurance, perseverance, persistence and selflessness: qualities well-suited to maintenance of the social status quo (Valentine 2001).

In a fascinating exploration of classic fiction for girls, Lois Keith (2001) showed that popular books such as *What Katy Did*, *Heidi* and *The Secret Garden* all featured a character who recovered from paralysis by being good. In light of the reality that a cure for paralysis remains an elusive goal at the time of writing (2005), the choice of this theme would seem to be more than coincidental. Using a feminist analysis of the cultural messages about correct behaviour these books delivered to girls, Keith makes some important observations: 'even as we failed to take account of it, we were storing up enough perceptions and ideas about disability to last a lifetime. We were learning that: (1) there is nothing good about being disabled; (2) disabled people have to learn the same qualities of submissive behaviour that women have always had to learn: patience, cheerfulness and making the best of things; (3) impairment can be a punishment for bad behaviour, for evil thoughts or for not being a good enough person; (4) although disabled people should be pitied rather than punished, they can never be accepted, and (5) the impairment is curable. If you want to enough, if you love yourself enough (but not more than you love others), if you believe in God enough, you will be cured' (p 7).

Congruent with the idea that cultures perpetuate and reproduce particular hegemonic beliefs, the same themes that Keith identified are readily identifiable in contemporary media accounts of disability, despite the passage of approximately one hundred years since these books were written. Barnes & Mercer (2003) identify a limited number of themes that dominate newspaper coverage of disability: primarily stories of personal tragedy, 'special' achievements, charities and 'cures'. Indeed, Biklen (1987 p 81) observed that 'when reporters approach any story, they bring with them one or a combination of standard "frames" for presenting it to the readers'. For example, the media celebrated the determination of actor Christopher Reeve to walk again despite his spinal cord injury, portraying this as a sign of heroism, willpower and the triumph of a positive attitude. There was a sense that because of amazing inner strength and personal drive, a 'miracle' was both imminent and inevitable (Keith 2001), despite the singular lack of evidence supporting this belief. Presumably, people who find a new way to live despite their impairments would be viewed as lacking inner fortitude and of having given up. Their resumption of ordinary lives is certainly not celebrated in the media and the cultural assumption that life with an impairment is not worth living goes unchallenged.

Valentine (2001 p 722) claimed that 'if your only images of certain people come from the media . . . and these representations tell consistent stories, then you are likely to have your view of these groups framed by media accounts'. Gold & Auslander (1999 p 709) observed that 'the modern-day media plays an important role not only in reflecting public attitudes and values, but also in shaping them'. For example, their research into newspaper coverage of disabled people indicates that the mainstream media colludes with Establishment interests by only rarely featuring military personnel who have been injured in combat, despite (or surely because of) on-going military conflicts producing thousands of casualties.

In artistic works such as the paintings of Pieter Brueghel the Elder, disability has traditionally been a visual metaphor for moral defects and depravity (Stainton 2004), if it has been portrayed at all. However, recent works such as Marc Quinn's *Alison Lapper Pregnant* – a sculpture of a heavily pregnant woman with absent arms and very short legs that has been displayed in London's Trafalgar Square – attempt to subvert the glorification of the "norm" (Guardian Weekly 2004).

'DESERVING' DISABILITY

So far in this chapter, it has been noted that disabled people are culturally stereotyped as pitiful or admirable, implying that there is a moral undertone to cultural beliefs. In the previous chapter it was seen that the 'pitiful' stereotype is both promoted and perpetuated in those books held to be holy by the major religions. It has also been suggested that specific, dominant beliefs are accorded 'common sense' status even when they are challenged by contesting evidence. This prompts consideration of why negative cultural beliefs about disability might have such universal appeal as to garner overwhelming literary and media support.

Pfeiffer (2003 p 98) noted the prevailing cultural view that impairment is a consequence of sinful activity, 'because God would not allow such a terrible thing to happen to good people'. Such pejorative beliefs and ignorance are not confined to religion and pulp fiction but are manifest in academia and public policy. Several historians report that this belief was strongly ensconced in the Reagan administration's policies in the USA (which is rather ironic in view of Reagan's subsequent dementia). Within Reagan's Department of Education, people described as "normal" and 'handicapped' were deemed to be 'higher' and 'lower' beings, respectively (Pfeiffer 2003), thus funds for 'special' education were deemed counterproductive. Reflecting the pervasive influence of Christianity on US society, in which disability is an external manifestation of internal, spiritual flaws (Devlieger et al 2003), the US Department of Education issued a statement contending that disabled people 'falsely assume that the lottery of life has penalised them at random' (Gardner 1983 p 22).

Wendell (1996 p 107) observed that 'most people are deeply reluctant to believe that bad things happen to people who do not deserve them, or seek them, or risk them, or fail to take care of themselves'. Indeed, to acknowledge this possibility would raise 'challenging religious or spiritual issues for people who believe that God is omnipotent, omniscient, and benevolent, for those who believe that one or more powerful transcendent beings are caring for them, and for those who believe (or just feel) that the universe is, if not benevolent, at least benign' (Wendell 1996 p 108). Murphy (1990 p 117) argued that disabled people 'serve as constant, visible reminders to the ablebodied that the society they live in is shot through with inequity and suffering, that they live in a counterfeit paradise, that they too are vulnerable. We represent a fearsome possibility'.

What better way to deny this 'fearsome possibility' than to perpetuate cultural images that reinforce how different disabled people are from 'us'; and especially if it can be shown that disability results from sinful actions or behaviour? Further, if disabled people are quite unlike 'us' and can be included within the social category of 'the undeserving', then their oppression is not only justifiable, but legitimate! Small wonder, then, that some disabled activists have sought to establish a disability counterculture.

DISABILITY CULTURE

Chapter 3 alluded to efforts aimed at promoting 'disability culture', in which impairment is perceived to be a source of pride (Swain & French 2000). Similar efforts to declare 'gay pride' or 'black is beautiful' have achieved some success in transforming a cultural hegemony that prized whiteness and heterosexuality and demeaned those deemed inferior to these valued "norms".

People who see themselves as part of a sign-language linguistic minority have achieved some success in affirming pride in their unique Deaf culture (Corker 1998b). Similarly, others with limb deficiencies assert pride and completeness in their bodily differences, equating these with the Venus de Milo: the famous, armless statue of the Greek goddess Aphrodite (Frank 2004, Snyder & Mitchell 2001). The artist Melina Fatsiou-Cowan (1997) creates flowing, sensuous paintings of women, like herself, who have profound scoliosis or other spinal 'deformities'. She believes that: 'people with disabilities have great aesthetic value – not less than one finds in standard "beauty"' (p 34) and also observed: 'unfortunately, in the field of art, scoliosis has been shown as a hateful deformity. But, as a person with scoliosis, I know that the curvature of the spine creates a magnificent flow of the body' (p 34).

Darke (1998) observed the paradox that some in the disabled community perceive 'positive' images of disabled people to be those in which disabled people most closely approximate "normal" people, arguing instead that such images validate "normality" and negate difference. Darke contends that this damages efforts to value difference and presents, instead, 'pseudo-normal images of abnormality' (Darke 1998 p 188). Disability theorists observe that "normals" believe the highest praise they can bestow upon disabled people is: s/he 'never seemed disabled to me' (Shapiro 1994 p 1). This implies that the key to social harmony is sameness – not the acknowledgement and acceptance of differences – through which deviants achieve acceptance through emulating the behaviour and characteristics of the dominant group (hooks 1995).

However, the notion of a unifying 'disability' identity on which to ground a shared culture is problematic (see Chapter 3) in that it posits disability as a totalizing identity and obscures – or ignores – important axes of differentiation (and identity) such as gender, age, "race", sexual orientation, class and age (Mulvany 2000, Shakespeare 1996b). This perpetuates – rather than contests – the dominant cultural representation of disability as a defining identity and tends to alienate and further marginalize those who are 'differently disabled' by virtue of multiple oppressions such as homophobia, ableism and racism and serves to marginalize and exclude those who are different from *this* "norm" (see Seidman 1995). Shakespeare & Watson (2001b) contend that denial of a specific 'disabled' identity may be based on the rejection of the ideal of "normality" and may constitute a refusal to be categorized. Many people do not self-identify as disabled because they refuse to see themselves as different but, rather, as part of the spectrum of normality. Further, Barnes et al (1999) observe that attempts to assert 'disability pride' seem problematic in the context of people who have painful and debilitating impairments that may result in premature mortality. It would surely be naïve to suggest that disability might be celebrated, for example, by those people who suffer pain from impairments caused by violence, abuse or torture or by those whose lives will be curtailed prematurely due to diseases such as motor neurone disease (MND) or amyotrophic lateral sclerosis (ALS). Barnes et al (1999 p 207) suggest the need to assert the value of people with impairments while 'refusing to glorify incapacity': to see disabled people as neither pitiful nor heroic, but as constituting one dimension of normal human experience.

IMPLICATIONS FOR REHABILITATION

The reality that few people now live in societies populated by people of a homogenous culture has led to an examination of ways in which rehabilitation practitioners might undertake their work in a culturally appropriate and respectful manner (e.g. Leavitt 1999b). However, while it is unquestionably laudable that therapists currently seek to understand and to respond appropriately to those from 'other' cultures (usually construed on the basis of ethnicity), Leavitt (1999c p 7) observes: 'it is not merely "the other" who has a unique culture, but each one of us. Understanding our own values, attitudes, beliefs and behaviours is a prerequisite to successful interventions'.

It has been suggested that rehabilitation professionals need to recognize that a focus on changing cultural attitudes towards disabled people might have a greater impact on their lives than teaching them exercise regimens (Leavitt 1999b). Yet therapists, too, are immersed in a culture that stereotypes disabled people as helpless or heroes, pitiful or inspiring. Those former clients who are attributed heroic and inspiring status frequently become part of the mythological stories retold in therapy departments. Those who appear to have acquiesced to the role of pitiful and helpless might be overrepresented in outpatient departments. However, due to therapists' preference for working only on weekdays, and only during those hours that they find convenient, they are least likely to see those former clients who have attained active and busy lives in the community. Disabled people who have jobs, families and active, fulfilling lives are those least likely to be able to attend mid-week, mid-day follow-up appointments and are therefore unlikely to present rehabilitation workers with a challenge to prevailing cultural stereotypes.

It has also been suggested that through the negative imagery frequently employed in health promotion and injury prevention campaigns, healthcare professionals actively contribute to reinforcing the 'stigma for people who already possess the attributes targeted for prevention' (Wang 1993). Clearly, a more sophisticated approach to injury prevention is warranted: one that does not perpetuate prejudice.

IDEOLOGY AND POWER

It has been claimed that 'society disables people with impairments, through negative attitudes, environmental barriers and institutional discrimination' (Stone 2001 p 51). Hahn (1993) outlined the equation that links ideology, power and social policy, observing: '(a) that social attitudes rather than physical inabilities are the primary source of the problems confronted by disabled men and women; (b) that all aspects of the social and built environment are shaped or moulded by public policy; and (c) that public policy is a reflection of pervasive social attitudes and values'. Ideology informs policy, such that segregation follows quite naturally from cultural beliefs concerning the inferiority and deviance of disability. Thus, policy making adheres to a value-laden agenda (Priestley 1999). As Thomson (1997a p 23) observed: 'While in the movement toward equality, race and gender are generally accepted as differences rather than deviances, disability is still most often seen as bodily inadequacy or catastrophe to be compensated for with pity and goodwill, rather than accommodated by systemic changes based on civil rights'.

In *Culture and Imperialism*, Said (1993) demonstrated that 'the institutional, political and economic operations of imperialism are nothing without the power of the culture that maintains them' (Ashcroft & Ahluwalia 1999 p 87). Said (1979) asks uncomfortable questions concerning the role of powerful intellectuals and professionals in perpetuating received ideas and in failing to challenge the authority of ideological straitjackets. This has clear relevance for the rehabilitation professions.

Priestley (1999) contends that it is inadequate to analyse culture without recalling that disabling cultural values reflect relations of power. He argues that we must ask 'why certain values remain dominant over others and whose interests are threatened when dominant values are challenged' (p 215), suggesting that these issues are best addressed by considering 'ideology' rather than 'culture'.

That ideology both reflects and reinforces power and powerlessness is a recurrent finding throughout this book. Because ideologies that disempower disabled people so successfully permeate our cultures, any analysis of the context in which disability is experienced must concern itself with both sociopolitical and cultural issues (Watson 1998). Such an examination has relevance, not solely for disabled people themselves, but for all members of society who could usefully learn from disabled people's knowledge (Wendell 1996). However, 'because disabled people's experience is not integrated into the culture, most newly disabled people know little or nothing about how to live with long-term or life-threatening illness [sic]' (Wendell 1996 p 65). Thus, Reynolds (2004b p 115) contends that 'conscientization – raising awareness of disabling cultural forces' is one of the most important skills that a therapist can bring to their partnership with clients.

Through the social/political model, disabled activists and theorists have identified *disability* as a form of discrimination and oppression, as has been seen. Although Wendell (1996) suggests that the fear of becoming disabled is exacerbated by the assumption that disability inevitably prohibits engagement in social life, even a cursory interrogation of culture suggests that it is not *disability* that "normates" fear, but *impairment* (Thomas 1999): the fear of bodily dis-integrity, and of deviance. The following chapter examines the ways in which the body has been addressed by social theorists, using these ideas to explore further the ideological representation of physical difference.

Chapter 6

The body and physical impairment

My life began in one body and will end in another . . . my life is bisected between its end points. It contains two beginnings and when death finally comes it will have a pair of ends.
(Hockenberry 1995 p 28; following his spinal cord injury)

INTRODUCTION: THEORY AND THE BODY

The previous chapter explored the role of culture in perpetuating prejudice against disabled people, noting that while the social/political model of disability has sought to redirect attention from bodily differences to hostile environments, it is on the *basis* of bodily difference that disabling attitudes and environments are constructed. Clearly, then, the body is the starting point for any theoretical contemplation of disability.

In recent years there has been a significant interest in the body among social theorists (e.g. Featherstone et al 1991, Shilling 1993, Turner 1992, 1995, 1996, Williams & Bendelow 1998a). Improbably, however, they have managed to generate a plethora of books and a journal – *The Body and Society* – that purportedly address 'the body' and 'physical difference' while scarcely mentioning disability (Marks 1999). This is a quite remarkable accomplishment, prompting Abberley (1997 p 37) to claim that 'for disabled people the much heralded advent of sociological interest in the body has been a disappointment' and Thomas (2002 p 46) to maintain that 'ideas in the field of the sociology of the body have yet to offer anything of significance on the subject of disability'.

As this chapter will show, some theorists' flights of fancy are not solely disappointing for disabled people, they are overwhelmingly ableist, frequently irrelevant and sometimes silly. Much that has been written by theorists of the body is couched in obfuscating language, being difficult to read, deliberately ambiguous and intellectually élitist. Indeed, some works constitute little more than what Oliver (2004 p 24) has termed 'intellectual masturbation'.

Although the majority of social theorists have written about bodies without acknowledging the existence of disability, disability theorists have been criticized, in turn, for their failure to incorporate the body and bodily experiences into their social/political model (Watson 1998).

Congruent with the stated intent of engaging with contemporary theories that provide different ways of thinking about disability – and thus about rehabilitation – this chapter outlines some contributions to theorizing the body and draws on the work of disability researchers to explore the relationship between the impaired body and the self.

THE SOCIAL/POLITICAL MODEL AND THE 'MISSING' BODY

One of the criticisms of the social/political model of disability that was outlined in Chapter 4 centred on the analytical division between 'impairment' and 'disability', and the exclusive theoretical attention focused by disability theorists on the impact of disabling social environments rather than on the physical body (Hughes & Paterson 1997).

Although most disabled people would acknowledge the disabling impact of physical and social barriers, some lament the theoretical neglect of bodily experiences such as pain, fatigue, paralysis and a reduced lifespan (see Chapter 4). For some, the analytical division between the problems associated with the body – impairment – and those imposed by society – disability – represent just another form of dualism in which the totality of the experience of living with impairment is carved up, and the bodily dimensions conceded to medical theory (Corker & French 1999, Thomas 1999, Williams 1999); and in which a focus on the 'public' occurs at the expense of the 'private' (Shakespeare 1999). This is an artificial division that makes political sense but fails to resonate with the experiences of those disabled people who encounter frustrations from both socially created barriers and their bodily limitations (Clare 1999, Thomas 2001a). Williams (1999 p 810) noted that 'in by-passing the body, disability theorists have tended to assume, implicitly if not explicitly, a homogeneity of interest between themselves and those whose interests they claim to represent'. This is a flawed assumption (Crow 1996).

A recurring theme throughout this book is that theories and knowledge are inseparable from ideologies (although this is seldom acknowledged by theorists). The social/political model, in contrast, is *explicitly* ideologically driven. This theory arose from the insights of activists and is designed to service an unambiguous political agenda: ensuring that disablist marginalization is seen in similar terms to racist, homophobic or sexist discrimination (Ahmad 2000). Allegiance to this ideology causes many theorists to reject claims for the integration of the experience of impairment into the social/political model of disability, believing this will dilute their political message (Barnes 1998b, Oliver 1996a).

However, attempting to eliminate the body from disability theory leads to an intellectual impasse, articulated by Corker and French (1999 p 2): 'if disability is indeed a form of social oppression, the questions then remain – *"Oppression of what or whom?"* and *"Why and how does this particular form of oppression occur?"'* They contend that one cannot adequately answer these questions without addressing impairment.

Some disability theorists query why the task of theorizing about the body should be conceded, exclusively, to medicine: a scientific discourse that has long been criticized for ignoring the experiential aspects of bodily aberrations (Hughes & Paterson 1997, Sacks 1991). Rehabilitation is perceived to have shared this propensity to objectify the body and ignore the subjective experiences of disabled people (Paterson & Hughes 2000), leading disabled people to claim that rehabilitation therapists know very little about living with impairments (Hammell 1998b).

Biomedical discourses depict the body as biologically determined. Social theorists adopt a more contextual approach, emphasizing the role of cultures, language and institutions in shaping the body (Priestley 2003), thus presenting a challenge to deterministic discourses. To explore the experience of impairment demands an exploration of taken-for-granted knowledge about the body and the place of bodies in cultures and societies.

THE BODY IN THEORY

Anthropologists have a long tradition of exploring the body in terms of evolution, symbolism, taboos and mythologies that provide evidence of the relationship between nature and culture (Turner 1991). They have found evidence of human interest in the body among ancient cultures – who enhanced the body with jewellery and fragrant oils, for example – and among contemporary global cultures, who adorn, augment, tattoo, pierce and sculpt the body with varying degrees of obsession. Bodies currently appear everywhere in Western society, glorifying 'an ideal of beauty that is crafted by special effects, computer-enhanced images or masking make-up' (Le Monde 2001 p 26) and the body has recently captured the attention of social theorists. It is beyond the scope of this chapter to summarize the ballooning theoretical work on the body emanating from academic traditions as diverse as geography, sociology and history. However, an important selection of ideas will be sketched to provide an introduction to a body of work that has arisen, seemingly unnoticed by the rehabilitation professions. Indeed, for the rehabilitation professions, the body remains curiously untheorized. Apart from tentative statements embracing holism and rejecting dualism, the rehabilitation professions have apparently accepted the body as a natural, taken-for-granted entity, conceding to others the work of theorizing about their central domain of concern. Social theorists demonstrate, instead, that the body is not solely a biological entity but one subjected to social, cultural, economic and political forces: that the body is central to power.

Power and the body

In Chapter 3 it was noted that there has been a long and global history of bestowing social power according to physique, with a hierarchy of physical traits – gender, "race", ability – traditionally determining the distribution of social privileges and economic opportunities (Hammell 2004g). The body is also a marker of social class (Bourdieu 1984). In Western societies, for example, rates of obesity are rising exponentially but this is not a phenomenon that occurs evenly throughout society. Obesity is predominantly associated with low levels of education and with low socioeconomic status (Mennell 1991), thus obesity has become a cultural signifier of "low class".

Kirk & Tinning (1994 p 605) note that 'like scripts, bodies are read and the signs they emit are interpreted by each one of us, in the normal course of our daily lives, as a means of discerning both the kind of person we are encountering and the kind of person we think we ourselves are'. Indeed, Hughes (1999 p 163) contends that bodies are 'read through categories which place them in a hierarchy of bodies'; thus skin colour, body shape, accent, eye shape and hair texture 'are read as indelible signs of the "natural" inferiority of their possessors' (Ashcroft et al 1995 p 321). The body is therefore more than the physical 'face' of the self; it is a visual display of social status, such that 'political struggles and social inequalities are inherently embodied' (Nettleton 1995 p 130). Bodies, therefore, are symbolic; a form of social currency, such that one's body signifies one's worth (Gerschick 1998).

Sociologists have explored bodily performance and the idea that the body represents a form of 'capital': that social power and status accrue to those whose bodies most closely adhere to an ideal (Bourdieu 1978). Bourdieu (1984) analysed social inequalities in terms of four forms of capital: economic capital (possessing money, wealth, property), cultural capital (education, knowledge of arts and literature), symbolic capital (demeanour, presentation of self) and physical capital (manner of speech, gait, body shape). Physical impairment reduces both symbolic and physical capital, thus reducing social status. Reduced opportunities for education and employment may additionally lead to reductions in economic and cultural capital. Physical bodies are therefore integral to social status and to power, being both receptors and generators of social meanings: arguments central to social constructionism.

Social constructionism

Social constructionism claims that all knowledge is socially constructed: that 'facts' are not true or real but inventions and interpretations (Berger & Luckmann 1966). This idea may be illustrated by studying the history of medicine, which has been governed by different constructions – or interpretations – of the body over time. Anatomical drawings from the Middle Ages, for example, reflected a prevailing, politicoreligious discourse – in which God invested the King with dominion over the common 'body' – and are markedly different from contemporary drawings of (presumably) the same physical form (Turner 1995).

Social constructionism contends that the body is 'a discursive product of power/knowledge' (Williams 1999 p 813), asserting that the body is 'a receptor rather than a generator of social meanings'; that is, 'that the body is somehow shaped, constrained and even invented by society' (Shilling 1993 p 70). Thus conditions classified as diseases and disorders are social constructs: they are the products of certain ways of interpreting the body. However, although it is all very well saying that disorders such as attention deficit hyperactivity disorder, Asperger syndrome or myalgic encephalomyelitis (chronic fatigue syndrome) are socially constructed – that specific constellations of symptoms arise in specific historical, social and cultural contexts as products of language, ideology or discourse – it is clearly inane to make the same claim for anomalies such as spinal cord injury or severe intellectual impairment. It is both naïve and disrespectful to contend that all impairments are socially constructed – that they are all the products of discourse – when some people with impairments would not survive, much less thrive, without the assistance and vigilance of others (Kittay 2001). By declaring that disability is socially constructed, postmodern theorists have ignored the reality that, for many people, life comprises a physical struggle for existence (Thomas 1999) and that some impairments entail intense physical suffering and emotional anguish (Meekosha 1998, Mulvany 2000).

Some critics have contested the exclusionary use of jargon in which social constructionists tend to engage. For example, Van Maanen (1988 p 27) suggested that 'the seemingly perverse practice of prefacing many nouns with the phrase "the social construction of" represents a writer's claim to membership in an intellectual club and a way of speaking only to well-versed members of that club'. He proposed that when one is at the mercy of mutual jargon, one is freed from thought.

Further, few theorists demonstrate an awareness of the contested term 'disability', glibly proclaiming that 'disability is socially constructed' without stating whether they are using the WHO's definition of disability, that of critical disability theorists, or whether they know the difference. Confusion also arises when theorists contend that the social/political model claims 'disability is socially constructed'. This demonstrates a fundamental misunderstanding of the idea of social constructionism, the social/political model, or both. Thomas (1999) observes that the model is based, instead, on the premise that disability is *socially created*: that disadvantages are the product of social relations and spatial structures, not that disability is some sort of idea or the product of discourse.

Foucault and the idea of discourse

Foucault, considered to be one of the most influential theorists of the body, sought to bring to the fore the crucial role of discourse in producing and sustaining power (Jones & Porter 1994). Foucault viewed scientific or specialized knowledge – discourses – as phenomena of social power and not simply a way of describing the world. A *discourse* is 'a system of statements within which, and by which, the world can be known' (Ashcroft & Ahluwalia 1999 p 68), embodying specific perspectives that a group of people consider to be knowledge and determining modes of thought (Fawcett 2000a). Discourses incorporate 'specific "grids of meaning" which underpin, generate and establish relations between all that can be seen, thought and said' (Shilling 1993 p 75). Discourses are historically and socially specific; thus their study links language to the study of society (Fraser 1992).

In Chapter 2 it was seen that the "normal" body is not precisely defined but constitutes a set of statistical averages. Hughes (2004 p 66) explains the phenomenon of "normality" in terms of discourse: 'in reality, the normal or non-disabled body does not exist. What does exist is the linguistic convention or discourse of normality that conveys something to us about bodies and helps us to make some sense of them'. Because the "normal" body does not exist, poststructuralists are able to contend that impairments – or ab-normal bodies – do not exist; that they are metaphors or cultural representations of defect and deficit (Hughes 2004).

Thus, poststructuralists contend that diseases are the effects of the discourses that describe them (Armstrong 1983). When a religious discourse was predominant, for example, anorexia was regarded as an expression of piety. Within a dominant medical discourse it is regarded as an expression of sexual immaturity; a psychiatric disorder (Turner 1992). However, like 'whiplash', myalgic encephalomyelitis, fibromyalgia and neurasthenia, anorexia is manifested only in certain, affluent, regions of the world (Mennell 1991) and among those social groups who 'share' the discourse, or 'script' (Malleson 2002): it is a 'textually' transmitted condition unknown in those cultures dominated by different discourses. In a similar vein the improbable transient paralyses, 'vapours' and hysterias manifested by many Victorian women are now perceived to have been learned expressions of resistance against the imposition of roles dictated by dominant sexist discourses (Turner 1995, 1996): ailments less literal than metaphorical. Silvers (2002) explained that in the nineteenth century, 'illness' represented a form of emancipation for women, by freeing them from domestic and reproductive roles to which they would otherwise be confined.

Although garnering considerable support within academia, Williams (2000 p 47) contends that a theoretical commitment to discourse 'has something of a hollow ring to it in the context of pain and sickness, disability and death: existential events *par excellence*'. It is apparent that the experience of profound suffering is willfully ignored by those poststructuralists who proclaim, for example, that mental illnesses are the products of discourse: that they are metaphors or myths (Mulvany 2000).

Feminist theories

Feminists have pursued the idea that the body is a medium for constructing and maintaining inequity, demonstrating that an ideology of biological inferiority has been used to justify discrimination (Nettleton 1995). Indeed, this line of thought has been central to feminist theory and might reasonably be expected to have been extended to bodies that are not only gendered, but impaired. Thomson (1997b p 279) noted, for example, that 'many parallels exist between the social meanings attributed to female bodies and those assigned to disabled bodies. Both the female and the disabled body are cast within cultural discourse as deviant and inferior; both are excluded from full participation in public as well as economic life; both are defined in opposition to a valued norm' (see Chapter 2).

However, the theoretical concern with the embodiment of social injustice that has preoccupied (white) feminists has only recently incorporated the experiences of black and colonized women (hooks 1984, Mohanty 1994) and has stopped short of including those of disabled women (Price & Shildrick 1998). Meekosha (1998) observed that although feminist discourses on the body lay claim to universality, this claim is 'corrupted by their unselfconscious exclusion of disability' (p 164).

This neglect is symptomatic of a more general exclusion of disabled women from feminist theory, research and politics (Begum 1992, Keith 1992, Morris 1991, 1993b, 1993c, 1995, Sheldon 1999); an exclusion that reflects not just ignorance but intent. Fine & Asch (1988 p 4) observed that because disabled women are perceived to be helpless, passive and dependent, 'nondisabled feminists have severed them from the sisterhood in an effort to advance more powerful, competent, and appealing female icons'. Despite feminists' rhetoric of inclusion, their ideology of autonomy and independence undermines the struggles of disabled women (Thomson 1997a). Thomson (1997b) claimed that: 'the disabled female figure occupies an intragender position; that is, she is not only defined against the masculine figure, but she is imagined as the antithesis of the normative woman as well' (p 288).

Critical debate at the intersection of feminist and disability theories flourishes among disabled feminists and because this is central to ideas of bodily difference it is worth sketching their central arguments here.

Primarily, Morris (1996) noted that disability provokes discrimination rather than solidarity from other women. For example, at the 1995 nongovernmental organizations' Forum on Women in Beijing, disabled women were excluded from full participation by physical barriers. Their issues were also relegated to the margins of discussion (Hershey 1997). Critics have astutely observed that, by identifying themselves as oppressed, white, able-bodied feminists attempt to overlook the ways in which they are oppressors (hooks 1981). Much feminist work portrays women as the victims of a patriarchal society that confines them to their homes and places them at the service of men. This ignores the situation of many disabled women who are prevented from having homes or partners. Further, women are not passive observers of societal practices that oppress and institutionalize disabled women and men but active participants in maintaining value systems that limit the opportunities of their disabled sisters.

Feminist activists have justifiably drawn attention to the metaphorical 'glass ceiling' of sexism that prevents women's ascent to the sort of high-paying jobs to which they, themselves, aspire but have been curiously silent about the literal barriers of ableism that prevent disabled women and men from gaining access to even basic levels of employment (Hammell 2004g).

Disabled women challenge the privileged, predominantly white feminist agenda that portrays motherhood as oppressive and equates reproductive rights with the right *not* to bear children, noting that their own history of compulsory sterilization, presumed asexuality and assumed incompetence has denied many of them the right *to* have and to care for their own children (Sheldon 1999, Thomson 1997a). Thus, many disabled women aspire to attain the stereotypical, traditional female roles from which they have been excluded (Lloyd 2001).

In 1981, Briggs observed that at any one time there were more women providing care for elderly and disabled dependents than for "normal" children; and it has been suggested that 'community care' might, in fact be a euphemism for care given by the nearest female relative (Finch & Groves 1980). Accordingly, when feminists first addressed disability, they championed the rights of those 'women' they perceived to be burdened by the care of 'dependent people' (e.g. Dalley 1988, Ungerson 1987). When mainstream feminists constructed the category of 'woman' as being non-disabled and non-elderly – identifying their interests with women who most closely resemble themselves – they failed to recognize that the majority of disabled and older people *are also women* (Lloyd 2001, Morris 1993b). From their ableist standpoint, feminist writers have portrayed disabled people not only as genderless but as passive, helpless, demanding, needy and burdensome (Barry 1995, Keith 1992); enabling them to claim that more residential care would alleviate the oppression faced by 'women' (Finch 1984, Parker 1993).

The assumption that disabled women and men are passive recipients of care has been challenged by researchers, who note that many are also involved in providing care for others (Lloyd 2001, Morris 1989, Walmsley 1993). The assumption that informal care-providers are almost always women is also challenged by research (Morris 1992). This is an oversimplification that ignores issues of "race" and class (Barry 1995) and renders 'men invisible in a one-dimensional gendered construction of caring' (Lloyd 2001 p 723). Many disabled people value the opportunity to care for other family members, challenging feminists' claims that providing care for others is onerous and oppressive (Fawcett 2000a, Morris 1995, Walmsley 1993).

Further, disabled women note that feminists often claim to be 'disabled' or 'handicapped' by their subordinate social status, demonstrating both ignorance and ableism (Meekosha 1998) and usurping negative images of disability to describe their own oppression (Thomson 1997a). While it *is* appropriate to contend, for example, that Chinese women whose feet were broken and bound were literally 'crippled' by sexist oppression, it is clearly inappropriate to invoke disability as an 'ugly' metaphor for the inequities experienced by able-bodied women.

The gaze

Feminists claim that 'women' (read 'able-bodied women like ourselves') are oppressed by an unremitting male 'gaze' (following Sartre 1956). Thomson (1997b) notes that disabled women, by contrast, are the objects of the stare; seen not as sexual but as deviant. Moreover, disabled women are not solely objectified by men. As Judy Heumann (cited in Thomson 1997b) noted, 'when I come into a room full of feminists, all they see is a wheelchair'. Neither is this experience unique to women. Both disabled women and men are objectified by stares that transgress gender boundaries and alienate them from those of all genders who perceive themselves to be normal (Shakespeare 1999). Indeed, it is through stares that disabled people are invalidated (Hughes 1999), continually reminded of their stigmatized status (Becker & Arnold 1986) and fixed as objects for others' value judgements (Hayim 1980).

The assumed right to stare at people with impairments and to experience a titillating mix of repulsion and fascination perhaps reached its nadir in the popular 'freak' shows of the nineteenth century, in which people with impairments and disfigurements were placed on display for the entertainment and excitement of 'normates' (Thomson 1996). Even today, many disabled people report that total strangers often demand information about their bodies, sexuality or the 'cause' of their impairments (Braithwaite 1991): questions they would not dream of asking "normal" people. This suggests that the assumed right to transgress private boundaries is not confined to the visual field and did not die with the Victorians. Clearly, the stare or gaze of ableism is qualitatively different from the sexualized gaze with which dominant feminists have been preoccupied.

Goffman (1963b p 86) noted that one of the greatest trials for people with physical impairments 'is that in public places they will be openly stared at, thereby having their privacy invaded, while at the same time, the invasion exposes their [perceived] undesirable attributes'. For many disabled people the stare – being looked down upon – produces overwhelming feelings of shame (Nijhof 1995, Toombs 1995). From her own experience with multiple sclerosis, Toombs (1995 p 18–19) described the physiological impact of feeling the negative appraisal of others: 'In neurological disorder shame manifests itself as an increase in the severity of symptoms. In the experience of the "gaze" of the Other an already existing tremor invariably intensifies, spastic limbs become more rigid, difficulty controlling movement is more pronounced'.

However, disabled people can choose not to be victimized by the gaze of others. The existential philosophers insisted that people can choose to ignore social norms and to refuse to feel shame in being different, thereby refusing to be devalued based on stigma (Coleman 1997). Frankl (1959 p 87) argued that humans always retain the ability to resist 'those powers which threaten . . . to rob you of your very self, your inner freedom'. Hughes (1999 p 162) claimed that to resist the stare 'is to refuse to be seen as one is supposed to be seen by the eye of power, to return the gaze and transform shame and humiliation into pride'. To resist the stare is also to reject the tyranny of "the norm". Accordingly, Tomlinson & Abdi (2003 p 918) contend that rehabilitation should be concerned with encouraging disabled people to realize 'they are equal to others and have a human right to be part of their community'. In reality, much of the rehabilitation enterprise has focused, instead, on striving to achieve closer proximity to physical normality: a quest central to 'the body as project'.

The body as a project

The rise of consumer culture in the West has generated a fascination with the representation, maintenance and performance of the body, encouraging individuals to strive to achieve a certain sort of appearance and to control their visual image (Featherstone 1991). In consumer culture the body is construed as a *project* to be worked at, to be continually acted upon and altered: shaped by actions (e.g. exercise, lifestyle choices), interventions (e.g. surgery), cultural expectations (e.g. cultivating specific gaits or accents) and biological processes (such as ageing) (Shilling 1993).

Because consumer cultures value youthful bodies, grey hair connotes a person of little social worth (especially if the person is female), compelling those who share – or do not resist – this cultural value to attempt to alter their hair colour to a more socially acceptable hue. The size of the market for hair dyes is testament to the power of the normalizing discourse and the attendant impulse towards conformity. Perpetuation of the belief that people – bodies – must appear youthful in order to have social value has overtly economic implications, fuelling the demand for cosmetics, plastic surgery, slimming regimens and exercise equipment. Thus, pursuit of specific bodily "norms" is integral to economic consumption and to capitalism (Priestley 2003). This is a political and value-laden discourse, with consequences for those who are unable or choose not to conform.

For example, Michalko (2002 p 22) observes that 'the contemporary obsession with health as well as with the purification and beautification of the body that defines the good life generates a particularly negative view of disability'. He suggests that any society with this obsession feels threatened by disability: a conclusion echoed in the previous chapter. The fantasy of the malleable, perfect body leads to increasingly intrusive interventions and to postmodernism's cyborg imaginings.

Cyborgs and postmodernism

Barnes & Mercer (2003 p 83) observed that 'the potential of science and technology to create new bodies or regenerate lost physical and intellectual capabilities has given rise to extravagant flights of academic fancy'. Perhaps foremost among these extravagant flights of fancy is Haraway's (1990) postmodern assertion that disabled people are *cyborgs*. Haraway (1990 p 190) claimed to use irony and a combination of 'humour and serious play' in decreeing that cyborgs are 'theorized and fabricated hybrids of machine and organism' (p 191). Cyborgs are said to exist when physical and non-physical boundaries are breached or transgressed. To undergo a joint replacement or spinal fusion, utilize an artificial limb, ventilator or cardiac pacemaker, operate a power wheelchair or a speech synthesizer is therefore to become a cyborg.

Williams (1997 p 1041) argued that there are 'already many "cyborgs" among us in society'. Clearly he is writing from an ableist stance: the cyborgs are *among* 'us'. They are explicitly not 'us'. Further, Williams (1997 p 1041–2) claimed that 'the next generation may well be the last of the "pure" humans': a particularly offensive proposition that denies pure humanity to those "cyborgs" already among 'us'. Discourses such as Haraway's might be lauded as playful (Haraway 1990), even 'exciting and witty' (Wendell 1996 p 169), but there are historical precedents of the collusion between ideologies and power that have profound consequences for those whom the 'pure humans' denigrate as the less human among 'us'. The Nazis, for example, exterminated those disabled children and adults they perceived to be less than 'pure humans' (see Chapter 3): a policy to which many intellectuals acquiesced.

Williams (1997 p 1047) enthused that human–machine couplings transform 'the accident victim in the intensive care unit' into a 'cyborg'; suggesting that it is: 'fruitful to conceptualize cyborgs along a continuum ranging from the all-too-human pole at one end to artificial intelligence (AI) devices at the other, with a broad range of human/machine couplings of varying degrees in between' (p 1047). It is tempting to query: fruitful for whom?

Said (1979 p 327) suggested, 'perhaps if we remember that the study of human experience usually has an ethical, to say nothing of a political, consequence in either the best or worst sense, we will not be indifferent to what we do as scholars'. Accordingly, Mulvany (2000 p 596) suggested that theorists must 'embrace with renewed vigour the practical and policy implications of their theorizing'. Even Williams (2000 p 47) admitted that 'the "playful" deconstructions of postmodernism are, in truth, really only an option for the healthy'.

'Owen', a young man with a high spinal cord lesion complained that since his injury: 'people don't look at you quite as a person anymore, but as a bit of an extension of the respirator' (Hammell 1998a). He was referring to the people he encounters in social spaces but his comments pertain just as insightfully to theoretical spaces. Equally problematically, postmodern theorists such as Williams (1997), who see the body's boundaries as fluid or permeable, contend that personal assistants are 'extensions' of a disabled person's body. This position ignores the often reciprocal nature of such relationships, denies personhood to carers (thereby denying to carers the agency that theorists value in themselves) and suggests that "normals" (Goffman 1963a) are bounded and complete whereas 'others' are not.

Mitchell & Snyder (1997) noted that cultural commentators seldom venture towards an elucidation of the experience of the population that underwrites their clever commentaries. Postmodern theorists such as Donna

Haraway celebrate technological enhancements of the body without any attempt to explore what it means to be reliant upon ventilators or artificial limbs in everyday life. Thus, to postmodernism's bodily playfulness, Williams & Bendelow (1998b p 132) announced: 'it is time to declare that the "emperor" has no clothes'.

It is also time to weigh the utility and merits of existent body theories.

Weighing theory

Few theorists have acknowledged the existence of impaired bodies, have sought to test their theories against the experiences of the physically 'different' or appear to expect their work to be read by disabled people. For example, Fox (1994), a postmodern theorist, attacked those theories of medical sociologists that 'merely serve to fabricate a subject who is effectively "trapped" by his/her body and its sensations of pain and disability, and is required to "adapt" to the limitations thus imposed' (p 146). It is evident that such attacks are ideologically driven and not informed by research or any insight into the experience of disability. Indeed, Kelly & Field (1996 p 247) observed that 'there are few accounts of chronic illness [sic] which do not acknowledge that basic to the experience of that illness is the disruption of the normal and usually desired routines of everyday life'.

Jean-Dominique Bauby (1997), for example, suffered a cerebrovascular accident in his brainstem: a condition formerly incompatible with life. For him, however, 'improved resuscitation techniques have now prolonged and refined the agony. You survive, but you survive with what is aptly known as "locked-in syndrome". Paralysed from head to toe, the patient is imprisoned inside his own body, his mind intact, but unable to speak or move. In my case, blinking my left eyelid is my only means of communication' (p 12). Bauby precisely describes a 'subject' – person – who is 'effectively trapped by his body' and 'its sensations of disability' (Fox 1994). Moreover, he must apparently adapt to the 'limitations thus imposed'. He explained: 'I would be the happiest of men if I could just swallow the overflow of saliva endlessly flooding my mouth' (Bauby 1997 p 20).

Although some theorists find postmodern and poststructuralist theories of the body to be 'exciting and witty' (Wendell 1996 p 169), their blatant ableism and alienation from the experience of people with impairments would seem to make them not only untested but astonishingly irrelevant.

THE BODY, IMPAIRMENT AND SOCIAL THEORY

Oliver (1996b p 19) observed: 'stemming from the influence of Foucault, sociology has recently rekindled its interest in the body, an area where it might reasonably be expected that "the disabled body" could be central to any theoretical or conceptual innovations. However, sociologists working in this area reproduce the disablism that sociology exhibits everywhere else'. For example, Featherstone & Hepworth (1991 p 376) claimed that 'to be an embodied person and to become a fully fledged member of society' requires a specific degree of physiological coordination to facilitate necessary movements, bodily gestures and other interpersonal responses. They contend that all these abilities 'are essential to becoming a person' (p 376). By definition, people like Owen and Bauby (above) are neither persons nor full members of society, nor, apparently, can they aspire to attain this status.

Shilling (1993 p 22–3) observed that: 'Our experiences of embodiment provide a basis for theorizing social commonality, social inequalities and the construction of difference'. It is surely because 'our' theorizing is undertaken by non-disabled scholars, whose objective is not social justice but academic advancement, that these theories have such limited value for the physically different: the uncontemplated victims of their theories.

On occasion, theory becomes dogma. For example, in 1991 Frank provided a comprehensive review of body theories. He carefully documented historical and contemporary theories of the body and illustrated his resulting typology with a model, or diagram. He then outlined the first-person accounts of Robert Murphy (an anthropologist who became a tetraplegic due to a spinal tumour) and Irving Zola (a sociologist partially paralyzed by polio compounded by injuries from a car accident) and observed that 'both their stories are about living in the fundamental conditions of the ill body . . . *it is not a condition which fits my diagram*' (p 87, emphasis added). However, he comforted himself by speculating that 'it is being residual to society, not to theory, which troubles Murphy and Zola' (p 87). In response, Oliver (1996b) observed that 'disabled people are not only relegated to the margins of society, they are relegated to the margins of sociological theory as well' (p 19). Notably, Frank (1991) did not revise his diagram in light of contesting evidence, choosing, instead, to ignore it. This illustrates the difference between theory and dogma: 'a model is revised or abandoned when it fails to fit all the data. A dogma, on the other hand, requires that discrepant data be forced to fit the model or be excluded' (Engel 1977 p 130).

It is remarkable that any theory of the body could be devised without consideration of how that theory could be tested or contested by impaired bodies, or, indeed, how theories can promote and perpetuate discrimination against certain people. To date, however, and with few exceptions, the major works concerning theories of the body have achieved publication without once contemplating impairment (although this has been attempted by Seymour 1989, 1998).

Following his brainstem stroke, Bauby (1997 p 79) watched his small son and bemoaned: 'I, his father, have lost the simple right to ruffle his bristly hair, clasp his downy neck, hug his small lithe warm body tight against me. There are no words to express it. My condition is monstrous, iniquitous, revolting, horrible'. Clearly, it is naïve to claim that the problems associated with disability are the products of discourse; fatuous to suggest that disability is wholly socially constructed; outrageous to attain academic prestige by inventing theories of the body that do not consider the experience of impairment.

DISABILITY, THE BODY AND THE SOCIAL THEORIST

Said (see Ashcroft & Ahluwalia 1999) claimed that work in the academy has retreated from the human realities of its subject matter and that in this 'priestly world' of theory, a 'precious jargon has grown up', characterized by 'formidable complexities' that obscure 'social realities' (p 50). This encapsulates the problem of the body in social theory.

To include the disabled body in social theory, 'our most basic conceptions of the body will need to be rewritten. Body theory will itself have to acknowledge its inadequate recognition of disability to date' (Porter 1997 p xiv). To do so requires also that the cause of this inadequacy be named and shamed. Abberley (1997 p 37) proposed: 'Even the merely amateur psychologist may feel that so systematic an absence of the disabled body is evidence of the strong feelings of repulsion, fear and disgust its prospect inspires in these theorists'. He argued that the origins of repulsion stem from deeply internalized ableism: an undercurrent with which 'body sociology must come to grips, if it is to develop a thoroughgoing theory, and, to me more importantly, if it is to be of potential use to disabled people' (p 38).

Fine (1994) noted that non-disabled academics exhibit an existential anxiety about body 'dis-integrity' that can be summed up in the perceived threat that a disability could interfere with valued capacities 'deemed necessary to the pursuit of a satisfactory life' (Hahn 1988 p 43). Indeed, Hahn argued that fear of disability outranks fear of (inevitable) death. He claimed that aesthetic anxiety results from a fear of succumbing to both a devalued physique and a minority, subordinate status. By maintaining the illusion of difference between 'us' (able-bodied academics) and 'them' (the cyborgs) theories of the body serve to quell this anxiety.

The following section explores the experience of succumbing to a devalued physique to illustrate what an evidence-based theory of the body might look like.

INCLUDING DISABILITY: THE BODY AND THE SELF

Western philosophy has largely rejected its dualistic Cartesian legacy, seeking instead to address the body/mind, or body/self, in which the body is understood to be an aspect of the self (Gadow 1982). This brings Western philosophy closer to those traditions of Eastern philosophy that understand the indivisibility and 'oneness' of existence (Kupperman 2001). It also provides a starting point for exploring the embodied experience of disability.

Giddens (1991 p 56) observed: 'the self, of course, is embodied', noting also that 'control of the body is a fundamental means whereby a biography of self-identity is maintained' (p 57). This prompts the question: What impact might physical impairment have on the maintenance of a sense of self? By focusing on disabling barriers, much disability theory has neglected issues of self and identity, yet these themes are central in documented narratives about the experience of impairment (Watson 1998). Many researchers have noted that disruption of one's physical condition is experienced as a disruption of one's self (e.g. Becker 1993, Carricaburu & Pierret 1995, Kaufman 1988a, 1988b, Kleiber et al 1995, Toombs 1992, 1994, 1995). It is also apparent that many people who lose the physical ability to undertake occupations that are important to them feel useless and valueless (Hammell 2004h, Lyons et al 2002, Reynolds 2003; see Chapter 11).

Three studies into the experience of spinal cord injury all identified the impact of body changes to a sense of self (Carpenter 1994, Taylor &

McGruder 1996, Yoshida 1993). Taylor & McGruder (1996 p 44) observed, for example, 'when a person sustains an irreversible injury, skills and unique qualities of the self that have taken a lifetime to develop are lost. When previous means of self-expression and areas of recognised competence and identity are taken away, the self must be re-defined'. This experience is frequently perceived to split the body from the self (Carpenter 1994, Ellis-Hill et al 2000), constituting the paradox of the embodied experience of disability. 'I am embodied' yet 'when bodily demands conflict with desired self-presentation the individual becomes acutely aware of the divergence between body and self' (Kelly & Field 1996 p 245). For example, a man with cerebral palsy explained his frustrations: 'I'm trapped inside this body that doesn't work' (cited in Shuttleworth 2001 p 86). While theorists may dismiss the idea of body/self dualism, they must also 'confront and account for the enduring power and qualities of these dichotomies at the *experiential* level of suffering' (Williams & Bendelow 1998b p 136). Thus, although the body and self are clearly indivisible, impairment makes the relationship between body and self more interesting (Gadow 1982), providing a largely untapped resource for exploring the nexus of bodies, selves and societies. Sartre's (1956) notion of the 'lived body' provides a useful concept for exploring this nexus.

The lived body

Toombs (1995) suggested that in considering the meaning of disability the phenomenological notion of the *lived body* is helpful in understanding the body as 'the basic scheme of orientation, the centre of one's system of coordinates' (p 10). (*Phenomenology* elucidates the existential meaning of an illness as a distinct human experience; the reality of illness as it is lived through by the individual; Kestenbaum 1982.)

The idea of the lived body proposes that 'I am "embodied" in the sense not that I "possess" a body but in the sense that I AM my body' (Toombs 1988 p 202). There is no question here of a dualism of body and self, or indeed of impairment and disability, but instead an interaction between the lived body and the world with which it engages and is engaged. It is because I am my body that a disruption to my body disrupts both my self and my life world (Gadow 1982, Toombs 1988).

Sartre (1956) observed that the body is taken for granted and forgotten when one's activities can be carried out with ease. By contrast, Toombs (1992 p 129) described the experience of neurological impairment, when the body suddenly 'refuses to yield to one's commands, frustrates one's intentions, and thwarts one's projects'. Far from being forgettable, the impaired body 'manifests itself as an *insistent presence* which remains always at the fringes of one's consciousness' (Toombs 1994 p 342). Indeed, many impairments continually intrude into daily life and require substantial periods of time to be devoted to body management (Williams & Wood 1988). Toombs (1992 p 333) discovered that the body can be experienced 'not merely as oppositional but as frankly malevolent, posing a constant threat to one's dignity and self-esteem'. The body can both humiliate the self and destroy future life possibilities (Gadow 1982).

Although exploration of the relationship between the body/self has evident merit for the rehabilitation professions, it is important to note that because the experience of disability emerges out of the interactions of people and society, exploration of the body/self cannot be undertaken in a decontextualized vacuum: a vortex of subjectivity and preoccupation with identity (Williams 1998). Just as bodies are inseparable from selves, so bodies/selves are inseparable from the context and circumstances of their lives. Indeed, the beauty of the concept of the 'lived body' is that it precisely addresses the interdependent triad of body/self/world. This would be a fruitful avenue of study for rehabilitation theorists.

THE RELEVANCE OF REHABILITATION

Traditionally, the rehabilitation professions have had little dialogue with the social sciences and humanities, aspiring to align themselves with the biological sciences and especially with medicine. Clearly, this exclusive allegiance to the biomedical sciences equips therapists to understand little more than the anatomy and physiology of the body: a singularly inadequate basis from which to understand the lived experience of impairment. To understand the social, cultural, political and economic worlds in which the impaired body is experienced and given meaning demands a wider intellectual engagement with the social sciences and humanities. However, the need for dialogue is bidirectional. Glaring inadequacies in the theories outlined in this chapter demonstrate the need for those disciplines with an awareness and understanding of disability to penetrate the ableist enclaves of academia. As Titchkosky (2003 p 28) observed: 'disability can teach us much about how the body shapes identity, how identity shapes the body, and how both have something to teach us about culture and its values'.

Although much of the work produced by theorists of the body is clearly unable to withstand critiques from the perspective of disability, this is an expanding and influential body of work concerning rehabilitation's central domain of concern that we can ill-afford to ignore. The insight that the body is so much more than an assembly of anatomy and physiology situates the rehabilitation enterprise in a broad social and cultural context. The experience of having/being a body is seen to be influenced, for example, by aesthetic ideals, economic and political imperatives, social values and powerful discourses, with the body centrally implicated in hierarchies of social power.

Rehabilitation is more than a physical endeavour. It is not about treating and curing, but about living. It is not solely about the body/mind but about life. Toombs (1994 p 351) contends that 'an important therapeutic goal is to assist those faced with physical disability in their efforts to reconstruct or redefine their changed selves. Indeed, to ignore the transformation of the self is to discount the major impact of disability'. Rehabilitation's traditional preoccupation with the physical body at the expense of the 'lived body' – the body as it is experienced and as it interacts with the self and the world – addresses only part of the body/self equation and would seem to miss much of the 'point' of being disabled.

Thompson et al (2003) proposed that people who have sustained a life-disrupting injury, such as a spinal cord injury, need to find a new 'I am' as well as a new 'I can'. To date, however, rehabilitation has focused entirely on the 'I can' – fostering abilities and facilitating functions – but has paid scant attention to redefining 'who I am' in the face of impairment. In this way, rehabilitation looks backwards to a dualistic era when the physical body was construed as extrinsic to the self and to an age when medicine was concerned with bodies, not people. Indeed, the self appears of little concern in the therapeutic endeavour (Toombs 1994).

In her exploration of women's experience of spinal cord injury, Morris (1989) reported that the overwhelming emphasis on sport, competition and physical achievement was not only perceived by women to be inappropriate but 'oppressive' (p 27). More recently, Kleiber & Hutchinson (1999) concluded from their own research that 'vigorous physical activity (and particularly sport involvement) is at best a temporary palliative to "the crisis" of physical disability for spinal cord injured men and at worst an impediment to a more complete personal transformation following the injury experience' (p 135–6). Kleiber & Hutchinson suggest that by promoting aggressive self-expression and celebrating physical prowess rehabilitation services seek to reinforce narrow hegemonic "norms" of suitable male behaviours and therefore limit their opportunities to explore other dimensions of themselves and other ways of being men. Indeed, this preoccupation with the masculine physique runs directly counter to substantial evidence that those people who make the best adjustments to life following spinal cord injury (for example) are those who can redefine their values, broaden the range of things that are cherished, expand their commitment to others and decrease the emphasis on physique as a measure of the self (Crewe 1996, Keany & Gluekauf 1993, Kleiber & Hutchinson 1999, McMillen & Cook 2003). Indeed, because adjustment to disability is found to be more difficult for men who are unable – or have not been enabled – to transcend dominant "norms" of masculinity (Gerschick & Miller 1995), a preoccupation with physical bodies may be completely counterproductive. Kleiber & Hutchinson (1999) suggest that adjustment to disability occurs not when the impairment is transcended but when the constraints of cultural norms, values and ideals are transcended.

Toombs (1994 p 356) observed that 'one does not simply RESUME life, following the onset of disability; one reconstitutes self-identity in integrating one's changed way of being into a new life plan'. This, the fundamental work of rehabilitation, will be explored further in Chapter 11.

Although centrally concerned with bodies in their physical, social, cultural, economic and political worlds, the rehabilitation professions have largely failed to challenge the idea of the body as a depersonalized and decontextualized 'shell'. This chapter has sought to present ideas that might destabilize that view and provoke a more rigorous and relevant approach to thinking about the body. The following chapter explores the experience of liminality – of being in limbo – that can result from moving from one bodily state to another.

Chapter 7

Disability, rehabilitation and liminality

Following a disruption, people experience a period of limbo before they can begin to restore a sense of order to their lives.
(Becker 1997 p 119)

INTRODUCTION: DISABILITY, REHABILITATION AND LIMINALITY

So far, this book has explored various ideas about "normal" and "abnormal" bodies, observing that social opportunities, privilege and status accrue to those whose bodies most closely conform to valued cultural norms. The present chapter further develops these ideas, drawing on the work of anthropologists to explore the experience of moving from a valued to a devalued bodily state following illness or injury, and focusing particularly on the 'in-between' or 'liminal' phase into which rehabilitation is inserted.

RITES OF PASSAGE

The Dutch anthropologist, Arnold van Gennep (1960) named and developed the concept of 'rites of passage' to describe the way in which people cross the boundaries from one social status to another. Van Gennep noted that people do not move abruptly between statuses, but tend instead to move through a three-phased process that includes a mediating period of 'liminality'.

Specific, culturally prescribed rituals, such as weddings, bar mitzvahs and graduations are undertaken to mark transitions between social states; or to mark the onset of puberty, admission to a warrior tribe, street gang, fraternity or the military, or to groups such as the girl guides. The common feature shared by all these rites of passage lies in their transformational nature: rites of passage signify a transition to a new social status with new rights and obligations.

Rites of passage are found in all cultures and in every region of the world and are all characterized by three successive and distinct phases that van Gennep (1960) identified as being: separation, liminality and reincorporation. *Separation* is a process of stripping away one's old status through physical removal from society. In a wedding ceremony, for instance, the bride and groom leave their everyday world and enter a special place – perhaps a civic or religious building – usually wearing special clothing. After undergoing specific rituals they leave this transitional, liminal place and are *reincorporated* back into their community with a new social status. Of particular interest to anthropologists – and to this chapter – is the middle phase of limbo: the *'ambiguous state of being between states of being'* (Barfield 1997 p 288): the *liminal* phase of transition. This is obviously brief in the instance of a wedding ceremony, but can be very prolonged in other rites of passage.

LIMINALITY

Turner (1967, 1969) furthered the work of van Gennep by exploring the liminal period in which people are in transition between culturally defined life crises or social states. Turner (1969 p 95) described those within this transitional period as being 'betwixt and between', cut off from their old status but not yet integrated into a new status: being neither one thing nor the other. This period of time is often marked by the receipt of special instruction. During puberty rites, for example, boys and girls learn from elders the practical wisdom they will need to function when they re-emerge as adult men and women (Barfield 1997).

Anthropologists note that this transitional stage frequently involves social isolation and the physical removal of the individual from their normal everyday life for a period of time. It is often characterized by endurance of certain unpleasant ordeals, being stripped of possessions, having an assumed asexuality or compulsory sexlessness and the enforcement of shared modes of dressing to emphasize common group identity. Anthropologists also note that those in the liminal stage experience powerlessness and a complete lack of autonomy, demonstrate an apparent equality within the group that transcends distinctions of class, age and gender, and are required to maintain utter subordination to those who hold complete authority over them and over their ability to exit this liminal phase (Ferraro 1995, Peoples & Bailey 1994).

Attaining a new social status might require a particular type of body. Thus, as a component of the rituals surrounding rites of passage, many cultures physically alter the body, for example through scarring, piercing, tattooing or performing female or male genital mutilation ('circumcision') to visually indicate the possession of a new social identity. The new body accordingly represents a new status and a new self.

DISABILITY AND LIMINALITY

It should come as no surprise that the experience of acquired impairment has been equated with van Gennep's rites of passage, with all that this implies concerning the transformation from one social status to another due to the possession of a changed body. It should be noted that rites of passage might not always be *from* a subordinate *to* a preferred social status. Someone who has been separated from his or her community for a criminal act, for example, will be reincorporated, following incarceration, into a lesser social status with a new set of obligations, such as regular contact with a parole officer, and new, diminished social opportunities.

The anthropologist Robert Murphy (1990) was one of the first to equate the experience of disability with that of liminality: an observation that arose from his own experience of progressive paralysis. Some anthropologists believe that certain groups of people, such as residents of refugee camps, remain in a life-long liminal state and Murphy subscribed to this perspective, claiming that 'most' disabled people 'dwell in twilight zones of social indefinition' (Murphy et al 1988 p 237): permanently suspended in a state of ambiguous social limbo. Pursuing the idea that those in a liminal state are neither one thing nor another, Murphy asserted that: 'the long-term physically impaired are neither sick nor well, neither dead nor fully alive, neither out of society nor wholly in it' (Murphy 1990 p 131). Murphy's contention has been embraced by others (e.g. Albrecht 1992), who view the concept of liminality as encapsulating what it means to be disabled in society.

However, the idea that impairment automatically reduces people to a permanent liminal status has been contested. Oliver (1990) criticized Murphy for failing to acknowledge that disabled people might be marginalized because of social restrictions rather than their own physical limitations.

For example, Murphy and his colleagues conducted a three-year anthropological investigation into the social relations of people with paraplegia or tetraplegia living in the New York metropolitan area and concluded, rather dramatically, that it is within 'sealed chambers at the edges or interstices of social systems that the disabled [sic] dwell' (Murphy et al 1988 p 238). Close scrutiny of their research reveals the physical reality behind these 'sealed chambers'. For example, many black paraplegics were living in walk-up tenements – the only housing they could afford – and were therefore only able to leave home when they were carried downstairs by van drivers to attend medical appointments.

There can be little dispute that these people were, indeed, stuck in a liminal state. However, this would seem to be due to poverty, powerlessness and the physical reality of being 'prisoners of their living quarters' (Murphy et al 1988 p 238). Indeed, this research would seem to encapsulate the social/political model and its assertion that disability is the social disadvantage imposed upon people with impairments (see Chapter 4). However, through their failure to tease out those problems caused by impairments and those superimposed by societal practices, the researchers implied that liminality is an inevitable consequence of impairment. Indeed, they claimed that disability is a permanent liminal state in which people 'have been made better, but not whole' (Murphy et al 1988 p 240). This conclusion recalls Goffman's (1963a) idea of 'spread', wherein a specific, stigmatizing attribute – such as an amputated limb – becomes a "master" status, serving to reduce all one's achievements and attributes to a single, stigmatized identity. Disabled people, according to Murphy, never regain a 'whole' status but are somehow always incomplete: 'neither dead nor fully alive' (Murphy 1990 p 131).

Further, Murphy et al (1988 p 241) applauded the liminality model for enabling analysis of cultural symbolism: 'the filter through which disability is perceived and given meaning' and lamented researchers' past neglect to attempt a 'ritual interpretation' of disability as a symbolic system. Critical disability theorists would contend that it is disability as a socially *created* problem that is at the root of the liminality experienced by this study population of housebound people with spinal cord lesions, rather than liminality as a socially constructed 'ritual interpretation' (Murphy et al 1988 p 241). Their liminality would seem to have been created and perpetuated not by interpretations but by steps, poverty and specific societal practices that serve to marginalize the physically different. Liminality might be triggered by an injury but it is maintained and perpetuated by society. It has nothing to do with whether people are 'whole' but with whether their human rights are respected.

However, while the premise that an impairment leads to a lifetime stuck in limbo is clearly contentious, the onset of impairment might certainly trigger a transitional, liminal period as a formerly taken-for-granted way of living is disrupted.

LIMINALITY AND BIOGRAPHICAL DISRUPTION

Oliver Sacks (1996) also described the onset of impairment as constituting a kind of 'limbo', characterizing this as a period in which the person has lost one world or way of living and has yet to reconstruct a new way of being in the world. This more nuanced and insightful observation reflects the findings of a large body of research into the experience of disability and suggests a process of transition through which individuals integrate the disruption of illness or impairment into their lives (Becker 1997). This clearly addresses the fundamental work of rehabilitation.

The sense of disruption to expectations, life plans and 'the seductive predictability' of everyday life (Hockenberry 1995 p 79) is a recurring theme in the life narratives of people who have experienced unexpected life events, such as illness or injury, and has been termed 'biographical disruption' (Bury 1982). Any unexpected event – such as the death of a life partner, an illness or injury, a marital breakdown, the loss of a valued job – can constitute a biographical disruption (Hammell 2004h). However, this may not be a simple, unidirectional equation. Biographical disruption might be implicated as a *cause* of illness, such as when bereavement leads to the development of cancer (Williams 2000).

Biographical disruption is said to occur when the routine activity and structure of everyday life is disordered (Bury 1982). Because it penetrates a biography, a disruption has repercussions for the body and self, has a temporal dimension and is indivisible from the individual's environmental context (Bury 1991). The onset of impairment, for example, constitutes an assault on the physical self – the body – and consequently also on a sense of identity and self-worth (Bury 1991), as noted in the previous chapter. It is also an assault on what Corbin & Strauss (1987) called 'biographical time': time as it is lived through activities, roles, routines, valued occupations, goals and life aspirations.

Biographical disruption can serve as a turning-point in one's life and is not inherently positive or negative. Rather, the meaning of the disruption is attributed by the individual (Nettleton 1995) and will be dependent on such factors as personal values, life stage, roles, interests and economic and social resources (Hammell 2004a). Research suggests that individuals who most successfully incorporate impairment into their ongoing lives are those able to redefine their values, broaden the range of things that are cherished and decrease the emphasis on physique as a measure of the self (Crewe 1996, Keany & Glueckauf 1993, McMillen & Cook 2003). However, no research appears to have been undertaken to determine how rehabilitation might assist in this endeavour.

Bury (1991) suggested that the meaning of a disruption will be determined by its potential *consequences* for everyday life – its impact on the practical aspects of life roles and occupations – and the symbolic *significance* of the event: its social connotations. The significance of an impairment will depend on cultural ideas concerning causation (blame), stigma, competence and social worth. Thus the experience of an impairment will vary depending on the biography of the individual, his or her values, circumstances and context (social, cultural, political, economic). Although both the consequences and significance of impairment can be changed through rehabilitation, interventions have tended to be focused exclusively on the practical consequences of impairment, with little effort to address either its symbolic significance or the potential impact of a diminished social status (Hammell 2004h).

Research that has explored the experience of impairments such as stroke, spinal cord injury and multiple sclerosis has identified common themes: a profound biographical disruption demanding an incorporation of the impaired body into a new sense of self, and an integration of one's changed circumstances to enable biographical continuity (Becker 1993, Carpenter 1994, Toombs 1995). Becker (1997 p 119) observed: 'following a disruption, people experience a period of limbo before they can begin to restore a sense of order to their lives'. This period of transition, or liminality, can take considerable time and is the space within which the major work of rehabilitation occurs.

RITES OF PASSAGE AND REHABILITATION

The profound biographical disruption precipitated by the onset of an impairment may require the individual to undergo a transition into a new way of being in the world (Sacks 1996). This process of rehabilitation epitomizes van Gennep's (1960) rites of passage: separation, liminality and reincorporation.

Separation, in this instance, occurs as one's old status is stripped away – either because of a physical inability to engage in former roles or because of a withdrawal of those social privileges and opportunities reserved for "normals" – and through physical removal from one's familiar world into a hospital or rehabilitation facility. Physically outside the boundaries of society, rehabilitation may constitute a sort of initiation process into a new, disabled, persona (Murphy et al 1988). People in this stage of their lives are in an ambiguous situation, cut off from their old status but not yet integrated into a new status (Marks 1999).

After a liminal period of social isolation and the receipt of specific instruction and 'practical wisdom' (Barfield 1997) disabled people may leave this transitional place to be reincorporated back into society. Although reincorporation, in theory, occurs upon discharge from an in-patient facility, many disabled people report that the process of learning to live in an altered physical form is not complete at this point but, rather, this is when their real learning begins (Becker 1997, Hammell 1995). Indeed, Bellaby (1993) suggested that the liminal phase continues long after discharge for those whose rehabilitation process has ill-equipped them for life in the community.

It is because rehabilitation is a transitional stage that this is an inappropriate time to be assessing outcomes. It is self-evident that outcome measurement can only be undertaken after reincorporation, once community living has resumed and an 'outcome' has occurred (see Chapter 8).

A few autobiographies penned by disabled people and a little qualitative research have enabled a glimpse of the experience of rehabilitation from the 'inside', and of its 'liminal' character. Perhaps because rehabilitation has often followed standard treatment regimens rather than being tailored to meet individual needs (Jorgensen 2000), clients have felt stripped of their former identities and histories, powerless and suspended in limbo (Clark 1993, Johnson 1993). People with a variety of impairments have all identified a loss of autonomy and sense of being in control following injury or diagnosis (Becker 1993, Carpenter 1994, Toombs 1987). Toombs (1987) claimed that this perception of helplessness and dependency was exacerbated by having one's activities and plans determined by 'powerful others': a characteristic of traditional rehabilitation programmes (Oliver et al 1988). In light of the reality that perceptions of choice and control are positive contributors to perceptions of quality of life (e.g. Crisp 1992, Fuhrer et al 1992, Krause 1992) it is paradoxical that the rehabilitation process is so often characterized as the experience of powerlessness (Dalley 1999, Johnson 1993, Morris 1991). Researchers have found that 'the feeling that the various aspects of life are under one's control is a major component of quality of life' (Tate & Forchheimer 1998 p 49). Powerlessness is incompatible with high quality of life. Murphy (1990 p 40) expressed the feeling of many who have undergone in-patient rehabilitation: 'my returns on Sunday evenings were marked by [a] sense of reimprisonment and depression'.

Of course, rehabilitation, by definition, represents an unwelcome interlude in a life that has been disrupted by illness or trauma and is a time of uncertainty, change and struggle. However, it is the specific nature of the powerlessness articulated by disabled people that characterizes this period of their lives. Congruent with anthropologists' observations, the liminal phase of rehabilitation is described as entailing unpleasant ordeals, a physical removal from normal everyday life, being bereft of most clothing and possessions and thrust into a sexually ambiguous or compulsorily sexlessness position. In addition, first-person and ethnographic accounts have reported that patients experience a sense of equality among themselves that transcends class, age, "race", gender and other previous social distinctions (Murphy 1990, Purves & Suto 2004). These accounts also describe a vulnerability to intrusive questioning and the experience of utter subordination to the dominance of those holding complete authority over them and over their ability to exit this liminal phase: the rehabilitation professionals (Cochran & Laub 1994). However, while there is always a limit to the time spent in rehabilitation, those with severe degrees of impairment or with few social and material resources may find themselves confined indefinitely within liminal, sequestered spaces.

LIVING IN LIMBO: THE EXPERIENCE OF INSTITUTIONALIZATION

Chapter 3 explored the practice of classifying people, noting that individuals categorized as 'deviant' by those wielding more social power have a history of being separated and excluded from society through institutionalization (Charlton 1998, Imrie 1996). Goffman (1961 p 11) defined a 'total institution' as a place of residence 'where a large number of like-situated individuals, cut off from the wider society for an appreciable period of time, together lead an enclosed, formally administered round of life'. A defining characteristic of the total institution is that inmates spend their lives under the control and surveillance of staff (Twigg 2000). For the vast majority of disabled people who find themselves in an institution, 'there is no alternative, no appeal, no remission of sentence for good behaviour, no escape except from life itself' (UPIAS 1981, cited in Hughes 1998).

Cultural imperialism – 'common sense' – has long decreed that those people who have severe physical impairments ought to be separated from society and placed within institutional settings because this is the only cost-effective and efficient means of ensuring their physical needs are met. (An argument that reduces human needs to bodily management and human rights to economics). However, common sense is an inadequate foundation for policy or practice and is often singularly lacking in evidence-based support! Instead, research evidence demonstrates a high incidence of pressure sores among institutionalized people (McGregor 1992) and shows that self-managed models of care (in which people with severe impairments receive money directly from the government with which to hire the personal assistants of their choice) are cost-effective, lead to high client satisfaction and to reductions in preventable – and expensive – medical complications (Beatty et al 1998, Mattson-Prince 1997, Zejdlik & Forwell 1993).

Writing from his own experience of institutional confinement, Hunt (1998 p 14) explained: 'there are staff who bully those who can't complain, who dictate what clothes people should wear, who switch the television off in the middle of a programme, and will take away "privileges" (like getting up for the day) when they choose'. French (1994c p 119) astutely observed that 'the many rules and regulations exist more for the benefit of the staff than the residents' and noted that because it is primarily created by staff attitudes and behaviours, an institutional atmosphere can be created in a small group home as readily as in a large facility. Goble (2004 p 42) also noted that it is every bit as possible to have institutionalized regimes and practices in community settings because 'institutions are made as much of thoughts, beliefs and institutional practices as of bricks and mortar'.

Many people with impairments are confined within institutions and marginalized from society, not because of the severity of their physical needs but because of their already marginalized social status. Duggan et al (2002), for example, noted a recent significant increase in the percentage of people with spinal cord injury being discharged to nursing homes in the USA. Their research revealed two particularly notable findings: (1) people are sent to nursing homes on the basis, not of the severity of their impairments, but of their lack of social and economic power, and (2) powerlessness and denial of the opportunity to exert any control over their own bodies or lives also characterizes their institutional experiences. This is, indeed, 'a kind of life sentence for bodily impairment' (Keith 2001 p 18).

Congruent with the physical restrictions frequently placed on novitiates in liminal situations, disabled residents in British institutions are often restricted to using the toilet at designated times and to accepting a bath or shower on a specified day each week (MacFarlane 1996). In Australia, Seymour (1998) found that some residents in institutions were granted the 'luxury' of a hair wash only three times in a five-week period. In the USA, Duggan et al (2002) reported that some people with spinal cord injuries who were confined in residential institutions had to lobby continually to get their teeth brushed at least twice a week, or their hair washed at least twice a month. Thus, the oppressive nature of 'care' within residential institutions is neither idiosyncratic nor localized within certain geographical, political, ideological, social or economic domains. Indeed, it is systemic.

For more than a century, healthcare professionals have quietly acquiesced to the segregation of disabled people into restrictive living environments 'that the professionals concerned would *never* have chosen for themselves' (Morris 1997 p 59). Further, few professionals have actively engaged with disabled people in their struggle to exit institutional liminality and live the sort of lives the professionals take for granted (see below). Although Hayashi & Okuhira (2001 p 855) noted that 'only two decades ago, Japanese society did not perceive confining disabled persons in institutions for life as a human rights violation', other nations apparently have not attained the same degree of insight.

In British Columbia, Canada it was formerly considered both inevitable and acceptable practice to send people with severe paralysis to residential institutions for the remainder of their lives. Indeed, by the 1990s many people who had survived the polio epidemic of the 1950s with severe impairments were still living in huge hospital wards in the same beds they had occupied for over 40 years (Hammell 1998a). A group of young men and women with high spinal cord injury (most of whom were also ventilator dependent) described their institutional experience in the following ways. 'It was hell really – they just warehoused us in an institution and we fought very hard to get out'; 'You weren't really treated like a real person . . . and just seeing how other people are treated . . . a lot of them had speech impediments and, you know, can't really fend for themselves and they're really at the mercy of the staff'; 'We were basically considered second- or third-class citizens and we were subject to a lot of denigration and abuse'; 'There was a penitentiary feeling . . . they didn't need actual bars on the windows because nobody was going to escape, but it was like a prison in every other sense' (Hammell 2004f p 611). Declaring that 'we wanted more of a quality of life', five of this group had lobbied for changes in social policy that would enable them to live in the community with self-managed care.

Since leaving institutional custody, their lives have come to resemble those of other members of society. Several have married, some have fathered children, some have attained university degrees or are currently studying for academic or professional qualifications. Some are employed full time, others volunteer or pursue artistic, literary or business endeavours. All these life-enhancing accomplishments were contingent on the opportunity to live in the community with self-managed assistance. Their achievements also highlight the flawed logic behind the cultural common sense: that people with severe impairments can only be properly 'cared for' in an institution.

Researchers have found institutional confinement to be characterized by powerlessness; dependence; low self-esteem; depersonalization; lack of choices and options; lack of privacy; constant surveillance; regulation and restriction; lack of legal rights; limited social contact; inflexibility of routines and menus; geographic, social and cultural distance from family and friends; recipient status and an inability to enact adult roles or contribute to others; assumed asexuality and enforced sexlessness; gender segregation; devaluation; loss of identity; lack of freedom; crowded conditions; a lack of opportunity to engage in meaningful or productive occupations; subordination and negative, disrespectful and belittling staff attitudes (Barnes & Mercer 2003, Dijkers 1998, Hammell 2004f, Lorimer 1984). Many of these findings precisely match the conditions endured by individuals within the liminal phase of rites of passage, as outlined above. Indeed, 'to be admitted to one of these institutions is to enter a kind of limbo in which one has been written off as a member of society but is not yet physically dead' (Miller & Gwynne 1972 p 80).

People with severe physical impairments understand 'the right to live in one's own home or accommodation within mainstream society and community without fear of incarceration in a residential institution' to be 'a fundamental human right' (Houston 2004 p 307); perceiving the interminable liminality of institutional living to be abusive, disempowering and profoundly oppressive.

LIMINAL STATUS AND OPPRESSION

Chapter 3 introduced the five 'faces' of oppression that were first delineated by Young (1990). Marginalization and cultural imperialism have already been discussed (Chapters 3 and 5) and this is an appropriate place to explore the other three dimensions of oppression: powerlessness, exploitation and violence. These are all interlinked concepts. Cultural imperialism perpetuates negative stereotypes, prejudices and discrimination against disabled people. Social and geographical marginalization, informed by cultural imperialism, create the sort of isolation that makes people easy prey for those wishing to abuse them (Westcott 1994). People who are powerless are especially vulnerable to neglect and abuse, exploitation and violence (French 1994c).

Feminists have worked hard to portray men as dominating and exploitative and women as caring and life-affirming and, indeed, the majority of health professionals are women who are paid to care. This ideology should not blind us to the reality that performing a paid, nurturing role 'does not necessarily mean that [women] value or respect that mode of relating as much as they may revere . . . the assertion of power', coercion and domination (hooks 1989 p 94). Twigg (2000) observed that research on nursing homes and institutions exposes darker, more manipulative dimensions; noting that 'care' is not always kind but can constitute an expression of power. Although critical of patriarchal domination and control over women's (able) bodies, feminists have failed to challenge the coercive control and domination by women over other bodies (hooks 1995), such as those of disabled people (the majority of whom are women). Power is central to all relationships between people in unbalanced social positions and is irreducible to simplistic gender dualisms. The health professions rather successfully portray themselves as benevolent, altruistic and client-centred – especially to themselves – yet little research has been undertaken to determine whether this equates with clients' experiences of rehabilitation and hospitalization. Intellectual rigour, ethics and accountability require that we continually challenge such hegemonies and seek to interrogate the evidence that supports or contests these ideologies.

Macfarlane (1996 p 13) notes that many disabled people define the care they have received as being 'oppressive, often of a custodial nature and provided in a controlled way'. Notably, those in residential institutions or rehabilitation facilities often have no control over who can touch their bodies or provide their personal care (Westcott 1994). Indeed, powerlessness is a defining characteristic of institutional care (Goffman 1961).

OPPRESSION: POWERLESSNESS

Powerlessness derives from a lack of decision-making power, the inability to enact choices and exposure to the disrespectful treatment that results from occupying a marginal status (Young 1990). Powerlessness is most likely to be experienced when there is a sharp divide between those wielding power and decision-making authority – like rehabilitation professionals – and those in subordinate statuses, like patients (Barnes & Mercer 2003).

Seligman (1975) developed the theory of *learned helplessness*, which states that unless people feel able to exert some control over their lives they will cease making the effort to try to do so. Institutional environments, such as hospitals and rehabilitation centres, that reward cooperative, compliant and passive behaviours and that do not permit clients to define their own problems nor engage in an interactive, problem-solving process actively contribute to clients' sense of powerlessness (Pollock 1993). To correctly attribute causality, this powerlessness is more appropriately termed 'taught helplessness' (Hammell 1995). When disabled people lose their freedom to control their own lives (for example by institutionalization or restrictive social policies), they may experience a 'threat to their whole life and purpose for living' (Maynard 1993 p 195). In addition, research has demonstrated a significant relationship between helplessness and depression (Seligman et al 1979).

Themes of loss – of choice, control and autonomy – were identified as being integral to their institutional experience by the people with high spinal cord injuries who were cited above. One man explained: 'I felt that everybody else had control' and another stated: 'I think all patients who've been in institutions for prolonged periods are quite aware of the overwhelming controls and attitudes'. When this group attained their right to live in the community it was: 'a *great* change. You get a lot more freedom. You're running your own life and there's no set schedule where you have to do certain things at certain times . . . it's back more to the way things were, when you can come and go and do whatever you like, eat whatever you like, eat *when* you like . . . you've got a lot more freedom' (Hammell 1998a). It was evident from these people's comments that institutionalization was inversely correlated with the ability to achieve a sense of autonomy and continuity in their lives. This is congruent with the concept of liminality, in which the person in limbo is caught in an ambiguous and transitional state that is not under their own volition or control.

OPPRESSION: EXPLOITATION

People who are powerless are vulnerable to exploitation. *Exploitation* is the social process by which work is organized to enact relations of power and perpetuate inequality (Charlton 1998). For example, structural barriers, such as lack of accessible and affordable transportation, serve to exclude disabled people from the paid labour market and perpetuate their economic dependence. These are not natural barriers but human creations.

The policy of providing 'care' in institutional rather than community settings is a useful example of the exploitation, or social process, by which work is organized to enact relations of power and perpetuate inequality. Critical disability theorists have observed that social policies and practices that create and perpetuate the dependency of disabled people – most particularly, policies that facilitate institutionalization – provide employment for significant numbers of the dominant population (Barnes et al 1999). In the USA, for example, nursing homes that warehouse disabled people provide employment for large numbers of people and are described by financial analysts as being a 'growth industry': a generator of economic capital for the dominant population. The owners of these 'homes' constitute a formidable and wealthy political lobby (Charlton 1998).

Healthcare workers' particular fondness for institutional models of 'care' stems not solely from employment opportunities but from power: the unfettered ability to control 'care'. In one's own home one can refuse to admit certain distasteful staff, resist professional domination and decline medications (Twigg 2000). In an institution, 'the space belongs not to the residents but the staff. It is they who are in charge and they determine the rules. Significant areas of the residential home – offices, rest rooms, staff toilets – belong solely to them' (Twigg 2000 p 84). When the young people with tetraplegia (mentioned above) fought to leave institutional custody and live in the community they expended a great deal of effort in challenging those hospital staff and medical personnel who resisted change and who benefited from the status quo. Notably, 'professional attitudes about the care and *control of care* of those who were severely disabled and ventilator-dependent had to be changed' (British Columbia Rehabilitation Society 1990 p 17, emphasis added). The location of 'care' has less to do with geography than with power.

In the USA, there has been considerable opposition to closing institutions from those unions who stand to lose both jobs and power (Shapiro 1993). In other countries too, healthcare unions oppose any move towards contracting out of work and their professional associations have skilled lobbyists working to preserve power (Hammell 2000a). The status quo benefits many in the majority population. A Canadian Minister of Health argued: 'Unions representing health care workers have expressed concern about job loss and contracting out of work ... If self-managed care is to be successful, these issues must be resolved to the satisfaction of the parties involved' (cited in Hammell 2000a). This intriguing insight suggests that disabled people are a commodity within health and social care systems governed by the demands of employees (who have a strong economic base and formidable lobbying powers) rather than by the rights of clients who do not appear to be among the 'parties involved' in the deinstitutionalization of their own care. Thus, the warehousing of disabled people within institutions is (apparently) acceptable if this provides secure employment for the able-bodied majority. This is the embodiment of exploitation.

OPPRESSION: VIOLENCE

The *violence* that Young (1990) identified as being a dimension of oppression constitutes those unprovoked assaults that serve to humiliate, torment and victimize those marked as vulnerable. Disabled people are prime victims of violence and have 'an inordinately high rate of abuse' (Davis 2002a p 147). Indeed, the fear of violence – of verbal ridicule, physical or sexual attacks – often conspires to restrict disabled people's life activities (Barnes & Mercer 2003).

The liminal space – as defined earlier – is a marginal zone wherein subordinate people have no rights, no status, no power and from which they do not have the ability to exit. Anthropologists characterize this as a time of danger and vulnerability (Ferraro 1995). Congruent with this theory, research has highlighted the high levels of sexual, physical, verbal and emotional abuse endured by disabled children and adults throughout the world; most particularly among those in institutions (French 1996, Philpott & Washeila 2001, Swain et al 2003, Wendell 1996). The reality that abuse and violence are most frequently experienced by those who are confined in institutions highlights their particular vulnerability. It is important to acknowledge, also, that the neglect that so pervades residential institutions is a particularly malignant form of abuse.

In some cultures it is believed that the rape of a young disabled virgin will cure the perpetrator of HIV/Aids (Philpott & Washeila 2001). In others, sexual predators have sought employment in those institutions where socially isolated disabled children and adults are especially vulnerable (Westcott 1994). Within institutions disabled victims are 'chosen because they cannot run away and there is nowhere to run' (Cross 1994 p 165).

However, abuse is not confined to institutions but pervades social care services in the community (Cambridge 1999) and private homes (Calderbank 2000). Hendey & Pascall (1998) note that disabled people may be least able to defend themselves in their own homes where they may be obliged to admit both acquaintances and strangers. Moreover, while rates of physical and sexual abuse are twice as high for disabled women than non-disabled women (Calderbank 2000, Shakespeare 1996c), few women's refuges have facilities for disabled women and their children (Calderbank 2000), electing instead to protect the rights and lives of "normal" women.

Because abuse is always perpetrated by the powerful against the powerless, Cambridge (1999) suggested that disabled men, women and children will continue to experience high levels of abuse as long as hierarchical structures of power are central to the provision of care and services. Just as physical impairments do not cause the disadvantage of disability, it is important to understand that it is a person's social position that creates their vulnerability to abuse, not their physical impairment, gender, age or "race" (Shakespeare 1996c). Because violence is about exerting and enforcing power, men may be victims (Shakespeare 1999) and women are frequently perpetrators (Kaminker 1997, Morris 1993a, Shakespeare 1996c).

The liminal, or transitional, period of institutionalization that can follow impairment has been characterized as a time of helplessness, dependency, powerlessness, loss of freedom and loss of control. However, it should also be recalled that the liminal period is a time of special instruction and the sharing of practical wisdom. The 'point' of the liminal period is not to entrap people in a lifetime of limbo but to prepare them to assume their new social status.

LIMINALITY: THE ROLE OF 'ELDERS'

Turner (1967) drew specific attention to the role of elders in facilitating the transition between two ways of being and in providing a model, or example, of how one might live in a new way. This crucial dimension of the process of transition to living in an altered physical form was mentioned frequently by those in the study into high spinal cord injury, who identified the need for peer models, or 'elders'. 'Alan' explained: 'What I'd have liked to have known [when I was injured] is that there *is* life after spinal cord injury!' He described a local research project that asked former spinal cord injury (SCI) clients what they felt was most needed in a 'high SCI' rehabilitation programme: 'and it was a peer mentor: a peer counsellor! They thought it was crucial'. When Alan had sustained his C3 lesion, he had been unable to meet anyone else who was in a similar situation. However, for those people who had been given the opportunity to do so this had been a critical experience. For example, 'Beth' claimed, 'my rehabilitation came from other people, with [high cord] injuries, who had lived the life'. Similarly, in response to a query about the relevance of his rehabilitation programme, 'Colin' explained: 'the only thing that really helped me was speaking with other 'quads' [tetraplegics] in the community. Right after you're hurt . . . the first thing you want to do is to find someone, and speak to someone that's in the same situation – preferably someone that's been in the community for a few years – so then you know what to expect'.

Anthropologists have identified the role played by elders in educating those in transition between states and it is apparent that this valuable role may be enacted for people with impairments by peer mentors. It is for rehabilitation professionals to ensure that this occurs.

REINCORPORATION AND REHABILITATION

Corbet (2000 p 4) described making a film about people's experience of rehabilitation. 'One thing common to everyone's story was that early on they'd been told more about what they couldn't do than what they could do'. Rehabilitation practitioners had elected not solely to convey their knowledge about physical impossibilities – the ability to walk after a complete spinal cord injury, for example – but also their beliefs about more general 'impossibilities': 'you'll never walk, or go to school or graduate or get married or hold a job. You can't fly a plane, you can't make music, you can't have children. You can't be a doctor or get elected to public office. Get real' (Corbet 2000 p 4). Clearly, Corbet's report almost precisely matches the experiences of David and others, described in the previous chapter.

Rather than providing clients with the knowledge and tools to resist the marginal status to which social norms strive to confine them, researchers have found that the process of 'getting real' comprises an effort to adjust clients' expectations downwards (Abberley 1995, Johnson 1993). This is believed to enable them to 'accept' or 'adapt to' their new, lowly status and its diminished opportunities and privileges. Murphy et al (1988 p 241) claimed: 'most rehabilitation establishments are ineffective in preparing people for the social conditions they will face . . . instead of being advised to become reconciled to their social condition, the disabled [sic] should be told to fight their way out of it'.

The finding that rehabilitation better enables people to assume a marginal, liminal social status than to attain the rights enjoyed by other citizens has been a recurrent theme in previous chapters. While this attempt to 'manage disappointment' might, at first blush, appear kind, it is clearly neither benevolent nor respectful. Rehabilitation is not about teaching exercises, mobility and self-care skills (although these might be useful for some people). Rather, rehabilitation is about enabling people to get on with their lives, to reconstruct their biographies and to attain a sense of continuity between their former and present selves. Fundamentally, it is also about assisting people to exit a liminal social status of diminished rights.

When disabled people organize to create their own support services their primary focus is not on exercises or self-care skills but on fostering self-esteem and self-confidence and on acquiring the skills and behaviours required to live with an impairment in a world inscribed with prejudice and discrimination (Shapiro 1993). Part of this process includes identifying the social norms of ableist society such that these "norms" can be transcended or negated (Hayashi & Okuhira 2001). This might usefully comprise one dimension of the mandate of relevant and useful rehabilitation services.

Further, Becker (1997) contends that by understanding the temporary nature of the liminal experience that so frequently follows the onset of impairment people are better able to endure their sense of life disruption and to comprehend that life will eventually continue. The desire for a sense of 'biographical continuity' – of getting 'back on track' – has been identified in the first-person accounts of people with various impairments (Becker 1997, Carpenter 1994, Hammell 1998; see Chapter 11). Boekamp and colleagues (1996) suggested that the concept of *continuity* might be a more useful avenue for rehabilitation than the traditional preoccupations with loss and change, enabling people to see 'that there are many important areas of their life that have been unchanged since the injury . . . By focusing on how things have remained the same, they are better able to cope with the areas that have changed' (p 343).

This chapter has explored the concept of liminality from two perspectives: the personal (following biographical disruption) and the social (the experience of rehabilitation and institutionalization). It has been suggested that rehabilitation could usefully focus on two areas: the personal (achieving biographical continuity) and the social (negating norms and contesting marginalization). The following chapter is wholly concerned with the fundamental practices of rehabilitation.

Chapter 8

Rehabilitation fundamentals

Rehabilitation cannot continue to be shaped by the norms of the physical world to which so few of its clients can aspire.
(Seymour 1998 p 126)

INTRODUCTION: THE FUNDAMENTAL PRACTICES OF REHABILITATION

Several themes have recurred repeatedly in the previous chapters. It has been seen, for example, that while "normality" – or "normal" function – is a culturally prized goal, this is both an elusive and often irrelevant aspiration for rehabilitation clients. It is also clear that rehabilitation has dual mandates: addressing the personal dimensions of impairment – enabling clients to get their lives 'back on track' – and the social dimensions of disability: contesting discrimination and striving to achieve equality of opportunity.

This chapter addresses the assumptions that underpin the fundamental practices of rehabilitation, interrogating these for their relevance to disability and to the findings of the previous chapters.

'OPTIMAL FUNCTION'

Rehabilitation practitioners often claim to be engaged in a process of maximizing their clients' physical and mental functions (Gadacz 1994). In light of the reality that few therapists have 'maximized' their own functions – few are élite athletes with PhDs, for example – this would seem to be an unlikely goal. It might, perhaps, be regarded as a useful slogan – a worthy yet unrealistic objective – if it could be shown to constitute an adequate response to disability. In reality, enhancement of function constitutes just one dimension of learning to live well with an impairment.

This again raises the critical difference between treatment and rehabilitation to which earlier chapters have alluded. Restoring movement following an acute sports injury, for example, is not rehabilitation; it is treatment: performed *by* someone *to* someone else, acutely focused and (hopefully) fully restorative. 'Rehabilitation does not provide a cure' (Reynolds 2005 p 229); rather, it is a *process* of learning to live well with an impairment in the context of one's environment (Trieschmann 1988); a process that might include – but cannot be limited to – enhancement of physical function. While a preoccupation with augmenting physical function through standardized treatment regimens might be both adequate and effective for people with minor, short-term problems such as torn cruciate ligaments, it is clearly inadequate for people with chronic or deteriorating conditions for whom enhancement of physical function is an insufficient goal (Hammell 2004a). Someone who has sustained a stroke, brain injury or spinal cord injury (for example) has disrupted not just a body but an entire life (Mattingly 1991). Although the torn cruciate ligament might reasonably be remedied through *treatment*, the *rehabilitation* endeavour is concerned not with treating and curing but with living. Thus disabled people want and need rehabilitation interventions to be tailored to their lives rather than to their bodies (Williams & Wood 1988).

STRUGGLING TOWARDS INDEPENDENCE

There has always been a pervasive idea that rehabilitation is the process of teaching skills to enable the highest level of physical independence (Swain et al 2003), as if this is a goal to which all clients aspire, or 'ought' to aspire, irrespective of culture, role demands or personal values. Stewart (1985 p 14), for example, asserted: 'nurses who are rehabilitation orientated know that the patient must *struggle towards independence*' [emphasis added]. This sometimes humiliating struggle is perceived by many disabled people to constitute abuse (e.g. Priestley 2003, Swain et al 2003). However, it is not only the attempt to justify making people struggle that disabled people challenge, but the very ideology of *independence*.

Physical independence is prized by the majority culture in the minority ("developed") world and is often unchallenged by therapists who assume that their belief in the importance of independence is universally shared (Penn 1999). Cross-cultural research shows that this is not a universal aspiration, thus imposing this as a goal reflects ethnocentricism (Wirz & Hartley 1999). People from South Asian cultures, for example, do not interpret 'dependence' and 'independence' in the same ways in which they are perceived by those from Western cultures (Katbamna et al 2000) but place much higher value on interdependence (Gibbs & Barnitt 1991). Similarly, researchers observe that within Arabic cultures and many countries of the South, interventions focused on a goal of independence rather than *inter*dependence are of questionable relevance or value (Chaleby 1992, Wirz & Hartley 1999). Although dependency is denigrated in the West, among those cultures that have traditions of reciprocity and mutual obligation, people in seemingly dependent positions are not devalued (Katbamna et al 2000). Thus, Atkin & Hussain (2003) observed that disabled Asian young people attempted to balance their need to exercise control over their own lives with their sense of interdependence and mutuality.

Bricher (2000 p 783) claimed that 'nurses consider independence to mean the ability to undertake self-care, rather than the ability to make decisions' and that this way of thinking is reflected in such nursing models as Orem's self-care deficit theory and Roy's adaptation model. Because the assumption that independence is a universally valued goal lacks evidence-based support, this ideology can be seen to reflect specific, dominant values – those of middle-class, Western-orientated therapists – rather than research evidence. Indeed, Whiteford & Wilcock (2000 p 332) observed that although physical independence in everyday tasks is a Western preoccupation it is 'a concept with which occupational therapists have become fixated'. Clearly, occupational therapists are not alone in their fixation. Research demonstrates that although rehabilitation professionals prioritize the ability to undertake activities without assistance, their clients, instead, value the importance of being able to make autonomous decisions: to be in control of their lives (Lund & Nygård 2004).

Contrary to Western, egocentric ideology, Reindal (1999 p 354) observed that interdependence is 'an indispensable feature of the human condition'. Although children are expected to be dependent on others for their survival and then to become more self-reliant and self-sufficient over time, Wehmeyer (1998 p 11) observes that 'this is a movement from dependence to interdependence, not a movement from dependence to absolute dominion'. While independence has been ideologically constructed as "the norm", it is evident that interdependence is the usual.

Throughout this book it has been observed that ideologies are insepara-ble from specific workings of power. It is evident that the ideology of inde-pendence serves particular political goals since it is easily challenged by anyone for whom marriage or partnership, friendships or family life demonstrate on a daily basis that we are all engaged in interdependent rela-tionships of reciprocal care. Walmsley (1993 p 131) observed that, 'caring and dependency, far from being dichotomous, are on a continuum. We are all dependent to a greater or lesser degree on others'.

Wendell (1996) suggested that once we understand all people as being interdependent we are less likely to place artificial divisions around the needs of disabled people and those of their informal carers. This enables the context of care and the reality of reciprocity to be acknowledged, and facili-tates the provision of appropriate forms of intervention and support to those engaged in networks of care.

An ideological preoccupation with physical independence, rather than with interdependence and reciprocity, reinforces normative judgements and cultural stereotypes that those who are 'dependent' are parasitic, needy and burdensome (e.g. Ungerson 1987). To many disabled people this ideology is offensive, yet by failing to contest it, rehabilitation professionals support it. To understand the offensive power of stereotypes, rehabilitation profession-als might ponder the stereotype that they, themselves, are 'parasitic' and 'dependent' on disabled people for their lucrative livelihoods, social status and professional power (Davis 1993, French 1994a, Oliver 1999, Swain et al 2003).

Importantly, a preoccupation with physical function and physical inde-pendence has often reduced rehabilitation to a process of relearning the skills that most four-year-olds have attained: self-care and mobility. This demeans adult clients, leaving them ill-equipped to re-engage with their complex lives or to transcend the marginal status to which social and cul-tural norms tend to confine them. As Murphy (1990 p 56) observed: 'there was nothing at all in my rehabilitation that prepared me for the psycholog-ical and social challenges I would face'.

In light of convincing evidence that humans, by definition, are social, interdependent beings it is evident that allegiance to a specific notion of independence reflects a particular alignment of ideology and power.

IDEOLOGY AND POWER

Critical disability theorists contend that 'professional thinking and action are embedded within complex social, political, economic, cultural, intellec-tual, and historical contexts' (DePoy & Gilson 2004 p 139): that rehabilitation professionals' approach to practice is 'value-based' (p 140). Thus, Marks (1999 p 106) recognizes 'the need for a certain amount of scepticism towards professional claims regarding their "disinterested" service orientation'.

Rehabilitation theory reflects dominant cultural values that are rarely challenged or made explicit. For example, current occupational therapy the-ory states that *occupations* comprise 'self-care, productivity and leisure' activ-ities (CAOT 2000 p 37): an ordering that is neither random nor alphabetical, but a hierarchy informed by the specific values and priorities of physically independent, employed theorists (Hammell 2004b, Suto 2004). Disability theorists would argue that by prioritizing self-care and productive activities – those that contribute to the social and economic fabric of communities (CAOT 2000) – occupational therapists act as agents of the State, actively promoting and perpetuating ideologies that denigrate those deemed 'dependent' or 'unproductive' (Hammell 2004h). Professional ideologies may support, rather than contest, dominant discourses. For example, Finger (1995 p 15) claimed: 'we need to argue against "productivity" . . . as a measure of human value'.

Although rehabilitation practitioners may prioritize physical independence in self-care activities, irrespective of the costs of time and effort for their clients (Marks 1999), research has demonstrated that disabled people often choose to live interdependently, preferring to use their time and energies in those activities that have personal value and importance (Holcomb 2000, Morris 1989, Yerxa & Locker 1990). A woman with multiple sclerosis remarked, for example, that she had learned not to waste her 'very limited energy on things that are boring' (cited in Reynolds 2004a p 21).

Some disabled writers claim that the pressure placed on disabled people to achieve physical independence is a form of oppression (e.g. French 1994a). The rehabilitation professions should therefore feel obliged to engage in active debate and critical reflection to interrogate the degree to which they are unwitting cogs in a specific political wheel, reinforcing ideologies of self-reliance and physical independence that may serve the interests of the state rather than their clients (French 1994a). Just as rehabilitation researchers are required to examine their social location with respect to their research assumptions (Hammell 2002a), so the rehabilitation professions must examine their location within those webs of power and political ideologies that shape their disabling practice assumptions.

Redefining independence

It is apparent that therapists and their clients do not share a common understanding of the concept of *independence* and that therapists rarely attempt to explore what independence means to their clients (Whiteford & Wilcock 2000). Rehabilitation practitioners tend to define independence as the ability to perform self-care activities without physical assistance (Reindal 1999), while for disabled people 'independence' is the quality of control they have over their lives and the opportunities they have to make decisions and enact choices (Clare 1999, d'Aboville 1991). Richardson (1997 p 1271) asserted that independence 'is about personal power and control over one's life rather than doing things for yourself, unassisted'.

Independence can be achieved by obtaining assistance when and how this is required (Reindal 1999). Indeed, independence is usefully defined 'not as the ability to perform necessary tasks but as the freedom to control one's own life and determine its course' (Williams & Wood 1988 p 132). This definition more closely aligns rehabilitation with disability theory, with the idea of autonomy and with clinical ethics.

Autonomy

Clinical ethics are informed by five central principles: respect for the person (such that all people are valued and treated with dignity), non-maleficence (the duty to refrain from causing harm), beneficence (the duty to assist those in need), justice (the duty to ensure fair and equitable distribution of benefits) and respect for autonomy (French 2004a, Jonsen et al 1998). Employed within early Greek writing to characterize independence from the tyranny of foreign rule (Reindal 1999), *autonomy* is defined as being both the moral right and the ability to act on particular desires and choices and to be in control of one's own life, unfettered by coercion, duress, restraint or deceit (French 2004a, Norman 1995). Autonomy therefore constitutes the power and right of self-government and of self-determination.

Clinical ethics constitute guidelines to protect individuals' fundamental human rights. Armstrong and Barton (1999 p 211) use the term *human rights* 'to mean a set of principles based on social justice; a standard by which the conditions and opportunities of human life can be evaluated'. Witkin (2000) explained that while human rights are obviously those rights to which every person is entitled, 'fundamental human rights are those rights which are primary, that supersede all others' (p 209). All people are entitled to two fundamental human rights: the right to well-being and the right to freedom. Witkin (2000 p 209) describes the right to freedom as entailing 'the right of individuals to act as they wish without interference from others, including the state'. The only limitation on such action is that it does not threaten or violate other people's rights to freedom or to well-being.

Thus the ethical principle of autonomy is central to human rights and is concerned with the moral right of clients to make choices and to follow their own plans of action and of life, in so far as these do not infringe upon someone else's rights or welfare (Jonsen et al 1998). Accordingly, healthcare ethics insist that clients' values and priorities 'trump' those of their service providers (Banja 1997). The principle of autonomy constitutes an ethical requirement for contemporary healthcare practice and is not an optional modus operandi.

Importantly, autonomy is dependent on possession of relevant information with which decisions can be made, indicating the considerable obligation for therapists to provide clear, comprehensive information (an argument central to evidence-based practice; see Chapter 10).

To suggest that autonomy is a specifically Western ideal, grounded in egocentric notions of individualism and independence (see Spiro 1993) is to misunderstand this basic concept. Autonomy refers to the fundamental human right to make choices, to enact choices, to be self-governing and to exercise self-determination (Wehmeyer 1998). This is as relevant for those who choose to accept assistance with daily living tasks and who choose interdependent modes of living as it is for those whose sense of self depends, instead, on accomplishing tasks alone. Autonomy refers, not to absolute control or domination, but to an ability to influence, direct, choose and manage one's life as situations and roles demand and personal preferences dictate.

It has been noted in earlier chapters that physical function does not have a demonstrable effect upon quality of life. However, researchers have found that autonomy – the ability and opportunity to make choices and exert control over one's life – *is* a positive contributor to perceptions of quality of life (e.g. Hammell 2004i, Treece et al 1999). Indeed, Johnstone (1998 p 65) observed: 'the exercise of choice and the opportunity to take control of the organization of one's own life is one of the first markers of quality'.

Conversely, research evidence demonstrates an association between perceptions of reduced control and low life satisfaction (Albrecht & Devlieger 1999, Krause 1997). Thus, while physical independence has little or no bearing on perceptions of life's quality (see below), it could be said that ethical practice – respecting clients' autonomy – is evidence-based practice and is a positive contributor to quality of life (Hammell 2004a).

PHYSICAL FUNCTION, INDEPENDENCE AND QUALITY OF LIFE

Rehabilitation practitioners often claim that by striving to improve their clients' physical functioning and physical independence they will somehow enhance their quality of life. This is an admirable goal, but not one that enjoys a supportive evidence base (Hammell 2004a). A large volume of research has demonstrated, counterintuitively, that perceptions of quality in living do not correlate with either the degree of physical function or the extent of physical independence (see Hammell 2004i). Further, neither the severity of an impairment nor degree of physical independence are predictive of psychological distress (e.g. Hartkopp et al 1998, Krause et al 2000, Post et al 1998). Indeed, quality of life can be improved irrespective of function, pathology or health (Johnston & Miklos 2002).

Although it is apparent that rehabilitation's claim to be enhancing the quality of lives through maximizing physical function and physical independence is not an evidence-based assumption, this belief persists among the rehabilitation professions (Hammell 2004a). This adds further support for the premise that beliefs and views that appear to constitute 'common sense' are singularly resilient to change, even when confronted with contradictory evidence (Taylor 1999).

EVIDENCE–BASED PRACTICE

Throughout the Western world, government policies and professional initiatives are demanding that rehabilitation practice be 'evidence-based'. This means that interventions ought to be informed by reference 'to a body of evidence about efficiency and effectiveness' (Gomm & Davies 2000 p x). Unfortunately, the rehabilitation professions have subjected relatively few of their interventions to rigorous research (Banja 1997), providing an unstable basis for their claims to knowledge and an uncertain basis for practice. Research revealing considerable variation in the provision of occupational therapy for total hip replacement across the UK, for example, suggests that services are not currently evidence based (McMurray et al 2000). The concept of evidence-based practice, its controversies and issues, will be discussed later (Chapter 10). However, I contend that *every* rehabilitation assumption should be interrogated with reference to the findings of research.

Research evidence has demonstrated, for example, that clients and therapists differ on the meaning of 'rehabilitation', the relevance and value of treatment services, their preferred approaches to service delivery, their priorities of treatment goals and their desired treatment outcomes (e.g. Clark et al 1993, Corring 1999). For professions claiming a client-centred orientation to practice and striving to demonstrate the evidence-based grounding of their theories, this is a rather shaky start.

ASSESSMENT

Central to the rehabilitation enterprise is the primacy of the assessment. Indeed, disability theorists contend that assessments are central to the exercise of professional power, defining problems and framing solutions in ways that suit the professionals' agenda (Gillman 2004). Therapists treat what they measure. Thus the ideological underpinnings of the forms of assessments used within rehabilitation establish the foundations for subsequent interventions and for outcome measurements. If therapists adhere to an individual/medical model of practice and focus on assessing specific skills, such as climbing stairs or performing transfers, these will be the targets for intervention, irrespective of their importance or relevance to individual clients' lives or environmental circumstances.

The nature of the questions in the assessment will determine whether the therapist will discern the client's goals and priorities or whether the assessment will be channelled along lines dictated by the therapist (Reynolds 2004b). "Standardized" assessments that reflect the priorities of therapists are popular among rehabilitation professionals, with very few assessments being designed to reflect the perspectives of clients (although Law et al 1998 and Stratford et al 1995 have developed tools for this endeavour). The emphasis of traditional assessments is on streamlined measures that are universally applied 'without reference to the disabled person's own perspective, the roles they occupy, the relationships in which they are embedded, the circumstances of their milieux or the wider political context of barriers, attitudes, and power' (Williams 1998 p 239). Indeed, streamlined assessments may be beautifully standardized yet, simultaneously, completely irrelevant.

The elements that are included in an assessment and the manner in which they are scored typically reflect societal norms (Johnston & Miklos 2002). Accordingly, the majority of assessments reflect the assumption that certain ways of performing activities are better than others – independence is 'better' than interdependence – and that each item on the assessment is of equal significance to the client. Assessments usually measure whether a client can perform a specified activity, irrespective of whether they wish to do so, or could do so in their own environment or within a span of time they consider to be reasonable.

Assessments are designed to determine needs, and definitions of need tend, coincidentally, to fall squarely within the remit of whichever profession is undertaking the assessment! McKnight (1981) claimed that a characteristic of disabling professionals is the practice of identifying in clients a problem for which *they – these* professionals – have the solution. He suggested that 'needs-assessments' should best be understood as a function of 'professionals in need of an income' (p 25).

Assessment constitutes part of the political role played by therapists: a contribution either to maintaining and perpetuating their own power, status and 'market share' or to empowerment of clients. Disabled critics contend that the very idea of 'assessment' is ideologically loaded, reflecting a mode of practice in which professionals not only define the needs of others but through which they actively ration resources and place limits on the rights of their clients (French 1994d, Zarb 1991). Assessment, then, can be less about determining the needs of the client than about preserving the fiscal and political status quo. Neither is this solely a function of resources or the economic climate (Stevenson & Parsloe 1993). Inadequate responses to disabled people's needs result 'as much from a failure of imagination as a shortage of resources' (Ellis 1993 p 19).

Marks (1999) observed that professional assessments of the needs of their disabled clients tend to be presented as if they are value-free, "objective" evaluations. Yet rehabilitation practitioners only rarely challenge the myth that "objectivity" – being uninfluenced or unbiased by personal values or opinions – is possible.

"Objectivity"

Despite claiming a scientific approach to knowledge development, the rehabilitation professions have largely failed to engage with insights from either the history or philosophy of science. Historians of science and medicine, feminist, postcolonial and postmodern philosophers have contested the belief that anyone can be objective – value-free – recognizing instead that the interpretations of what we perceive will always be influenced by contemporary beliefs and by our 'location': our perspective as the member of a particular gender, sexual identity, class, ethnicity, education, profession and so forth (Alcoff 1991, Haraway 1988, Said 1993). Science is the product of the interpretations and perceptions of humans; thus claims to objectivity are not sustainable (Kuhn 1962, Latour 1987).

Many scholars acknowledge that all analysis is a form of interpretation; that a researcher's own values and views have important effects on how they interpret data, and that neutrality or objectivity are always impossible (e.g. Armstrong et al 1997, Haraway 1988, Shakespeare 1996a). Indeed, postmodern theorists contend that it is impossible to achieve either "objective" knowledge or "truth" (Fawcett 2000b): an insight central to Buddhist, Confucian and Taoist philosophies, which acknowledge that knowledge is always inadequate and partial. Further, Jeffreys (2002 p 32) observed that 'many of the most egregiously oppressive and even genocidal practices of the modern era, including race laws, eugenics, and the Holocaust, have been buttressed and defended by the authoritative rhetoric of objective science'.

Science has always been a social product: 'its projects and claims to knowledge bear the fingerprints of its human producers' (Harding 1986 p 137). Irrespective of whether researchers adopt a quantitative or a qualitative approach to collecting information, data will always be interpreted through the filter of the researcher's past experiences and present beliefs, making claims to "objectivity" impotent. Slevin et al (1988), for example, showed that assessments of a patient's quality of life demonstrated a wide variability in scores between different physicians and health professionals, even on ostensibly "objective" scores.

Ferrarotti (1981) noted that because people who are being observed or assessed will continually modify their own behaviour according to the behaviour of the observer, it renders 'any presumption of objective knowledge simply ridiculous' (p 20). To suggest that an assessment is objective because it is made by an outside observer is fundamentally to misunderstand and misappropriate the word 'objective'. Mor & Guadagnoli (1988 p 1056) astutely observed: '"objectivity" is not bestowed upon a measure merely because another person makes it'. Nonetheless, this is the precise way in which "objectivity" is usually employed by rehabilitation professionals, implying that 'our' perceptions are objective; clients' perceptions are subjective. This is erroneous. Dockery (2000 p 98) notes that 'the "outsider" is no more able to offer value-free or neutral knowledge than the "insider"; rather, they speak from different positions'. Regrettably, 'the dominant experience of disabled people when they place themselves in the hands of professionals is one of "knowledge denial" rather than knowledge enhancement (. . .) as their ways of knowing and accounting for their experience are devalued as insufficiently "dispassionate" and "objective"' (Dorn 1998 p 198).

It has been noted that therapists treat what they measure. The nature of the assessment thus dictates the nature of subsequent interventions.

INTERVENTION

Previous chapters have identified the need for a two-pronged approach to rehabilitation: the personal (achieving biographical continuity) and the social (negating norms and contesting marginalization through environmental interventions). Therefore the term 'intervention' is preferred instead of 'treatment', not solely because 'treatment' implies client passivity but also to reflect a mode of practice that will focus on environmental changes – such as access to public transportation – in addition, perhaps, to modifying individuals' abilities (Hammell 2004a).

The consequences of an impairment depend not solely upon specific dysfunctions but upon the context in which the impairment is experienced, and on the meaning of dysfunction within the individual's life (Oliver et al 1988). As Reynolds (2004b p 111) explained: 'medically similar illnesses may have widely different meanings and implications for individuals, depending upon their social context, personal priorities and resources'. The experience of living with a stroke (for example) will be determined by a range of environmental variables (such as income, social support, physical access to the home and community, and social policies and services), personal variables, for example, one's age, role expectations (such as worker, wife, mother), interests and beliefs (such as fate or divine will) and the meanings or values that the person attributes to all these factors (Hammell 2004a).

These personal dimensions will determine the priorities for intervention and cannot, obviously, be addressed by a generic, prescriptive approach to stroke 'management'. The objective of rehabilitation is not to 'manage a stroke' but to assist someone to manage their life, given the occurrence of a stroke.

OUTCOME MEASUREMENT: COUNTING OUTCOMES OR OUTCOMES THAT COUNT?

Outcome measurements ostensibly evaluate the effectiveness of interventions. By definition, they should assess outcomes after clients have 'come out' of rehabilitation. Outcome measurements have traditionally focused on functional achievements, yet these are superficial outcome indicators, at best. As Woolsey (1985 p 119) observed, while 'some functionally independent patients are happy, productive and socially active . . . others are not'. Clearly then, assessment of physical function is an inadequate gauge of the usefulness, relevance or value of rehabilitation services.

Although widely employed and seldom challenged, quantitative outcome indicators are neither objective nor absolute measures but are reflective of social norms and expectations (Keith 1995). Indeed, although outcome measures are often deemed to be 'standardized', they are inevitably culturally biased, reflecting the values the dominant culture regards as 'standard' (Spencer et al 1993). In most instances, outcome measures reflect the normative values of their developers and users. For example, assessment of accomplishments in activities of daily living (ADL) has long been a staple component of occupational therapists' professional repertoire, yet ADL scales are usually biased, with scoring systems reflecting value judgements about how an activity 'ought' to be performed (Hammell 1995). Those disabled people who choose to live interdependently, or to use equipment to accomplish their daily tasks will receive a low score, while people with severe physical impairments who live independent lifestyles by managing and directing others in their care will usually receive no score at all (Law 1993).

Scoring systems can therefore be seen to reflect the values of the dominant population. For example, the Craig Handicap Assessment and Reporting Technique (CHART; Whiteneck et al 1992), a widely used rehabilitation outcome measure, decrees that any assistance with self-care activities deserves a low score, yet someone who elects to receive assistance in dressing (for example) might have chosen to conserve their time and energy for more productive and personally valuable activities. Clearly, denigrating this as 'dependence' reflects a specific value system and the role expectations of the dominant culture, with no reference to the values or priorities of those being assessed. The importance of this argument is not to claim that "standardized" outcome measures are deliberately discriminatory, but rather to observe that if someone with multiple sclerosis, for example, is satisfied with directing others in her personal care then a high score should be attained and the outside observer's values discounted.

Von Zweck (1999 p 212) argued that occupational therapists need to utilize evidence in their decision-making to enable them to define approaches for service delivery that will achieve 'optimal client outcomes, promote consistency, continuity and cost containment, and validate the role of occupational therapy to clients, payers and other health professionals'. But what are *optimal client outcomes*?

In the scramble to demonstrate the efficiency and effectiveness of rehabilitation services it is tempting to generate evidence based solely on therapists' views of 'optimal' outcomes. 'It is comparatively simple to demonstrate, for example, that *x* number of clients with C6 tetraplegia can dress themselves or that clients with stroke have improved *x* points on the Bartel Index, thereby demonstrating the "effectiveness" (but not the relevance) of interventions' (Hammell 2001b p 231). Clearly, the impact and outcome of rehabilitation cannot be derived from the viewpoints of service providers because we do not have to live with the outcomes.

In light of considerable evidence showing that disabled people neither share the same priorities, preoccupations or perceptions of problems as their healthcare providers (e.g. Clark et al 1993, Corring 1999) it has been queried whether the purpose of judging 'successful' outcomes by measuring those skills prioritized by therapists is simply a means to justify and validate customary rehabilitation practice (Eisenberg & Saltz 1991). As Ray & Mayan (2001) observed, a 'clinically significant' outcome may be significant only to a clinician. Evidence also suggests that rehabilitation services tend to 'skim off the top', concentrating on people with minimal functional impairments rather than those most in need of their services (Kemp 2002, Seymour 1998); electing to serve those clients most likely to achieve impressive outcome statistics. This is not only misleading, it is unethical (see Chapter 9).

It is surely perverse that the healthcare professions wield the power to administer and interpret those assessments that gauge the effectiveness and value of their own work? In his analysis of the ways in which professional services are disabling to clients, McKnight (1981) noted the tendency of professionals 'to define the output of their service in accordance with their own satisfaction with the result' (p 32). He observed that 'the important, valued and evaluated outcome of service is the professional's assessment of his [*sic*] own efficacy' and that professionals assert that 'only we can decide whether the solution has dealt with your problem' (p 32).

It should be self-evident that the most important question in evaluating outcomes is: 'What outcomes are important to clients?' Secondary questions include: 'To what extent have specific rehabilitation services enabled clients to get their lives "back on track"?' and 'How successfully have specific rehabilitation services enabled clients to challenge those discriminatory attitudes and societal practices that reduce their life opportunities?' These questions demand consideration of how outcomes can be assessed such that they reflect clients' priorities. In addition, clients should determine the most appropriate time for assessing such outcomes (Needham & Oliver 1998).

Many medical researchers now recognize the self-evident need to understand clients' perceptions of outcomes, and the importance and meaning of specific outcomes to their lives (Fischer et al 1999). Yet, despite a declared client-centred orientation to practice (e.g. COT 2000), the rehabilitation professions do not consistently permit clients to prioritize those outcomes that are most relevant to their lives. Further, despite an espoused commitment to enhancing quality of life, rehabilitation practitioners have often limited their assessment of outcomes to such decontextualized minutiae as measurements of range of motion or strength, assessments of stair-climbing or the ability to dress without assistance, as if they believe these accomplishments somehow enhance the quality of one's life (Hammell 1998b). In reality, such measurements as range of motion, exercise capacity or 'functional independence' are surrogates for what rehabilitation really ought to assess: the effect of interventions on our clients' lives (Guyatt et al 1997).

ASSESSING QUALITY OF LIFE

Quality of life has justifiably become both the ultimate goal of rehabilitation and a key outcome in determining the effectiveness of rehabilitation programmes (Whiteneck 1992). However, the concept of *quality of life* lacks a clear definition, being used within medical research to refer both to the measurable, material *conditions* of life and to the *experiences* that make life meaningful and valuable (Roy 1992). Because there is no consensus among healthcare professionals as to what 'quality of life' actually means, no unified approach has been taken towards its 'measurement' (Gill & Feinstein 1994), there is no agreement about whether it should be measured by healthcare professionals or patients (Hammell 2004i), or, indeed, whether measurement of quality is possible (Dijkers 1999). Perhaps because of these difficulties, assessments of quality of life have infrequently been used to gauge the efficacy or value of rehabilitation's interventions, despite an espoused commitment among the rehabilitation professions to enhancement of quality of life (Johnston & Miklos 2002).

Although the way in which quality of life is defined is inherently value led, neither the values that underlie its definition nor the operational definition of the term are usually made explicit (Priestley 1999). Reflecting a belief that the quality of a life can only be appraised by the person whose life it is, within this book, the term 'quality of life' is conceptualized as *the experience of a life worth living* (Hammell 2004f).

The majority of research into quality of life has used quantitative methods, including various rating scales and questionnaires (Post et al 1998). However, quantitative research into quality of life is inherently problematic for several reasons. Clearly, attempting to quantify a qualitative experience erases the difference between the quantitative and the qualitative (Hammell 2004i). Indeed, the belief that *quality* of life can be *quantitatively* measured (Kennedy & Rogers 2000) is an obvious oxymoron. Thus, Leplège & Hunt (1997 p 47) claimed that many quantitative instruments 'tell us something about life, but nothing about quality'.

Further, the categories that researchers choose to include in their surveys or scales inevitably reflect the researchers' beliefs, values and culture (Dijkers 1999) and can be deemed neither "neutral" nor "objective". By prioritizing independence and paid employment, for example, quality of life assessments can be shown to reflect the norms and values of the dominant culture and privileged classes (Johnston et al 2002, Wolfensberger 1994). These are culturally specific and not universal values (Whyte & Ingstad 1995); indeed quality of life measurement is not a value-free endeavour but one that is inherently political, being informed by assumptions, values and convictions with which research subjects might not agree at all (Dijkers 1999).

Many variables contribute to the formation of values, such as education, material wealth, gender, "race", age and social class/caste and there may be a poor match between the values and priorities of researchers and their 'subjects' (Hammell 2004i). In addition, researchers have reported that a serious injury or illness can prompt a revision of values and a re-evaluation of the dimensions that are considered to be personally important and to be contributors to quality of life (Boswell et al 1998, Gill 2001, Wright 1983). Despite this, Dijkers (1997) noted that many researchers appear to assume that their own judgements about what contributes to quality of life are shared by others; that everyone wants the same out of life that they do. This is not only naïve but produces research results of questionable validity or relevance. (*Validity* has to do with whether a research instrument is measuring what it is intended to measure.)

It is evident that research scales are prone to embody the researchers' view of what is relevant to quality of life. Moreover, 'once this view is built in to the item construction, studies that subsequently use the scale can do no more than confirm or not confirm these preconceptions' (Stenner et al 2003 p 2162).

Perhaps unsurprisingly, a great deal of research has demonstrated serious discrepancies between the "objective" (i.e. the researcher's) assessment of quality of life and the subjective satisfaction with that life (e.g. Albrecht & Devlieger 1999, Johnston & Miklos 2002, Loew & Rapin 1994, Woodend et al 1997). Indeed, 'life satisfaction can be remarkably unrelated to activities defined by researchers or even clinicians' (Johnston & Miklos 2001 p S53), making much quality of life research invalid.

Researchers have been cautioned against an over-reliance on objective indicators of quality of life – such as measures of functional independence – because it is the relative importance of these indicators to each individual that is of greater significance (DeLisa 2002). In reality, however, respondents are only rarely provided with the opportunity to rate the importance of various factors to their own lives (Gill & Feinstein 1994), making the validity of research findings questionable.

Some researchers claim to be assessing 'subjective' quality of life using "standardized" questionnaires that are completed by research 'subjects'. However, using quality of life criteria that have been selected by researchers constitutes forced 'choices' and not a subjective appraisal of the factors that are important to individuals' lives, based on their own values and priorities. Leplège & Hunt (1997 p 48) explain that this practice ignores the relative meaning and importance given to various dimensions of life by the individual and that 'the guise of obtaining patients' perceptions acts to preserve the supremacy of professional judgments, leading to the suppression of what is supposed to be under scrutiny'. Indeed, how a researcher or clinician attempts to 'measure' quality of life reveals more about their own values, priorities and fundamental orientation to life than it does about the quality of life perceived by the people whose lives are ostensibly being studied (Hammell 2004i).

Quality of life: measuring what counts

Glass (1999 p 123) stated that 'the primary goal [in rehabilitation] must be achieving the highest level of quality of life. Implicit in such a statement is the involvement of the individual in deciding the parameters of quality'. Indeed, Gill and Feinstein (1994 p 624) noted that if researchers persist in using instruments developed by "experts", 'quality of life may continue to be measured with a psychometric statistical elegance that is accompanied by unsatisfactory face validity'. Clearly, quality of life can only be measured by the individual whose life it is because perceptions necessarily reflect personal values and specific contexts (Dale 1995). For this reason, Dale (1995) argued that any claims to have measured the quality of life experienced by a patient using existing standardized 'objective' tools are 'false' and the results of no value.

The difficulty of assessing quality of life centres on the problem of understanding a life different to one's own and of its value to the person whose life it is (Walsh 1993). Acknowledgement of this difficulty, and of the reality that 'the subjective experience of a life is more important than its outward expression' (Walsh 1993 p 144), has prompted many researchers to argue that an understanding of subjective experience requires qualitative research methods that can probe both the content and the context of that life (e.g. Batterham et al 1996, Whiteneck 1994).

It is clear that an 'analysis of the factors that are likely to influence quality of life may help to focus interventions that could maximize quality of life outcomes' (Consortium for Spinal Cord Medicine 1999 p 24). Because enhancement of quality of life is ostensibly the ultimate objective of the rehabilitation enterprise (Glass 1999, Whiteneck 1992), rigorous analysis of the factors that contribute to the subjective experience of quality of life is of central concern to rehabilitation researchers (see Chapter 11). Indeed, such research must be the foundation for the process of reasoning that informs clinical practice.

CLINICAL REASONING

During the past decade there has been considerable interest in clinical reasoning among the rehabilitation professions (e.g. Harries & Harries 2001, Mattingly & Fleming 1994). Clinical reasoning is more than the application of theory to practice; it is a cognitive process of critical analysis and reflection that underpins decision-making and guides action (Hammell 2004a). Applying standard treatment protocols to specific diagnoses requires little intellectual effort or reasoning skills, being a technical rather than a professional endeavour (Richardson 1999). However, because rehabilitation is concerned with people, not diagnoses, rehabilitation interventions must be tailored to suit the skills, needs and priorities of each client. This demands a high degree of reasoning, with client input at every stage to ensure both relevance and accountability.

A vast body of work on reasoning has been generated by researchers with diverse academic orientations. The following outline provides a brief overview of the clinical reasoning process as this pertains to everyday rehabilitation practice.

Clinical reasoning blends theoretical knowledge, research evidence and clinical expertise with the client's knowledge and experience (Hammell 2004a).

Theoretical knowledge

Theories – conceptual frameworks encapsulating specific knowledge – guide all clinical practice and every research inquiry, informing what we believe should be done in various situations (Hammell & Carpenter 2000). Clinical reasoning therefore requires the therapist to decide which theoretical approaches are appropriate to understanding and addressing each client's situation. For example, an approach to a client's physical state might be informed by theories of neuroplasticity, while concern for how he or she will resume a meaningful life in the community might draw on person–environment theories informed by the social/political model of disability.

Research evidence

Clinical reasoning is central to evidence-based practice and requires both the identification of relevant current *research* and the critical appraisal of this evidence for its applicability and usefulness, given the specific circumstances of an individual client (Hammell 2001b). Without recourse to research evidence, the reasoning process is dependent on intuition, trial and error, the perpetuation of formerly fashionable routines (Ritchie 1999), on the therapist's 'best guess' or 'whim' (Banja 1997 p 53), increasingly out-of-date primary training or the overinterpretation of experiences with individual clients (Rosenberg & Donald 1995). This accounts, in part, for the vast diversity of interventions experienced by clients with similar impairments and similar circumstances in different clinics.

Clinical expertise

The reasoning process will also be guided by knowledge the therapist has derived from reflective practice and *clinical expertise* and from the lived experience of the client's peer group. Importantly, clinical expertise is not the accumulation of clients treated over many years (Richardson 1999) but is defined as the 'thoughtful identification and compassionate use of individual patients' predicaments, rights and preferences in making clinical decisions' (Sackett et al 1996 p 71). Drawing from the insights of postmodernism, Fook (2000) suggested that the concept of professional expertise might be usefully reframed in terms of 'the ability to work in, and with, the whole context or situation' (p 116).

Clients' knowledge and experience

This brings us to the most important dimension of clinical reasoning: the *client's experience, values and priorities* (Sackett et al 1996). Without grasping the meaning and consequences of impairment to clients' lives or their particular social, cultural, economic, legal, political and physical circumstances, therapists do not have the necessary information with which to ensure the relevance of their interventions.

Reasoning and context

Physiotherapists and occupational therapists acknowledge the importance of environmental context in their theories of occupational performance (CAOT 1997) and of movement (Cott et al 1995). In an effort to determine whether theory is translated through reasoning into practice, Jorgensen (2000) undertook research to discover what physiotherapists knew about the social and cultural lives of their clients with total hip arthroplasty and how such information served to inform and shape their clinical practice. Sadly, Jorgensen's findings demonstrated that physiotherapists nurtured a mechanical view of the body and a perception that the role of the physiotherapist is to teach clients a standard treatment regimen rather than to tailor interventions to meet individual needs. However, studies investigating "expert" practice in physiotherapy (Jensen et al 2000) and occupational therapy (Strong et al 1995) have demonstrated that "expert" clinicians are those who strive to understand clients, the context of their lives and how these are affected by illness or impairment. (Clearly, the élitist term "expert" is problematic for professions that aspire to client-centredness and to non-hierarchical client–therapist relationships, as discussed in Chapter 1). Because clients are key sources of knowledge, collaboration and communication are central to the process of clinical reasoning (Jensen et al 2000). Communication, by definition, is a two-way process and therapists clearly need to communicate their reasoning to the client to illuminate the links between their interventions and the client's goals (Peloquin 1990).

Effective clinical reasoning occurs within the context of client-centred practice (Higgs & Jones 2000), being wholly concerned with clients' values and priorities and with the contexts of their lives. An approach to rehabilitation that focuses on the physical dimensions of an impairment may initially be appropriate, for example, after the onset of a stroke. Subsequently, however, interventions at the sociopolitical level will be required to maximize opportunities and minimize discriminatory barriers. As Shakespeare & Watson (2001b) contend, one approach cannot be a substitute for the other.

REHABILITATION: PRACTICE AND POLITICS

Napoleon Bonaparte is reported to have said that 'ability is of little account without opportunity' (Wehmeyer 1998 p 12). This has considerable relevance for the mandates of the rehabilitation professions. Shapiro (1993) claimed that segregation of disabled people because of a lack of access to education, employment, transport and the built environment constitutes a form of 'apartheid'. Clearly, then, when rehabilitation professionals strive to change a dimension of the environment (physical, cultural, social, political, legal, economic) to counter discrimination and to equalize opportunities this is a political act. What is important to understand is that when rehabilitation professionals strive instead to change dimensions of individuals so that they can better fit within segregated environments *this is also a political act.*

Acquiescing to the inequities of the status quo might be politically conservative, but it *is* political.

However, in reality, rehabilitation practices are typically oriented towards implementing, not inclusion, but a version of inclusion (Titchkosky 2003). Schriner (2001) observed that adhering to modes of intervention that are focused on changing individuals and avoiding confrontations with the structural and attitudinal barriers that discriminate against disabled people is not only politically conservative but attracts to the rehabilitation professions those people who are more interested in modifying individuals than achieving social justice. Perhaps this is why many therapists are content to teach new wheelchair users to 'jump' kerbs, for example, yet do not perceive lobbying for kerb cuts to be an integral part of their mandate. These are political choices.

Adhering to the individual/medical model of disability is *as* political as adopting the social/political model (see Chapter 4). Therapists play an active role in maintaining and perpetuating disabling environments, or an active role in changing them. Both roles are political; there is no neutral stance.

This chapter has explored the assumptions that underpin the fundamental practices of rehabilitation, noting that relevant interventions can only follow relevant assessments, and that assessments, interventions and outcome measurements can only be useful if they are relevant to the meaning and context of disability for individuals' lives. The following chapter explores an approach to practice that respects clients, their values and priorities and supports their rights to autonomy: client-centred practice.

Chapter 9

Client–centred philosophy: exploring privilege and power

The challenge for professionals is that, from the experiences of disabled people, they have been part of the disablement of people with impairments.
(French & Swain 2001 p 751)

CHAPTER CONTENTS

INTRODUCTION: CLIENT–CENTRED PHILOSOPHY, PRIVILEGE AND POWER

It is claimed that disabled people on both sides of the Atlantic perceive their relationships with rehabilitation professionals to be hierarchical, with professionals intent on reinforcing their own power and the powerlessness of disabled people (Barnes & Mercer 2003). Regrettably, these perspectives have been unaffected by two decades of self-professed 'client-centred' practice.

In the quote with which this book began, Mike Oliver (1996a p 104) argued that the central problems within rehabilitation are 'the failure to address the issue of power and to acknowledge the existence of ideology'. Much of the previous chapters has been concerned with issues of ideology: acknowledging its existence among the rehabilitation professions and exploring its contours, content and consequences. Thus far, however, the book has largely failed to address the issue of power within rehabilitation and so this must be the central focus for the present chapter.

POWER AND POWERLESSNESS

When Foucault (1980) observed that knowledge, operating through discourse, is inseparable from power he drew attention to the reality that the work of rehabilitation – categorizing, assessing, measuring and adjusting individuals towards a valued norm – is an expression and assertion of power. Because Foucault demonstrated that nothing can be considered to be outside power, Rossiter (2000 p 31) claims that Foucault's legacy highlights the 'caring' professions' 'lost innocence of helping'. Nonetheless, it is evident that these professions have barely begun the work of understanding their construction within power, choosing instead to promulgate 'notions of innocent helping by dedicated professionals' (Rossiter 2000 p 32).

It is curious that the rehabilitation professions have expended little effort in exploring issues of power, when *powerlessness* is central to the experience – and even the definition – of disability (Barnes & Mercer 2003). Indeed, to *disable* is 'to deprive of power' (Chambers Twentieth Century Dictionary 1972). Although many rehabilitation professionals do not *feel* powerful (especially in the presence of professionals accorded higher status, such as physicians, or as a consequence of sexism), it is important to recognize the distinction between feeling powerful and having power (Peace 1993). *Power* is not a commodity that is concentrated in the hands of a few – like wealth – but is widely dispersed and a function of dynamic processes of interaction. Thus decision-makers may be agents of power despite lacking privilege (Young 1990).

In Chapter 7 it was seen that powerlessness derives from a lack of decision-making power, the inability to enact choices and exposure to the disrespectful treatment that results from occupying a marginal status (Young 1990). It was also suggested that powerlessness is most likely to be experienced when there is a sharp divide between those wielding decision-making authority (like rehabilitation professionals) and those in subordinate statuses, like patients (Barnes & Mercer 2003). Far from being issues of peripheral concern it is evident that issues of power and powerlessness are central to discussions of disability and rehabilitation.

Resisting power: naming power and powerlessness

Swain et al (2003 p 136) observed that professional rhetoric is generally expressed 'in terms of altruism and acting in the best interest of disabled clients'. In light of the reality that the rehabilitation professions perceive themselves to be altruistic and to be acting in the best interest of their clients, I have been advised to avoid provoking resentment and hostility by contesting these beliefs and to focus instead on exemplars of good practice that might enable our professional self-images to remain intact. To do so, however, would be selectively to ignore the biographical reports of former rehabilitation clients, research evidence and the critiques of disability theorists, so much of which portrays professionals as coercive, dominating and manipulative (Abberley 2004) and 'as controlling, distant, privileged, self-interested, domineering and the gate-keepers of scarce resources' (Swain et al 2003 p 133). It must also be acknowledged that locating evidence of excellence *from clients' perspectives* is inordinately difficult.

Although I concede that many – perhaps most – rehabilitation professionals believe themselves to be acting in the best interests of their clients, it is important to acknowledge that believing something does not make it true. In reality, sincere intent, hard work and clinical competence do not, in and of themselves, guarantee positive outcomes. To ignore rehabilitation's location within frameworks of power that disempower our clients is to maintain a status quo that can be profoundly oppressive to disabled people. I believe that, as rehabilitation professionals, we need the courage to confront and acknowledge our critics, a sincere resolve to challenge professional privilege and a commitment to 'speak truth to power' (Said 1996 p 102). Indeed, I believe that the nature and context of our work demands precisely this degree of critical self-reflection. After all, the rehabilitation professions ostensibly exist to benefit rehabilitation clients, not to make us, the rehabilitation professionals, feel good about ourselves.

Far from extolling the virtues of rehabilitation services as a whole, or specific therapists in particular, the disability literature – almost without exception – describes rehabilitation services that are oppressive (e.g. Northway 1997), irrelevant (e.g. Johnson 1993), decontextualized (e.g. French 2004b), dehumanizing (e.g. French 1994d) and that reinforce status differences and powerlessness (Abberley 1995, Corring & Cook 1999, Dalley 1999). In turn, therapists are described as being pessimistic and negative (Cant 1997, Corring & Cook 1999), controlling (Kemp 2002), unaware of the realities of living with an impairment (Hammell 1995), indifferent to clients as human beings and untrustworthy (Corring & Cook 1999), slavish adherents to procedural 'red tape' (Finkelstein 2004) and as striving to dictate clients' lifestyles (Kemp 2002). Regrettably, those disabled people who have managed to accomplish their goals claim to have done so 'in the teeth of opposition from professionals' (Campbell & Oliver 1996 p 187); 'in spite of, rather than because of, the involvement of social workers and other "caring" professionals' (Priestley 1999, p 73). This is discouraging.

POWER AND THE PROFESSIONS

Ideologies of professionalism justify, legitimate and privilege professional knowledge and authority in ways that assert the domination of professionals and reinforce their power. Rehabilitation professionals, with their ideology of "normality," their claim to "expert" status and their pretence of objectivity are perceived to contribute to the oppression experienced by disabled people (French & Swain 2001). Indeed, disability professionals are perceived to be involved in just two endeavours: the pursuit of professional self-interest, and the maintenance of the status quo in their role as agents of the State (French & Swain 2001) (i.e. the economic and political élite [Illich 1976]).

Such critiques prompted Coleridge (1993 p 75) to ponder: 'professional rehabilitation therapists are generally well-meaning and committed people: they are not blatant agents of social control, and do not sign up for their jobs with the intent to oppress disabled people. So what has gone wrong?' In attempting to answer his own question, Coleridge suggested that therapists are unwitting cogs in an oppressive system: a system in which professionals see themselves as "experts" (an élitist concept that was deconstructed in Chapter 1); and a system in which they 'relate to disabled people from a position of power and dominance, not equality' (p 75). Fundamentally, however, this is a system which rehabilitation practitioners have largely failed to challenge because they are the beneficiaries of a status quo that accords them social status, prestige and power over those who must use their services.

In a stated attempt to dismantle their disempowering, hierarchical relationships with clients, the rehabilitation professions have long claimed an allegiance to client-centred practice (e.g. CAOT 1983, COT 2000, Chartered Society of Physiotherapy (CSP) 1996). However, little evidence exists – in the biographical accounts of former clients, in client-centred research or in the analyses of disability theorists – to suggest that this espoused philosophy has manifested itself widely in professional rehabilitation practice.

As long ago as 1990, Jongbloed & Crichton (1990a) observed that the rehabilitation professionals had an inauspicious record in the struggle to change social policies that might benefit disabled people, tending to reserve advocacy in the political and institutional arenas for issues pertaining to their own professional self-interests. Little has changed. Schriner (2001) notes that professionals are more likely to engage in political dialogues to protect their own turf than to advocate for fundamental changes that would benefit disabled people. The recent decision in North America and Australasia to require a bachelor's degree as the minimum entry to the educational programmes of the rehabilitation professions perfectly illustrates this point.

Those (primarily academics) who have advocated masters' degree entry programmes have claimed all manner of potential benefits for stakeholders, with 'stakeholders' being explicitly delineated as the 'profession' and 'students' (Allen et al 2001). This implies that *clients* are neither stakeholders nor likely beneficiaries of the professions' efforts to elevate their own prestige and status (Hammell 2002b) and is not an accidental oversight. Indeed, it reflects the professions' self-interest, desire for self-aggrandizement and efforts to entrench and reinforce power with little or no demonstrable benefit to clients. (In reality, little effort has been expended to ascertain the potential impact on clients). Client-centred practice, it seems, is all very well for clinicians but is not a philosophy to trouble decision-makers in the higher echelons of the rehabilitation professions. Indeed, Abbott (1994 p 304) has argued that a profession's claim to a 'unique' client-centred focus is part of a 'professionalizing strategy' to consolidate a professional identity, distance themselves from other care-givers and increase status.

Professional aspirations are not unproblematic. As Namsoo & Armstrong (1999 p 36) observe: 'professionalism may easily transform into the oppression of "expertise" through the colonization of knowledge'. Abbott (1994) described how an aspiration to 'élite' professional status has similarly led nurses to claim a 'unique', holistic approach to practice that enables active patient participation in care. Further, Abbott observed that nurses' claim to professional expertise and status is enhanced by having unqualified staff working under their direction. In light of these observations it is, perhaps, more than a coincidence that the growth of training programmes for rehabilitation assistants has occurred concurrently with the move to graduate-level entry programmes for rehabilitation professionals.

Aspiring to professional status has little to do with service excellence and everything to do with power. As French (1994d p 109) observed: 'professionals usually receive above-average pay, high status, and autonomy in their work. They have the power to control the encounter with their patients or clients; setting the agenda, managing time to suit their own schedules, defining problems and the appropriate solutions to them and making all the decisions'. Professional power is seductive and sometimes irresistible.

It is important to note that while the word 'professional' is deemed praiseworthy by some people (notably, professionals), for clients the observation that a therapist is 'just a professional' (French 2004b p 101) is used in a derogatory manner, denoting someone perceived to be cold, detached, 'neutral' and 'just doing her [sic] job' (French 2004b p 101).

It is easy for the healthcare professions to claim to be client-centred (indeed, the professions possess the power to make any claim they choose). This is both politically expedient and beneficial for the professions' public image. However, it is important to engage in a sceptical analysis of whether the professions 'walk the walk' or whether they just 'talk the talk' (to use a popular expression). If the rehabilitation professions' everyday practices, research practices, theories, education programmes, modes of service delivery and professionalizing strategies do not place clients' expressed needs at their centre, then they are not client-centred professions, despite assertions to the contrary. Townsend (1998) has argued that those professions, such as occupational therapy, that claim to be client-centred must actually *be* client-centred not just in their talk but in their actions and their everyday practices. This requires a challenge to the organization of power within our own professions and educational programmes, as well as in our work environments.

Although the professions choose to view and portray themselves as benevolent or p/maternalistic, Stalker & Jones (1998 p 174) suggest that the professions' real agenda might instead be the maintenance 'of power, prestige and the financial rewards associated with professional status'.

POWER AND COLONIZATION

The relationship between disabled people and professionals has been equated to that of colonized people and their colonizers, with the colonizers determining what services are in the best interests of those who are 'incapable' of determining this for themselves (Hirsch & Hirsch 1995). Rehabilitation professionals hold the power to determine 'desirable' goals for their disabled clients and to choose their preferred modes of service delivery: activities which serve to keep disabled people 'within the constraints of the inferior and dependent role' (Safilios-Rothschild 1981 p 6), like colonized peoples. Jorgensen (2000) noted that physiotherapists frequently believe they know what is best for their patients. The basis for this 'knowledge' is unclear but Jorgensen observed that those recipients of physiotherapy services who challenge this view are characterized as 'bad patients'.

Like colonized people, disabled people are often subjected to endless professional and bureaucratic interventions in their lives, ostensibly to administer to their needs (as these are defined by the professionals and bureaucrats). Like colonizers, the professions often seem preoccupied with justifying their privilege and status (Davis 1993).

Power and privilege: the selection and education of future professionals

Swain et al (2003) note that medical and rehabilitation education does not occur in a social vacuum but reflects existing relationships of power in society. Indeed, the more advanced a professional education programme becomes, the wider the social gulf between service providers and many of their clients. Davis (1993) has noted that disabled people are not permitted to define the sort of workers they want or need; rather, these choices are made by professionals in university departments. Thus the sort of qualities that disabled people value in their service providers, such as kindness, warmth, genuineness, empathy, openness, equality and a willingness to share power and work in partnership (French 2004b, Marquis & Jackson 2000, Reynolds 2004b) are trumped in the selection process by the qualities valued by the professions, notably academic and technical excellence and social conformity. Further, 'the rise of professionalism and attractive career paths for service workers may . . . attract workers into human services who have not internalised the value system necessary to operate with humanitarian principles' (Marquis & Jackson 2000 p 414).

Although surprisingly little effort has been expended to determine the attributes that rehabilitation clients value in their therapists, it is apparent that therapists' abilities to work in collaborative partnerships and to share power and control are valued more highly by clients than are practical and technical expertise (French 2004b, Marquis & Jackson 2000). Indeed, what clients appear to value most in their therapists is not their professional skills but a sense of being valued as a human being (Corring & Cook 1999, French 2004b).

Relinquishing power

Although the nursing and rehabilitation professions sometimes see themselves as 'allied' to medicine, Stone (1999 p 3) has argued that 'professionals should be allied to disabled people and the community, not allied to medicine or administration'. Some rehabilitation professionals are already committed to challenging the status quo and working alongside disabled people, not as prescribers and dictators but as partners and enablers (e.g. Rebeiro 2004, Silburn et al 1994). Visionaries within the rehabilitation professions advocate precisely this mode of practice. For example, Mary Law (1991 p 178) envisioned an approach to practice in which occupational therapists 'will give up power, acknowledge the political nature of our role and work together with clients and others to resolve environmental problems'. Similarly, Sally French, a physiotherapist, argued that 'to be truly effective health and welfare professionals must relinquish their power and control and work closely with disabled people under their direction' (French 1994d p 111).

It is noteworthy that both Law and French identified the first step towards practice excellence as *relinquishing power*. As Priestley (1999 p 158) observed: 'it is impossible to discuss user participation without reference to power. If providers are committed to increasing user power then they must contemplate a corresponding reduction of their own power'. A former rehabilitation client also claimed that therapists need to relinquish their power, but observed: 'there's an awful lot of people with a lot of vested interests' (French 2004a p 106). Sadly, there is little evidence to suggest that the ideology of client-centred practice has led therapists to relinquish power.

COLLABORATIVE PRACTICE

In Chapter 8 it was suggested that professional expertise is characterized by the ability to work in and with the whole context and situation of each client. Fook (2000 p 114) expands upon such exemplary practice: 'rather than entering situations with superior and fixed notions of desirable outcomes . . . practitioners engage in a mutual process of discovery with service users, in which, together they create and experience the conditions which assist the person . . . [Thus,] the traditional professional/service user hierarchy is upset. The professional does not use specialised knowledge or expertise to legitimate a powerful position, but rather to create a situation for mutual benefit'.

Finkelstein (1991 p 36) claimed that 'workers in rehabilitation services should see themselves as a resource, to be tapped by disabled clients, rather than as professionals trained to make highly specialized assessments of what is appropriate for individual disabled people'. The belief that professionals might usefully view themselves as a *resource* is shared by many commentators (e.g. Coleridge 1993, Finkelstein 1981). This does not mean that professionals' knowledge and skills are not valued. 'Quite the contrary: acting as a resource actually requires a higher degree of skill than treating someone who is merely an object in the process' (Coleridge 1993 p 78). Indeed, while applying standard treatment techniques to specific diagnostic categories requires rather rudimentary skills, the ability to meld one's knowledge, skills and experience to a client's unique needs is the hallmark of a true professional.

Once professionals see themselves as a resource rather than an "expert", 'they do not attempt to dominate, to take control or to *manage* disabled people, but rather to act as supportive enablers, actively sharing their expertise and knowledge while recognizing the expertise of disabled people and learning from them. Such a change of relationship requires a radical shift in the balance of power, making the traditional professional role untenable' (French 1994d p 115). Regrettably, many health professionals like to cling to their traditional role, seeing this 'as "allowing" disabled people to have a say in their treatment' (Hasler, cited in Khanna 2004 p 4); as if empowerment constitutes some sort of gift from the powerful to the powerless.

IDEOLOGY AND POWER

Oliver (1996a p 104) has argued that 'rehabilitation is the exercise of power by one group over another' and that 'the exercise of power involves the identification and pursuit of goals chosen by the powerful . . . these goals are shaped by an ideology of normality, which, like most ideologies, goes unrecognised, often by professionals and their victims alike'. Titchkosky (2003 p 37) also claims that the professions actively perpetuate and sponsor the cultural perception of disability as a lack of "normality", 'which, of course, requires professional remedy and thus leads to the self-perpetuation of the status and power of the helping professions'. Ideologies are integral to the perpetuation of power.

Pursuit of "normality" (see Chapter 2) informs those rehabilitation programmes that focus on teaching disabled people skills to function in a world created and maintained for the needs of others. In reflecting on her experience of rehabilitation, 'Kate' (cited in French 2004b) observed: 'what concerns me most of all is this focus on trying to make me "normal". I get that from all the therapists . . . I want them to say, "What sort of things would help you to lead a full life in the context of your impairment?"' (p 103).

It has been argued by Brechin (2000) that healthcare professionals are so much a part of the status quo that they inevitably play a part in the disadvantage and oppression of less powerful and minority groups. However, if disability professionals possess the power to support the status quo, they possess the power to challenge the status quo. Change is always possible and 'the questioning of dominant ideologies can be a starting point for changing power relations' (Swain 2004c p 86). Clearly, if the rehabilitation professions are seriously committed to reducing the oppression of disabled people then we need to be open to criticism, prepared to challenge existing hierarchical power structures, dominant ideologies and vested professional interests (Northway 1997). Client-centred practice is part of this endeavour.

CLIENT–CENTRED PRACTICE: CONTEXT

Consumers' criticisms of traditional modes of healthcare practice and their demands for services that are accountable, responsive to their needs and appropriate to their individual circumstances have prompted governments throughout the Western world to take a new 'consumer-orientated' approach to service delivery (Department of Health 1997, 1999, Neistadt 1995). Healthcare practitioners are exhorted to embrace active patient participation and partnership (NHS Executive 1999), facilitate greater patient choice (Department of Health 2000) and empower people to become key decision-makers in their own care (Chief Medical Officer 2001). Indeed, government policy on clinical governance in the UK *requires* user involvement in the planning and implementation of health services (Cusak & Sealey-Lapeš 2000). Accordingly, client-centred practice is required by the Codes of Ethics and Rules of Professional Conduct governing some of the healthcare professions, such as occupational therapy (COT 2000) and physiotherapy (CSP 1996). The CSP, for example, emphasizes the right of clients to a significant degree of involvement in all treatment decisions (Mead 2000).

These innovations have prompted the claim that 'rehabilitation is user and community centred, with an emphasis on the rights of individuals to make choices and control their own lives from a range of options' (NHS Executive 1997 p 7). However, research suggests that this claim should be regarded as a goal rather than a reality, with changes in rehabilitation practice lagging behind changes in political and professional rhetoric (e.g. Abberley 1995, Dalley 1999, Johnson 1993).

Nonetheless, the ethical and legal principle of informed consent (which arises from the right to autonomy, discussed in Chapter 8) requires at least a degree of shared decision-making between clients and service providers. Indeed, the Canadian and American governments currently endorse the principle of informed choice rather than mere consent (Charles et al 1997, Towle & Godolphin 1999), favouring active engagement over passive submission. This 'evidence-based patient choice' is an important model for client–provider interactions that has emerged from the intersection of two important contemporary healthcare initiatives: evidence-based medicine and patient-centred care (Ford et al 2003).

Client-centred practice is congruent with postmodern challenges: to traditional power hierarchies, to the exclusive authority of professional knowledge and to the de-legitimizing of the knowledge and experience of service users (Fook 2000).

Client-centred practice is sometimes portrayed as a mode of service provision to which the professions might aspire if and when they so choose. However, in a political context of government policies, professional standards and ethical imperatives it is apparent that 'the decision about whether to involve clients actively in their own care is no longer optional' (Hughes 2002 p 12). Client-centred practice is not an optional modus operandi. It is a requirement.

WHAT IS CLIENT–CENTRED PRACTICE? THE PROFESSIONS' PERSPECTIVES

Client-centred practice is said to be characterized by collaborative approaches to practice that encourage and respect clients' autonomy, and that support and advocate for clients' rights to make and enact choices

(Law et al 1995). Client-centred practice requires therapists to respect each client's values, work collaboratively towards the client's goals and assess the achievement of outcomes that matter to the client. Fundamentally, client-centred practice is concerned with a realignment of power and with ensuring that the rehabilitation process is useful and relevant to the client's life, values and priorities (CAOT 1997, Law et al 1995, MacDonald et al 2001).

Occupational therapists, who have discussed client-centred practice for over two decades, have defined this as practice that emanates from the client's perspective (CAOT 2000). It is therefore particularly ironic that although occupational therapists have debated and refined their own definitions of client-centred practice (e.g. CAOT 2000, Sumsion 2000), little effort has been expended in exploring the meaning of client-centred practice with clients. This exposes the unstable basis for the profession's claims to this philosophical orientation to practice (Hammell 2001b); a situation that is not unique to the occupational therapy profession.

WHAT IS CLIENT–CENTRED PRACTICE? CLIENTS' PERSPECTIVES

So, how do clients define client-centred practice? This is practice undertaken by therapists who clearly value clients and who seek and respect clients' experience and knowledge: therapists who choose closeness over distance and detachment, who demonstrate respect for clients, who create supportive and accepting relationships with clients, and who are kind (Bibyk et al 1999, Blank 2004, Corring 1999, French 2004b, Marquis & Jackson 2000, Rebeiro 2000). Indeed, client-centred practice appears to be more about the calibre of client–therapist relationships than it is about professional intervention. This is egalitarian practice undertaken by therapists who: strive to reduce power inequalities and to work in collaboration with their clients; understand the link between control and confidence and therefore strive to enable their clients to make choices and to be in control of their decisions and lives; are neither authoritarian nor judgemental; do not tell their clients what to do, and work on behalf of, for and with their clients towards those goals that are identified by, and of importance to, their clients (Bibyk et al 1999, Blank 2004, Corring 1999, French 2004b).

A consistent research finding is that clients view the interpersonal qualities of their therapists as being more important than their technical skills in that their interventions are responsive to the individuals rather than to their 'conditions' (French 2004b). Following their research among people who had strokes, Pound et al (1995) reported that the quality of interactions between patients and health professionals impacted the patients' self-esteem and enhanced their rehabilitation outcomes. Thus clients' preferences have evidence-based support.

The client–centred therapist: the evidence base

Research demonstrates that when people are treated as equals they feel involved in their rehabilitation; when they are respected, they feel inspired and motivated (Johnson 1993). When clients are actively involved in making decisions, have their perspectives and goals acknowledged and their questions answered they not only become more knowledgeable about their conditions but are more committed to participating in therapy, express more confidence in the competence of those providing care and greater satisfaction with the therapeutic process and outcome (Ford et al 2003, Ley 1988, Steele et al 1987). Indeed, understanding clients' perceptions and identifying their life goals has been found to offer 'an optimal condition for therapeutic success' (van Bennekom et al 1996 p 293).

Rehabilitation relationships that are characterized by respect, acceptance, trust, empathy and equality are found to contribute positively to clients' feelings of confidence, self-worth and self-esteem (Blank 2004, Marquis & Jackson 2000). Research also demonstrates that the opinions of healthcare professions are unreliable guides to the sort of working relationships their clients' prefer. For example, nurses have argued that clients in the community prefer their personal care to be undertaken by nurses rather than by workers who have less training and status. However, no evidence can be found to substantiate this claim (which can be seen as a machination for 'turf' and for professional power). On the contrary, clients express greater satisfaction with the service provided by those with less professional status, who are seen as friendly, approachable, helpful, flexible, warm and client-centred rather than cold, distant and hierarchical, like the professionals (Abbott 1994, Twigg 2000). These findings reflect those of many researchers, such as French (2004b p 102), who found that in comparison to professional occupational therapists, occupational therapy assistants were perceived by clients to be 'better', 'more aware of the person', 'more aware of relationships', more 'person-centred' and 'much more concerned about the person's needs'. (This has relevance to the earlier discussion about graduate-level entry and its potential impact on clients).

The dynamics of difference

Swain and French (2004 p 54) observed that 'to engage with questions of enabling relationships is to engage with questions of power, both between therapist and client, and within the social worlds of which both are a part'. Leavitt (1999c) has argued that a crucial component of competent rehabilitation practice is an awareness of the dynamics of difference: of how cultural assumptions, power differentials and the various social positions of people may affect communication between them. Differing social positions confer unequal access to resources and power and enable different life chances.

Because therapists' value systems are informed by their personal and cultural backgrounds, these will not necessarily be compatible with those of their clients, nor will their priorities, goals or visions of desirable rehabilitation outcomes. Sartre observed that values '"spring up around us like partridges" when we take a step in any direction' (Warnock 1970 p 99). Because values are shaped by a complex interaction of variables such as education, professional and employment status, material wealth, gender, "race", ethnicity, age, social class/caste, sexual orientation, [dis]ability and religion there will often be a poor match between the values of therapists and their clients (Hammell 2004i). While rehabilitation therapists reflect homogeneity on many of these variables, their clients are likely to be more diverse and thus unlikely to share their therapists' value systems. Indeed, an early study of women with spinal cord injuries found that their values and interests least resembled those of physiotherapists, occupational therapists, nurses, social workers and psychologists (Rohe & Athelstan 1982). This demonstrates the futility and irrelevance of interventions informed by therapists' values (Hammell 2004a).

It is important to recall not only that different perspectives exist, but that people have the right to hold different perspectives. Therapists do not possess the "correct" values or opinions, and interventions based on therapists' values are not only irrelevant but constitute an abuse of power.

On the record

Current concerns about accountability and liability have led to a preoccupation among rehabilitation workers with documentation: of assessments, intervention plans, outcomes, recommendations, incidents and so forth. Of particular concern to clients is the inclusion in these records of material *that has no bearing on the rehabilitation process*. As Cant (1997 p 301) recalled: 'you realize after a while that you need to exercise great care in what you say. Even casual "throw-away" remarks made in normal social interaction can end up "on record"'.

Clients identify the breech of trust that occurs when comments made during relaxed and informal conversations with therapists are recorded as part of the regulatory processes of the system, understandably viewing this as inconsistent with client-centred practice (Marquis & Jackson 2000).

TURNING CLIENT–CENTRED RHETORIC INTO REALITY

In light of a worldwide disability movement that affirms the rights of disabled people to make choices about their own lives, it is evident that moves towards collaborative service delivery are neither culturally-specific (Neufeldt 1999) nor represent a form of ethnocentrism or cultural imperialism in which Western values are foisted onto the rest of the world. Indeed, disabled people all over the world advocate for forms of service delivery that are consumer-controlled and demand an end to professional conflicts of interest (Neufeldt 1999).

Translating client-centred rhetoric into client-centred practice requires a transformation of the ways in which assessments, interventions and outcome measurements are undertaken and services are delivered. Because the activities of assessment, intervention and outcome measurement have been discussed in the previous chapter they will be addressed here only in regard to their fit with client-centred philosophy. The intersection of client-centred philosophy, theory and research will be the subject matter of the next chapter.

Assessment and intervention planning: informed choice

Within a client-centred modus operandi this is a process in which therapists enable clients to identify their problems, catalogue their skills and resources and prioritize their needs; and in which they provide sufficient breadth and depth of information to enable clients to establish relevant and achievable goals (Law et al 1995). This is the basis for informed choice (Chapter 8) and is a process that brings the meaning and context of the life disruption occasioned by impairment or illness into sharp focus, for both client and therapist, 'including the resources – physical as well as social, temporal as well as financial, medical as well as cultural – available to individuals and their families in the face of their adversity' (Williams 2000 p 43). Leavitt (1999d p x) suggested: 'it may be less important to teach a patient exercises than it is to understand what having an impairment or disability means to the patient'. Clearly, teaching patients exercises is *always* less important than understanding their needs and priorities.

Client-centred assessment requires client-focused tools (Dalley 1999) because 'the use of a set protocol of assessments and interventions for diagnostically defined types of clients is not supported within client-centred practice' (Law et al 1995 p 253). A therapist-centred approach to practice uses standardized forms of assessment to identify problems from within a specific and predetermined range of issues that are important to the therapist (Chapter 8). The opinion of the professional "expert" is privileged (Foster 2001) in a modus operandi that benefits the professions by reinforcing their professional dominance (Basnett 2001).

French (1994d) observed that professional dominance can be seen in those forms of assessment wherein therapists' perceptions are deemed "objective", while those of clients are viewed as "subjective". Privileging objectivity over subjectivity reflects a specific, pseudoscientific world view that has been challenged by critical theorists, antiracists and feminists, together with scholars from such diverse backgrounds as biology, medicine and sociology (see Chapter 8). Examples of client-centred forms of occupational therapy and physiotherapy assessment are provided by Law et al (1998) and Stratford et al (1995).

Intervention

This is the phase in which therapists maximize both their own skills and resources and those of the client in striving to achieve the goals the client has established (Law et al 1995). Central to the philosophy of client-centred practice is the right to take risks and to experience the negative outcomes that might result from specific choices. Of course, not every decision a client makes turns out to be an optimal decision. Indeed, some people appear to lurch through life making one poor choice after another (Wehmeyer 1998): a right that is not forfeited due to impairment. However, a client-centred mode of practice does not mean that therapists abandon their legal and ethical responsibilities for identifying and seeking to avoid harm. While adult clients have the same rights as other adults to pursue actions that place themselves at risk, therapists have the obligation to identify and examine risk, enabling clients to understand the implications of their decisions and to anticipate and deal with possible consequences (Hammell 2004a). Therapists can refuse to cooperate with clients' wishes if these are believed to be unethical or would constitute malpractice (e.g. CAOT 1997).

P/maternalism is an expression of power that negates clients' rights to risk and that seeks to restrict their rights to autonomy. This is not just unethical (see Chapter 8); research demonstrates that it is counterproductive (Cook 1981).

Locus of control

It is claimed that those people who believe they have both the ability and opportunity to control their lives have an 'internal locus of control'. Conversely, those who believe that their life circumstances are due to luck, fate, divine will or powerful people have an 'external locus of control' (Rotter 1966). Research has indicated that while people with an internal locus of control assume more responsibility for self-care and enlargement of their life opportunities, those with an external locus of control experience more distress following neurological injury and exhibit less adaptive behaviours (e.g. Frank & Elliott 1989). External expectancy of control is closely affiliated with learned helplessness (see Chapter 7): this is a learned expectation. Accordingly, research has demonstrated that internal control can be increased simply by providing information to clients about their own role and potential impact upon treatment outcomes (Johnston et al 1992).

People who have spinal cord injuries, strokes or multiple sclerosis have all identified a loss of autonomy and sense of being in control following injury or diagnosis (Becker 1993, Carpenter 1994, Toombs 1987). Toombs (1987) claimed that this perception of helplessness and dependency was exacerbated by having one's activities and plans determined by 'powerful others'. In light of these observations it is argued that a client-centred approach to assessment, intervention and decision-making may be intrinsically therapeutic, irrespective of the intervention that ensues (Hammell 1998a).

Motivation

Those behaviours traditionally viewed as characterizing 'good' patients – acquiescence, submission, cooperation, obedience, deference, compliance – are not those required to live successfully with an impairment. However, while assertiveness and self-directiveness *are* behaviours that enable people to live well with impairments (Gadacz 1994), rehabilitation professionals often perceive those disabled people who are assertive to be 'manipulative', preferring clients who are passive and grateful (French 1994d). Pollock (1993) noted that when clients are not permitted to define their own priorities the overwhelming sense of powerlessness and loss of self-determination may, in fact, appear as non-compliance. Indeed, 'non-compliance' might reflect a form of resistance: the exercise of power.

Abberley (2004) observed that therapists are quick to blame their clients for any problems encountered during the rehabilitation process. Blame is generally couched within specific professional discourses and pseudodiagnoses, such as denigrating clients as 'unmotivated'. Traditionally viewed as an inner drive, motivation is frequently equated with cooperation, with the implicit assumption that if clients are cooperating with their therapists' prescribed activities and objectives, they must be well-motivated. By default, those clients perceived to be uncooperative have often been subjected to pseudodiagnostic and derogatory labelling, such as 'unmotivated', 'non-compliant' or 'unrealistic' and have been referred for psychiatric assessment (Caplan & Shechter 1993, Steinglass et al 1982). Indeed, clients who choose not to work towards goals dictated by others are promptly discharged (Kemp 2002).

Researchers have demonstrated that people who are unmotivated to participate actively in their rehabilitation programmes are those for whom rehabilitation is offering no personally meaningful rewards for which they choose to work. Further, if clients have learned that their rehabilitation goals are determined by other, more powerful people they are less likely to strive towards attaining these goals. Indeed, motivational levels can be expected to be low if the 'change cost' – the amount of effort required to effect change – is disproportionate to the client's value of the potential outcome (Hammell 1998b, Jordan et al 1991). Low motivation is a reflection of low commitment to a seemingly irrelevant rehabilitation process; thus it is clearly incumbent upon rehabilitation professionals to focus their interventions on outcomes that matter to their clients.

Outcome measurement

A client-centred orientation to practice requires that rehabilitation outcome assessments reflect the values, priorities and goals of the client (see Chapter 8). However, there is little evidence to suggest that current outcome assessments address those issues that are important to clients, that assessments are undertaken at an appropriate time (i.e. *after* discharge) or that outcome measures developed from a user perspective are used to inform patterns of service delivery. The issue of *who* evaluates outcomes is rarely addressed, yet there are clear conflicts of interest when services are evaluated by those who also provide those services (Abberley 1995, and see Chapter 8).

Client–centred services: delivery and evaluation

Scullion (1999 p 540) observed that although interventions might be of a reasonable standard 'their manner of delivery may primarily serve the interests of institutions or staff'. Rehabilitation services have tended to be 'provider led' rather than 'consumer led', being 'based around pre-existing skills, techniques and facilities which are only available at specific times' (French 1994d p 108). By contrast, client-oriented service provision enables access to rehabilitation services in local areas when needs are identified and at times that suit clients (Hammell 1998b, Rebeiro 2004). This requires a new approach to working practices because rehabilitation therapists have traditionally worked only on weekdays, and then only during social hours.

Although working social hours might be viewed as a privilege (and congruent with professional power) it does not fit well with a philosophy of client centredness (Hammell 1995). Indeed, client-oriented service provision requires a dismantling of traditional hierarchies of power in which therapists dictate the hours and modes of service provision to suit their own convenience and lifestyles.

Recognizing that mental health systems work better for professionals than for the clients they are ostensibly created to help, Rebeiro (2004) engaged in participatory research with individuals diagnosed with severe mental illness, using qualitative methods to explore clients' perspectives of their needs. It was evident that service delivery can only be effective if it is addressing the problems perceived by service users and grounded in their experiences and perspectives. In collaboration with mental health service users, Rebeiro used the findings to inform new approaches to service delivery that assisted the clients to establish more satisfying lives in the community and also significantly reduced hospital re-admissions.

If clients are to be involved in planning services that are relevant to their lives and responsive to their needs then it is probably redundant to observe that they must also be centrally involved in evaluating the effectiveness of those services. However, although service users with a diversity of physical and mental health issues have successfully been involved in service evaluation, such involvement is rare (Salmon 2003). Thus Finkelstein (2004 p 209) spoke for many rehabilitation clients when he queried: 'where other than in the health and social welfare service could workers actually maintain so many illusions about the quality of the work they were providing?'

Client–centred practice: the evidence base

Research evidence derived from diverse client groups has demonstrated that a client-centred approach to health-service delivery leads both to improved client satisfaction and to improved outcomes, with time and resources maximized when attention is focused on those issues of greatest importance to the client/family (Law 1998, Towle & Godolphin 1999).

Research has demonstrated a link between shared decision making and positive client outcomes (Charles et al 1997) and has indicated that client–therapist collaborations on goal setting, and on intervention planning and implementation, result in better client outcomes, such as shorter hospital stays, reduced symptoms, reduced anxiety, greater sense of control and satisfaction, better goal attainment, greater adherence to treatment plans, and statistically and clinically significant gains in clients' abilities to perform or direct self-care and community living skills (Ford et al 2003, Guadagnoli & Ward 1998, Neistadt 1995, Towle & Godolphin 1999). Conversely, a treatment environment that overrides clients' goals and imposes goals valued by therapists results in ineffective rehabilitation (Cook 1981). Because research evidence supports client-centred service delivery, it can be claimed that client-centred practice is an evidence-based mode of practice (Hammell 2001b).

STRIVING FOR NON-DISABLING PROFESSIONALISM: THE ETHICAL DILEMMAS

Working in a client-centred mode of practice is both challenging and complex, due to two ethical issues: an unwillingness to relinquish professional power and a conflict of accountability.

'Professionalism' or equality?

'The process of giving more power/control to the client threatens the traditional view of the therapist as expert' (Law et al 1995 p 255). While the therapy professions have often been preoccupied with *gaining* the respect of others – notably the medical profession, administrators and the government – client-centred practice is a mode of practice that *accords* respect: to service users (Hammell 2004a). Observing that 'society has been constructed by able-bodied people in ways which serve and perpetuate their own interests', Davis (1993 p 199) observed that disability professionals are preoccupied not with a struggle for social change or equalizing opportunities for disabled people but with enhancing their own career opportunities and power.

This chapter has demonstrated that professional power can be reinforced in every activity in which professionals engage: education, research, assessment, intervention, outcome measurement and the manner in which services are delivered and evaluated. Illich (1977) claimed that healthcare professionals have misappropriated and monopolized knowledge, disregarded social injustice and mystified their expertise. More recently, Rossiter (2000) argued that there are profound ethical questions surrounding the contradictions between 'professionalism' and commitments to social equality. These are not the sort of ethical questions with which the rehabilitation professions have elected to wrestle. Indeed, Rossiter et al (2000) claim that 'professional ethics' has traditionally been an innocent endeavour, untroubled by attempts to discern the ways in which the professions exert and perpetuate their power, or by examination of whether professional practices and discourses are consistent with social justice. Small wonder, perhaps, that the rehabilitation professions' espoused commitment to client-centredness is regarded by critics as a rhetorical device (McKnight 1981).

Conflicting accountability

Therapists claim that their client-centred intentions are difficult to sustain within those hierarchical, restrictive and policy-bound environments in which they have chosen to work (e.g. Townsend 1998). From his observations of occupational therapy, Abberley (2004 p 242) noted that 'failure [of intervention], in so far as it is acknowledged, tends to be attributed to forces beyond the therapist's control. These fall into three categories: lack of financial resources, "the system" and . . . the client'.

The rehabilitation professions have given little attention to the practical and ethical implications of serving two "masters" – the system in which they are employed, and their clients – yet this is an area of profound conflict of interest. Stalker & Jones (1998 p 182) have observed that rehabilitation professionals such as occupational therapists 'act as "agents of the state" (or insurance companies), i.e. employed within and accountable to bureaucratic organizations'. While undoubtedly true, this is incompatible with professional discourses of accountability to clients. It is also perverse. Politicians, policy makers, bureaucrats and administrators are mere intermediaries between those who fund social and healthcare services (tax payers who are past, present and potential service users) and present service users. Unresolved, however, this conflict of interest profoundly diminishes the possibility of attaining even a semblance of client-centred practice. Private practices, by offering restricted services to specific people, constitute an additional dilemma, being incompatible with the fundamental ethical principles of both beneficence and justice (see Chapter 8) and also with the rehabilitation professions' duty to ensure equity of service provision (e.g. COT 2000). For example, in South Africa, 80% of physiotherapists work in the private sector, serving 20% of the population: the privileged élite (Cornielje & Ferrinho 1999).

If the rehabilitation professions are seriously committed to translating client-centred rhetoric into client-centred practice, all these ethical dilemmas will require sustained debate.

This chapter has explored the ideology of client-centred practice and has exposed some of the ethical issues that arise from various professionalizing strategies. Clients and therapists both require a significant quantity of quality information with which to inform their decisions and it is client-centred research that the next chapter needs to address.

Chapter 10

Researching disability and rehabilitation

Much research on disability has contributed little or nothing to improving the quality of life of disabled people, though it might have substantially improved the career prospects of the researchers.
(Oliver 1987 p 10)

INTRODUCTION: RESEARCHING DISABILITY AND REHABILITATION

The need for rehabilitation interventions to be 'evidence based', and the requirement for therapy students to undertake research projects, has led to a flurry of research activity within the rehabilitation professions. However, although much attention has been focused on research methods, little appears to have been given to the politics of research. Perhaps even more perturbing, rehabilitation researchers have rarely engaged with the substantial body of scholarly criticism that challenges their work. Although researchers are not obliged to agree with these critiques, intellectual integrity does require them to acknowledge an awareness of the arguments and to frame some sort of informed response.

This chapter seeks to apply client-centred philosophy to research and the development of knowledge and theory by drawing upon critiques articulated by postcolonial, feminist and disability theorists. It builds on the work of these theorists to propose a *disability methodology* that incorporates an engaged and committed dedication to countering inequalities of power, congruent with the widely touted client-centred orientation to practice.

METHODOLOGY AND METHODS

It should be noted that the terms 'methods' and 'methodology' are not synonymous. A methodology is a specific philosophical and ethical approach to developing knowledge; a theory of how research should, or ought, to proceed given the nature of the issue it seeks to address, and an analytic approach to the political issues involved in the research process. Thus, a methodology incorporates and reflects the values that underpin research. Research methods are the actual techniques, tools and strategies employed to acquire knowledge and manipulate data, congruent with the chosen methodology (Harding 1987, Maynard 1994, Stubbs 1999). Skeggs (1995 p 2) advises that 'a methodology is a theory of methods which informs decisions about such things as what to study, how to analyse, which theories to use, how to interpret, how to write'.

Thus, 'different research methods are not simply different *ways of doing*, they also represent different *ways of seeing* and *ways of thinking*' (Sidell 1993 p 108). This chapter is concerned with issues of methodology.

REHABILITATION RESEARCH: THE CLIENT–CENTRED IMPERATIVE

Critics claim that researchers of all methodological persuasions have consistently misunderstood and distorted both the phenomenon of disability and the experiences of disabled people. However, Oliver (1992) noted that because similar criticisms are made by black people, minority women and by rural poor people in the majority ("third") world it is apparent that the problem of researching disadvantaged people is somehow inherent in the research process itself and is not unique to disability research. Oliver (1992 p 102) claims it is only by addressing the 'social relations of research' that research can become more useful and relevant. Once again, this concerns power.

A change in the social relations of research can be achieved by dismantling hierarchical research relationships that accord researchers an élite role; by validating the experience and knowledge of *both* the researcher and the researched; and by enabling ill, injured, impaired and disabled people to decide what topics should be researched and how research should be undertaken and the findings publicized. In short, for disability research to become more authentic, relevant and useful it must adhere to a more client-centred format.

Chapter 9 demonstrated that the rehabilitation professions claim a client-centred approach to their work and that this philosophy of practice is now an ethical requirement for rehabilitation practice. It is also a legal requirement. Legislation in countries such as Australia, Canada, the UK and USA requires service providers to ensure that clients have direct input into the planning, development and evaluation of services (Clark et al 1993, Twible 1992), i.e. they must be involved in research. It is self-evident that the research that informs client-centred practice should reflect a client-centred orientation. 'Clearly, the philosophy underpinning the development of the evidence base destined to provide guidelines for practice should be ethically consistent with the espoused practice philosophy' (Hammell 2001b p 229). It should also be recalled that client-centred practice is not a fad but an evidence-based mode of practice (Chapter 9).

The rehabilitation professions recognize that research ought to reflect client-centred rhetoric. For example, the British Occupational Therapists' Research and Development Strategic Vision and Action Plan (Ilott & White 2001) states clearly: 'researchers are . . . expected to act collaboratively, involving consumers at all levels and stages of the research process' (p 270); and 'research and evidence-based practice is expected to incorporate a user perspective; this means involving consumers and carers throughout the research process and as partners in quality-enhancement initiatives' (p 275). In light of these legal, ethical and professional expectations it is important to ascertain whether rehabilitation research consistently reflects a client-centred orientation.

EXPLORING THE CONGRUENCE BETWEEN CLIENT–CENTRED PHILOSOPHY AND RESEARCH

Disability theorists contend that although there is no shortage of research 'on' disabled people, this is usually completely divorced from their everyday experiences (Oliver 1990), with very little research contributing to changing the conditions of their lives (Zarb 1992). They contend that this is an inevitable consequence of the inequitable relationships of power between those who research and those who are researched (Oliver 1992).

Disabled theorists observe that irrespective of whether researchers employ qualitative or quantitative methods, 'the power of the researcher-as-expert is enshrined in their control over the design, implementation, analysis and dissemination of research findings' (Barnes et al 1999 p 217). This reality sits uncomfortably with a client-centred philosophy and contributes to the disempowerment of research participants. For example, disabled people have complained of being exploited by the research process, 'their knowledge and experiences "mined" by the researcher(s), who were then never heard of again' (Kitchin 2000 p 33). Often they receive no feedback from researchers and are unable to discover what conclusions and recommendations arise and what actions will be undertaken in light of the study findings (Kitchin 2000). Far from being included as respected partners in the research process, disabled people are often 'merely the lubrication of someone else's research agenda' (Stubbs 1999 p 276). Oliver (1992) called this the 'rape' model of research.

Researchers often like to speculate that their research subjects value the research experience and find it somehow empowering, cathartic and meaningful (e.g. Patai 1991, Wolf 1996). Empirical investigation challenges this assumption, demonstrating that the research process can be disempowering and the absence of tangible results can provoke anger and frustration (Barnitt & Partridge 1999, Brannen 1993). Indeed, although research can lead to the achievement of a respectable academic thesis or paper, the work might make 'absolutely no positive, but plenty of negative, difference to those whose interests it claims to have at heart' (Moore et al 1998 p 20).

Disability theorists have argued that when "experts" undertake research with powerless 'subjects' the research relationship will remain the same, irrespective of whether the chosen methodology is quantitative or qualitative (Oliver 1992, Ward & Flynn 1994). (Indeed, by definition, a *'subject'* is a subordinate, a person of lower power and lower value, one who is under the control of another, Chambers 1972). Despite the 'liberal trappings of the qualitative paradigm' (Ward & Flynn 1994, p 31), qualitative methods do not inevitably ensure respect or egalitarianism, but can support the status quo just as effectively as traditional, quantitative studies (Lawson 1995, Matysiak 2001). Thus 'a well crafted quantitative study may be more useful to policy makers and cause less harm [to the study group] than a poorly crafted qualitative one' (Fonow & Cook 1991 p 8).

Thomas (1999 p 152) observed: 'in the way it has been conceived, organized and conducted, as well as in the nature and use of results, traditional disability research in medicine, rehabilitation, psychology, sociology and social policy has been carried out by representatives of professional groups with little or no consultation with, or involvement of, disabled people themselves (other than as research subjects)'. It is argued that the consequence of much of this research has been 'not just to alienate disabled people but to positively reinforce disablism in society' (Thomas 1999 p 152). This is a poor foundation with which to inform client-centred practice or client-oriented professional theories.

EXPLORING THE INTERSECTION BETWEEN CLIENT-CENTRED PHILOSOPHY AND THE DEVELOPMENT OF REHABILITATION THEORY

'All health care and research are influenced by theories' (Oliver 1998 p 1446). *Theories* are systems of explanatory principles that inform professional actions. Evidence-based practice promotes the importance of establishing interventions that are informed by dependable theory. Claims to dependability require that theories are firmly grounded in research evidence (Hammell 2004b). Claims to client-centred philosophy require, in turn, that this research reflects clients' priorities and perspectives. This raises some important issues.

Are rehabilitation interventions always informed by dependable theory? Researchers who have examined rehabilitation practice report that approaches to intervention often appear to be devoid of a theoretical basis and that when therapists do lay claim to a governing theory, this theory, itself, is found to be devoid of a supporting evidence-base (e.g. Davidson & Waters 2000, Walker et al 2000). There is, in short, a theory–practice gap (Carpenter 2004a).

If theory informs practice (as it should), then theory should be grounded in research evidence that is informed by clients' priorities and perspectives. Is it? Occupation is central to the conceptual foundation of occupational therapy, yet despite the profession's declared allegiance to client-centredness there has been little effort to include the perspectives of diverse client groups in the development of theories of occupation. It should therefore not be surprising that recent efforts to enable a client-centred approach to theory building (e.g. Hammell 2004b, Law 2004, Suto 2004) have exposed the normative and ableist assumptions that underlie existing professional theory. Similar efforts by the physiotherapy profession are still pending. Indeed, while many clinicians have embraced client-centred practice, those professionals centrally concerned with building knowledge – academics and researchers – have been slow to loosen their grasp on power.

POWER/KNOWLEDGE

Critics contend that research and the production of knowledge are not neutral activities but are located within contexts of power. Brechin & Sidell (2000 p 20) observed: 'knowledge and the development of knowledge is not value-free. Research is a powerful and power generating tool'. The French philosopher Michel Foucault explored the dynamic of knowledge and power, claiming that knowledge 'is linked in a circular relation with systems of power which produce and sustain it' (Foucault 1980 p 133).

Negating the possibility of objectivity and detachment, Foucault (1980 p 132) proposed that 'the intellectual is not the "bearer of universal values"' but a person occupying a specific position relative to power. This is relevant to research and the process of generating knowledge, because 'no one has ever devised a method for detaching the scholar from the circumstances of life, from the fact of his [sic] involvement (conscious or unconscious) with a class, a set of beliefs, a social position, or from the mere activity of being a member of society' (Said 1979 p 10). As Griffin & Phoenix (1994 p 288) pointed out, 'research is never value-free or apolitical. We can claim to be distanced, objective observers, but this simply obscures the potential impact of our own theoretical and political preferences, the role of our own career strategies, and the wider context in which research is funded and resourced'.

Chapter 8 alluded to the epistemological debates that have 'shattered the traditional picture of science as neutral, disinterested, and value free' (Riger

1992 p 737), demonstrating that research is not a neutral, objective undertaking but, instead, an exercise of power: a political act. Thus Mohanty (1994 p 197) observed: 'scholarly practices exist within relations of power– relations which they counter, redefine or even implicitly support. There can, of course, be no apolitical scholarship' (p 197). Mohanty draws attention to the reality that research is not a depoliticized process but one implicitly located within contexts of power.

Neither is research, by definition, a humanistic, altruistic endeavour. Rather, it is an activity with rich rewards for its protagonists, being a commodity by which students attain degrees and professional accreditations, and academics accumulate papers, books and conference presentations, thereby achieving peer recognition, promotion, research grants and tenure (Hall 1992, Hammell 2000b). Thus, Oliver (1997 p 27) referred to the 'inescapable fact' that researchers, like himself, 'are the main beneficiaries of our own research activities'.

Rehabilitation researchers have not generally engaged with philosophical debates about power nor subjected their research to a great deal of critical analysis, beyond simplistic and out-dated arguments about the relative merits of quantitative and qualitative methods. Indeed, rehabilitation researchers' good intentions appear to have been so taken for granted that little attention has been given to the nature of their work. However, because many theorists and researchers *have* engaged in critical reflection, rehabilitation researchers have an opportunity – and obligation – to draw from their insights.

POWER AND PARTICIPATION

'All research has the potential to exploit and oppress participants if attention is not paid to the power imbalances between researchers and research participants' (French et al 2001 p 244). Indeed, the asymmetrical relationship between researchers and researched is cited as a major reason for the alienation of disabled people from research (Barnes & Mercer 2004).

The work of postcolonial, feminist and disability theorists has contributed critical insights into the research process, raising concerns about power, and highlighting the need for constant self-criticism, especially among those who undertake research with marginalized groups. It is no coincidence that these particular theorists, for whom oppression is a central domain of concern, have been especially influential in reassessing research paradigms and methods. 'Researchers in these areas are acutely aware of the potential for research to constitute an oppressive practice, or to contribute to oppressive social structures and processes' (Thomas 1999 p 153). The following sections outline the contributions of theorists who advocate collaborative, non-hierarchical research relationships that are congruent with the rehabilitation professions' espoused client-centred orientation.

Postcolonial theorists

Originating in critiques of colonialism – wherein the powerless are controlled, defined, described and represented by the powerful – postcolonial theory is associated, philosophically, with postmodernism and poststructuralism while retaining a political edge: highlighting power and disempowerment (Selden & Widdowson 1993). While postmodernism is detached, postcolonialism engages with political imperatives (Ashcroft & Ahluwalia 1999). Although postmodernists usefully critique dogma, challenge authoritarian assumptions, contest ideologies of normality and recognize the possibility of multiple viewpoints (Cheek 2000) they have been criticized by some disability theorists for undermining the foundation of social justice through their assault on universal values (Watson 2004) and for celebrating difference and diversity while having no committed vision of how things could, or ought, to be (Oliver & Barnes 1998). As Linton (1998) observed, speaking about diversity can be a comfortable substitute for speaking about equality and oppression.

Primarily a product of literary criticism, *postcolonial theory* is concerned with empowerment of the dispossessed; the establishment of minorities' rights; and achieving just and equitable relationships among people. It challenges privilege and power, critiques domination and control, resists all forms of exploitation and oppression and encourages cross-cultural dialogue (Said 1979, Young 2003). Postcolonial theorists examine how marginalized and disempowered people (those considered "inferior" on the basis of normative judgements about physical appearance, colour, behaviour, physical ability, etc) are represented by those in more powerful positions; hence their relevance for disability research.

When a research issue is defined by the researcher, the research process is controlled by the researcher and the findings are analyzed and disseminated according to the researcher's perspectives and priorities, this is a *colonial* methodology (Ryen 2000): inherently inequitable. Edward Said pondered how marginalized people might instead be studied from a non-repressive and non-manipulative perspective, proposing that 'one would have to rethink the whole complex problem of knowledge and power' (Said 1979 p 24). This would require a *post*colonial methodology.

Postcolonial critics draw attention to the reality that certain opinions are usually granted authority, like researchers', and others are always spoken for, like research subjects (hooks 1990, Mann 1995). For example, university students and academics are authorized/authorize themselves to engage in research and to use their findings to generate theories. This is not unproblematic. Alcoff (1991 p 7) observed: 'we are authorized by virtue of our academic positions to develop theories that express and encompass the ideas, needs, and goals of others. However, we must begin to ask ourselves whether this is a legitimate authority'. Accordingly, Childs & Williams (1997 p 89) called for an awareness, not only of 'who speaks, from where, and for whom' but also of whose knowledge is discounted, suppressed or unacknowledged. It is this knowledge – of marginalized and subordinated people – that postcolonial researchers seek to privilege.

In contrast, *theoretical imperialism* is said to occur when researchers (i.e. those wielding more power) frame the experiences of their 'subjects' within their own perspectives, privileging their own interpretations over those of the researched (Mann 1995). Theoretical imperialism is a reflection of specific relations of power/knowledge. Therefore, to assess research from a postcolonial perspective is to ask what knowledge has been produced, under what conditions, about whom and for whom (Mohanty 1994); and in what ways the knowledge produced is returned to the community from which the research participants are drawn (Patai 1991). Feminist theorists have asked similar questions.

Feminist theorists

Feminist theories are centrally concerned with inequalities of power. Originally focusing solely on an ideological dualism of genders, feminist theorists have more recently sought to probe inequalities constructed on the basis of age, "race", sexual orientation, class, economics, ability/disability and First/Third world citizenship (Sherwin 2002); hence their relevance for disability research. Because of this preoccupation with power, it is claimed that the central dilemma for contemporary feminists engaged in research 'is power and the unequal hierarchies or levels of control that are often maintained, perpetuated, created and re-created during and after field research' (Wolf 1996 p 2).

Feminists claim that all knowledge is 'situated': that it is imprinted by the time, context and social 'positionings' of its creators (Haraway 1988, Thomas 1999). In an attempt to contest inequalities of power, feminist theorists have sought to expose the role of various positions within the research relationship and their impact on knowledge creation. It has already been noted that 'positioning' refers to the gender, class, "race", sexual orientation, age, religion, (dis)ability, language, nationality, citizenship status, education, professional status, economics and other dimensions of differentiation associated with different distributions of power between the researcher and the researched. (In non-Western societies, positioning and status might be dependent on other variables, such as marital status and reproductive success.) The researcher's positioning cannot be left unexamined for to do so suggests that it is possible for knowledge production to be value free, neutral and objective: a suggestion that feminist theorists do not support (see Chapter 8).

Feminists contend, however, that positioning is not just about one's biography but also about one's chosen philosophical, political and theoretical position: the standpoint from which one works (Kelly et al 1992). Their argument – that researchers must *take* a position – is supported by those disability researchers who contend that researchers must choose to align themselves with disabled people rather than the status quo. For example, Barnes (1996c p 110) argues: 'researchers should be espousing commitment not value freedom, engagement not objectivity . . . there is no independent haven or middle ground'.

Further, feminist theorists claim that researchers should seek to engage in non-exploitive research relationships that are characterized by reciprocity, cooperation and collaboration; striving to minimize power imbalances in the relationships between researcher/researched, and between data/theory (Oakley 1981, Punch 1994). Clearly, this stance is congruent with the fundamental principles of client-centred practice.

Although articulated in different ways by different theorists, feminist research methodology has certain defining principles:

- Participants' lives are studied using their own priorities and perspectives.
- The research uses methods that are not oppressive and do not reproduce hierarchies of power.
- The research contributes to the interests of marginalized people through producing knowledge that can be used by the people themselves.
- The research utilizes a critical perspective that questions dominant intellectual traditions, examines the role of the researcher's positioning and is reflexive about its own assumptions and development (e.g. Acker et al 1991, Bhopal 2000, Cancian 1992, Kirsch 1999).

These principles are echoed and expanded by a rising tide of disability theorists.

Disability theorists

Like postcolonial and feminist theorists, disability theorists have critiqued the power imbalances between those who research and those who are researched. They bemoan the quality of much disability research, the theoretical models used, the questions posed, the vocabulary used, the modes of analysis, the absence of tangible results and the propensity to ethical abuse (e.g. Barnartt & Altan 2001). In a blistering attack, for example, Oliver (1992) claimed that disabled people have come to see research as a violation of their experience and as irrelevant to their needs; in fact, 'nothing more than a "rip-off"' (Oliver 1997 p 15). Similarly, Pfeiffer (2001 p 45) has claimed that 'most of the research done on people with disabilities in public health, medicine and rehabilitation is worthless'. Barnes et al (1999 p 217) are also critical of much research into disability, noting that many researchers 'move between research fields like "academic tourists", using disability as a means of advancing their own status and careers'.

Hunt (1981) referred to those researchers who further their own professional and academic interests while ignoring the priorities of the disabled people they study as 'parasites'. Disability theorists have proposed that in order to avoid 'parasitic' research, researchers must give up the pursuit of 'objectivity' and engage with the thoughts, actions and structures that oppress disabled people (Oliver 1999). Further, they must challenge traditional hierarchies of power, striving for partnerships in the research process, and respecting and valuing the expertise of disabled people. Most importantly, any research undertaken should be of practical benefit and relevance to disabled people (Stone & Priestley 1996, White 2002).

Observing that 'most research' among disabled people is 'at best irrelevant, and at worst, oppressive' (Oliver 1996a p 139), a few, predominantly disabled researchers have explored alternative modes of research that have a more 'emancipatory', participatory or *action orientation*.

Action orientation

Punch (1994) noted that several contemporary impulses advocate participant input into the research process, notably feminist scholarship (outlined above), action orientation and institutional concerns (outlined below).

Action research has been defined in many ways by many researchers. Fundamentally, it is concerned both with solving concrete problems in real situations ('action') and with trying to further knowledge ('research'), particularly among marginalized people (Robson 1993). An action orientation to research insists that the interests of participants must be taken into account at every phase of the research process. Research participants are understood to be 'stakeholders' in action research; thus, action orientated research is described as being 'humanizing', enabling marginalized people to speak for themselves and empowering them to initiate positive changes (Bogdan & Biklen 1992).

Fonow & Cook (1991 p 5) claimed that an action approach to research 'is reflected in the purpose, topic selection, theoretical orientation, choice of method, view of human nature, and definitions of the researcher's roles'. Recognizing that because it occurs within contexts of power, research always has political consequences, action research demands interrogation of the purpose or outcome of research: Whose agenda dictated the research issue? Who will benefit from the research? How will changes occur?

One of the most sustained criticisms of academic research is that many researchers fail to advocate and work for change, apparently hoping instead that other people will read their research report and act on it (Kitchen 2000). An action orientation to research is committed to working towards positive change and ensuring that research findings are translated into real results. Robson (1993) notes that an action orientation constitutes the embodiment of democratic principles in research and it is thus clearly consistent with the philosophy of client-centred practice.

Institutional concern for human rights

The final impetus for participatory modes of research to be explored here arises from an institutional concern for the protection of human rights (Punch 1994). This concerns ethics.

Rehabilitation researchers and students will all be familiar with both the formal process of ethical review required by universities and health administrations and the imperative for informed consent that seeks to protect human rights. This concern for human rights requires researchers to be explicit about the purpose and agenda of research when attaining 'informed consent', such that participants' rights to privacy, confidentiality and protection from deceit and harm are protected (Carpenter & Hammell 2000). Researchers have a duty and moral obligation to make clear the real purpose of the research to those who are asked to participate. 'Informed consent' has not occurred if potential participants have not been fully apprised of the nature and intent of the study.

However, ethical obligations go beyond these routine concerns for consent, confidentiality and respect for participants' rights. Robson (1993) claimed that an action orientation towards research demands a commitment to genuine participation in the research process such that research is a collaborative effort. This same conclusion has been reached by the postcolonial, feminist and disability theorists outlined above, who collectively advocate a new understanding of the concept of accountability in research.

Accountability

Disability theorists contend that 'there should be meaningful input by research subjects, at all stages of the investigation process, including adequate monitoring and accountability' (Barnes et al 1999 p 217). In light of the power imbalance within the research relationship, some also propose that: 'disability research should be judged solely in terms of whether it has contributed to the process of enabling disabled people to empower themselves' (Barnes et al 1999 p 219). This resonates with the philosophy that informs client-centred practice – 'essentially, client-centred practice re-defines and shifts power' (CAOT 2000 p 50) – but is not consistently reflected in rehabilitation research.

As members of a profession and as employees we are required to be accountable to our profession and to our employers. However, in critically examining the purpose and likely beneficiaries of our research a client-centred orientation requires that we strive also for accountability to research participants and the population from which they are drawn. This is most likely to be achieved when researchers and disabled people are engaged in collaborative research practice.

People with impairments require relevant information in order to make truly informed choices about their rehabilitation interventions, including open discussion about alternatives, existing gaps in knowledge and areas of uncertainty (Mead 1998, Needham & Oliver 1998). Clearly, both clients and therapists need access to relevant research evidence. Indeed, Needham & Oliver (1998 p 89) note that because of access to the internet 'health professionals will find themselves dealing with an increasingly informed public and this will contribute to the pressure for them to keep abreast of emerging evidence'.

EVIDENCE-BASED PRACTICE

'Government policy and professional guidance insist that professional practice should be "evidence-based"' (Gomm & Davies 2000 p x). *Evidence-based practice* is currently one of the most influential concepts in rehabilitation (Law 2002), being claimed to enhance client outcomes, provide consistency and continuity, facilitate cost containment and financial accountability, and validate the role and efficacy of interventions (Law & Baum 1998, Von Zweck 1999). 'The argument for evidence-based practice is simple: If there is a better way to practice, therapists should find it' (Law 2002 p 5).

Evidence-based practice is frequently (mis)construed as 'the implementation of credible research in clinical practice' (Atwal 2002 p 335). This reflects an incomplete and simplistic understanding that mistakes *research utilization* for the more complex process of clinical reasoning that is intended by the term *evidence-based practice*. Clients have the right to expect their therapists to do more than select effective interventions based on empirical evidence, requiring instead that they use interventions that are appropriate to the needs of the client and consistent with the client's stated goals (Rogers & Holm 1994). Thus, professional practice entails far more than a wholesale application of research to practice because 'even "best" evidence can lead to bad practice if applied . . . uncritically' (Carpenter 2004a p 8).

Surprisingly, although 'evidence-based practice' and 'client-centred practice' are the two most influential paradigms in current healthcare practice (Ford et al 2003), these terms are rarely used by the same authors. Indeed, less than 2% of published papers concerning evidence-based practice also mention client-centred practice (Bensing 2000). However, evidence-based practice, properly administered, is not incompatible with client-centred practice (Law 2002).

Evidence-based practice evolved from the problem-based approach to learning medicine in which research findings are located and critically evaluated to aid rational decision-making (Carpenter 2004a). Sackett et al (2000) subsequently promoted the idea of a hierarchy of evidence that privileged randomized controlled trials (RCTs) as a sort of 'gold standard'. Thus 'best research evidence' has tended to be defined as the product of experimental, quantitative research (Carpenter 2004a). Inevitably, this has served to restrict the sort of questions it has been possible to ask and the sort of issues it has been possible to investigate (Hyde 2004).

Unfortunately, proponents of the evidence hierarchy have failed to acknowledge that RCTs are not value-free, objective measures but inevitably incorporate the values and beliefs of their developers (Pieters 1998). As Stubbs (1999 p 272) observed: 'statistics and data do not speak for themselves: they will always have an underpinning philosophy and interpretation which may or may not be overt'. Indeed, the claim that RCTs are 'objective' disguises the degree of interpretation involved in producing results (Ballinger & Wiles 2001). It is hardly surprising that interpretation of the findings from RCTs has led to opposing conclusions, or 'evidence' (Hyde 2004). Further, the evidence of RCTs can be 'misleading, reductionist, and irrelevant to the real issue' (Greenhalgh 1997 p 743). Most importantly, 'RCTs are *not* patient-centred' (Bensing 2000 p 19). Indeed, because much medical 'evidence' is statistical and derived from groups it can only be crudely applied to a specific patient.

Just because a certain hierarchy of evidence is privileged within medicine does not mean this same hierarchy has any relevance for rehabilitation therapists, whose concern with context and whose focus of inquiry are very different from that of medicine (Bithell 2000). Thus, Canada's Joint Position Statement on Evidence-based Occupational Therapy (Townsend & Rebeiro 2001 p 8) recommended that the profession should 'determine what kinds of evidence are appropriate for client-centred, occupation-focused occupational therapy'.

Writing in the *British Medical Journal*, Hodgkin (1996 p 1568) observed that 'an evidence-based approach will only work for as long as we all view medicine as "modern" – that is, as making statements about an objective, verifiable external reality. To the postmodernist the question is whose "evidence" is this anyway and whose interests does it promote?' Moreover, critics within medicine have challenged the exclusive emphasis sometimes given to research evidence and the apparent neglect of other forms of knowledge, such as clinical expertise and patients' priorities and values (e.g. Maynard 1997). It is now generally acknowledged that evidence-based practice depends not solely upon research results but upon 'the integration of *best research evidence* with *clinical expertise* and *patient values*' (Sackett et al 2000 p 1). However, the idea of clinical expertise was shown to be problematic in Chapter 1, with research evidence suggesting that therapists often equate expertise with 'patient miles' – the number of clients/patients treated over many years (Richardson 1999) – and further evidence suggesting that misperceptions of clients' problems by rehabilitation professionals may actually worsen with the length of clinical experience (e.g. Bodenhamer et al 1983, Ernst 1987). Indeed, it should be noted that 'experience' is not necessarily a positive term and is not a synonym for 'expertise'. The foundations for claims to 'expertise' must always be subjected to considerable scrutiny and scepticism.

Proponents of evidence-based practice recognize the importance of 'patient-centred clinical research' (Sackett et al 2000 p 1) and acknowledge that research evidence can, and indeed must, include greater methodological diversity, notably by including qualitative methods (Bithell 2000, Miller & Crabtree 2000, Pope & Mays 2000, Ritchie 2001, Townsend & Rebeiro 2001). Because 'the key to the evaluation of evidence rests on the ability of the method to answer the question asked' (Hyde 2004 p 92), the idea of a hierarchy of evidence is clearly unsupportable.

Writing in the *Journal of Clinical Epidemiology*, Holman (1993 p 35) observed that 'the almost sole recognition given to quantitative methods has trained [medical] students inadequately, established flawed standards of practice and research, and delayed the development of essential medical knowledge'. This is an important observation for physiotherapy researchers, given their profession's 'close alignment with medicine and enthusiastic commitment' to a positivist [i.e. quantitative] form of research inquiry (Carpenter 2004a p 2).

Basnett (2001) argued that while evidence-based practice has much to recommend it, the evidence-base itself is currently flawed because it has been developed from research undertaken without consideration of the outcomes that matter to disabled people. It is important to recall that clients require interventions that are not only effective but *appropriate to their needs and preferences* (Law & Baum 1998, emphasis added), if evidence-based practice is to achieve any degree of congruence with a client-centred ethic. Achieving this calibre of evidence requires modes of research that incorporate clients' views, values, priorities and preferences at every stage.

CHOICES

Research is not, by definition, valuable, meaningful, useful or relevant; thus Germon (1998 p 251) contends that if the work of researchers and academics is to be relevant, 'it has to be made relevant'. The research process is shaped by a series of choices. These choices, in turn, reflect the philosophy, ethics and values of the researcher. The following section briefly outlines some of the choices facing researchers from the inception of research to its dissemination.

Identifying a research issue

Who should set the agenda for research into disability and rehabilitation? How should research issues be identified? Disability theorists contend that 'the very idea that small groups of "experts" can get together and set a research agenda for disability is . . . fundamentally flawed' (Oliver 1992 p 102). Disabled people have criticized the way in which research agendas are usually determined, not by those who are the espoused beneficiaries of research, but by academics, clinicians and funding bodies (Barnes et al 1999). This is an expression of power, for as McKnight (1981 p 31) observed: 'there is no greater power than the right to define the question'.

In response to the imperative for 'consumer-orientated' approaches to service delivery (see Chapter 9), some major funding agencies invite disabled people to help identify issues that require research and actively involve them in reviewing grant applications to ensure the relevance of the research and the potential value of the anticipated outcomes (White et al 2001). Some agencies also insist that projects incorporate significant consumer involvement and demonstrate a clear potential to improve the lives of disabled people (Mercer 2004).

Responding to Canadian physiotherapists' frustration that little published research appeared relevant to clinical practice, Miles-Tapping et al (1990) undertook a study to determine physiotherapists' research priorities. Similar research was undertaken by Walker (1994) in the UK. There was significant agreement between the groups in the two countries, revealing shared concerns about the areas of research that clinicians believed required prompt attention by their profession. Adopting a more client-oriented approach, Weaver et al (2001) created a research agenda for people with spinal cord injury by drawing from the perspectives of people with spinal cord injuries, in addition to their healthcare professionals. However, such innovations are rare.

The participation rate in a study can be used as one method to gauge the relevance of the study to those it purports to be about. If a minority of potential participants agree to participate in a study this suggests that a minority of people perceived the research issue to be of sufficient importance or relevance to warrant their input.

Data collection, analysis and interpretation

A great deal of attention has been given to data collection tools, such as interviews, questionnaires and standardized assessments. Fundamentally, the choice of tools used to collect data reflects the priorities, values and assumptions of the researcher and determines the nature of the findings. For example, asking whether someone's impairment prevents them from going out as often as they would like will generate very different data from asking whether there are any transportation or access problems that prevent them from going out as often as they would like (Oliver 1992). Answers to the first question will catalogue individual 'flaws'; the second may generate an agenda for environmental intervention (Bochel & Bochel 1994). Involving participants in the choice of research tools ensures that the resulting data will reflect their priorities. Bonell (1999) notes that all human research – quantitative or qualitative – should flow from the participants' own accounts rather than being imposed by researchers' prior assumptions and categories.

All research data – whether qualitative, in the form of words, or quantitative, in the form of statistics – require interpretation. Without checking interpretations with study participants there is a danger of merely fitting data into existing theories with which we are comfortable (Borlund 1991). Frequently, the views of the researcher are presented as if they are definitive, with no reference to the participants' perspectives (Acker et al 1991, Stubbs 1999). The strategy of involving all or some of the participants in analysis ensures that the researcher has accurately translated the participants' perspectives and decreases the chances of misrepresentation, appropriation or stereotype (Opie 1992). The purpose of member-checking is not to achieve consensus. There may be conflicts between the researcher's interpretations and those of the participants. This is not unacceptable. The aim of incorporating the perspectives of participants or their peers 'is not necessarily to achieve consensus but to highlight the points of difference and the tensions between competing accounts as well as shared interpretations' (Opie 1992 p 63). An exchange of views reveals differences in perspective, enabling assumptions to be challenged and existing theories to be questioned (Ribbens & Edwards 1998). Harris (1996 p 154) suggested that if the researcher states clearly his or her personal location and says: 'this is what I think is going on, here are the contradictions and complexities, from my point of view it could mean this', there is room for recognition that each analysis is but one of several possibilities. As Stone (1997 p 224) contends: 'the point is to make sense of difference not distort or disregard it'.

Rather than seeking reasons *for* the inclusion of participants in data analysis and interpretation, a client-centred orientation to research would surely demand: if participants were not involved, why not?

Disseminating findings: the politics of publication

Although a significant body of literature addresses issues of participation in the research process, little attention has been paid to concerns about retaining the voices, perspectives and priorities of the research participants in the phases of data analysis, writing up and subsequent publication (Edwards & Ribbens 1998).

Disability theorists observe that 'university based researchers are far more likely to write for other university based researchers than they are for their research subjects – disabled people' (Barnes 1996c p 108–9); and to publish in locations that will further their own careers rather than informing disabled people of the research findings (Shakespeare 1996a). These theorists contend that 'academic and professional writing is tied to and shaped by prestige and privilege' (French 1993b p 129). Noting that academic advancement is associated with publications in peer-reviewed journals and with papers presented at academic conferences, Goodley & Moore (2000 p 880) observe: 'it remains convenient for academic researchers to stick with the production of research outputs that are not noted for either their accessibility or their potency for bringing about change'.

Kitchen (2000 p 31) contends that 'the failure of academia to translate findings and recommendations into the public sphere is disenfranchising to those whom the research seeks to represent'. In professions espousing a client-centred ethic it is not good enough simply to acknowledge the competing demands of academia and of accountability to research participants and thereafter to defer to academia (and careerism). Instead, researchers must commit to disseminating their findings to a much wider audience and in a variety of formats. The language we choose to use, the ideologies and assumptions we subscribe to, the theories we employ and the production and location of written reports all declare who it is we place at the centre of our research (hooks 1989). These are political choices. 'The extent to which knowledge is made available, accessible, etc. depends on the nature of one's political commitments' (hooks 1990 p 31).

Bonell (1999 p 118) argued that research findings should be provided to the group being researched for ethical reasons and to ensure 'that the research is not mindlessly parasitic'. Publishing research findings in an accessible language and in publications that are read by disabled people ensures that these people have access to information that *they* can use to influence policy and attain more control over their lives (Shakespeare 1996a). In light of the reality that the impetus for social changes that benefit disabled people tends, almost without exception, to originate with disabled people themselves (rather than from able-bodied researchers, therapists, theorists or policy makers), Shakespeare's suggestion should surely be taken seriously.

Barriers to participation

Although participation cannot be tokenistic and should constitute more than consultation, it must also be acknowledged that participants have other commitments and constraints on their time and energies and this may limit their desire or ability to participate throughout the research process. Further, while most professionals receive financial remuneration for their research endeavours (and most students hope to gain a degree), disabled people are often expected to participate in research without any compensation at all (Priestley 1999). If for no other reason, this should compel researchers to ensure their research is relevant and useful to those they choose to study!

Braye (2000 p 23) identified two further barriers to participation: the politics of organizations (policies, procedures and practices) and the politics of professionalism: i.e. 'the patterns of power ownership upon which professional status is constructed, achieving role security from the use of specialist expertise and function'. The difficulties in translating an intent to be inclusive and collaborative into practice can be expressed in terms of knowledge and power: 'the power differences among researchers . . . , the various knowledges they bring, and the authority afforded to different kinds of knowledge' (Campbell et al 1998 p 95). Indeed, Campbell et al's research findings indicate that this disjuncture between intent and accomplishment in research perfectly mirrors the disjuncture between intent and accomplishment in healthcare practice.

Although it is naïve to imagine that all disabled people will possess the necessary skills and knowledge to direct the research process from its inception, Stewart & Bhagwanjee (1999) demonstrate that through a process of education and empowerment, group members can assume ownership of a project over time, transforming this from a professionally led to a peer-led endeavour.

SKETCHING A DISABILITY METHODOLOGY

Jenny Morris (1991 p 130) has argued: 'as long as an unequal power relationship exists between disabled people and the non-disabled academics and professionals who make a living out of our needs ... disabilism will continue to characterize the nature of the research done and the service provided'. How might things be different?

It has been stated already that a methodology is a philosophical and ethical approach to developing knowledge: a theory of how research should, or ought, to proceed given the nature of the issue it seeks to address. Drawing upon the work of feminist theorists (e.g. Cancian 1992, Kirsch 1999) and disability theorists (e.g. Barnes 2004a, Morris 1992) it is possible to sketch the beginnings of a disability methodology.

A disability methodology primarily addresses the nature of the relationship between researchers and those being researched. It exemplifies the following principles:

- Research is built on respect, contests traditional hierarchical, 'colonial' research relationships and requires collaboration with participants.
- Research is based on the priorities of disabled people and service users.
- Research contributes to the evidence base required by disabled people through producing knowledge that they can use.
- Research recognizes that disabled people are disadvantaged by social, cultural, political, legal, economic and physical structures and that these inequalities intersect with others constructed on the basis of, for example, gender, "race", class, age and sexual orientation.
- Research incorporates a reflexive, critical stance to conventional assumptions about disability (and about rehabilitation).
- Research focuses on person/environment interactions to enable the contextual nature of disability to be acknowledged.
- Research includes an action component, ensuring that research has the potential for meaningful outcomes for disabled people; and it includes an accountability component, with a commitment to work with disabled people to *achieve* meaningful outcomes.
- Participants are involved in evaluating the research process.

It is noteworthy that participatory, collaborative research such as this reflects the basic ethical principles underpinning healthcare practice (see Chapter 8): respect for the person (such that all people are valued and treated with dignity), non-maleficence (the duty to refrain from causing harm), beneficence (the duty to advance the good of others), justice (recognition that all people are equal, and the duty to ensure fair and equitable distribution of benefits) and autonomy (a respect for each person's right to autonomous decision making) (Stuart 1998). Thus, collaborative research is ethical research.

EXEMPLARS OF DISABILITY RESEARCH

At the end of a lengthy examination of the problems of disability research and the possibilities offered by a more client-centred approach it is important to translate theory into practice and highlight some exemplary and rigorous client-oriented studies.

Mary Law (2004), for example, engaged in participatory research with the parents of children with physical impairments with the shared goal of identifying those environmental barriers that presented the most substantial challenges to the children. The participatory and collaborative nature of the study assured its relevance, facilitated the translation of research findings into action (e.g. attaining accessible recreation programmes) and empowered the parents to undertake further research themselves (for which they have successfully attained funding).

Karen Rebeiro (2004), an occupational therapist, engaged her co-researchers (mental health service users) in a series of studies that led to the development of a collaborative, occupation-based mental health programme that has been enormously successful in meeting their needs. Together, they have evaluated this initiative on an ongoing basis. The programme, and the research that informed it, required Rebeiro to develop trusting, reciprocal relationships with her partners, to redefine professionalism and to work in a client-centred way. As an example of this non-hierarchical approach to research, all members of the research team have been involved in writing about the studies and the programme and in disseminating the research findings (e.g. Bibyk et al 1999, Rebeiro et al 2001). Their names appear as equal colleagues on these publications.

Clinicians often complain that much research is irrelevant and that the only outcome of most studies is a published paper calling for further research. Rebeiro and Law demonstrate that when researchers undertake research in a manner that reflects their deep commitment to client-centred philosophy, the study is inevitably framed within a relevant issue and is more likely to produce positive change. They provide evidence-based support for the premise that 'collaboration . . . encourages researchers to develop research that is both rigorous and relevant' (White et al 2001 p 32).

Oliver (1992 p 111) claimed that a change in the social relations of research would occur when researchers 'learn how to put their knowledge and skills at the disposal of their research subjects'. In an innovative project, Chris Carpenter, a university-based physiotherapy researcher, was contracted by the British Columbia Paraplegic Association (an advocacy organization) to collaborate in a systematic, client-focused evaluation of its role and services in an effort to ensure that the organization meets the needs of its members (Carpenter 2004b, Carpenter & Forman 2004). The organization decided the nature of the issue to be explored and the specific areas to be addressed. In turn, Carpenter contributed her experience of working with spinal cord-injured people, and her specific skills and abilities as an experienced researcher and facilitator, to ensure that the research was conducted in a rigorous manner. Choices about the way in which the research would be conducted – whether it would use qualitative or quantitative methods, which geographic areas would be included, how potential participants would be informed of the study, and so forth – were collaborative decisions. The project demonstrated that client-centred research can be used successfully to generate the evidence with which to evaluate and inform client-centred models of service delivery (Carpenter & Forman 2004). The study participants made frequent comments that the research process was both useful and enjoyable (Carpenter 2004b) and the findings have been of direct value and relevance to their organization, to whom the researcher was ultimately accountable.

These three examples lend support to the suggestion that if researchers and disabled people pool their expertise, there is the potential to achieve better research (Ward & Flynn 1994).

This chapter has examined the process of undertaking research within a client-centred ethic; and has sketched a disability methodology to provide client-centred guidelines for generating the evidence with which to inform professional theory and practice. The final chapter seeks to translate research and theory into practice, drawing from the previous chapters to suggest ways in which challenging assumptions might inform changes in rehabilitation practice.

Chapter 11

Contesting assumptions; challenging practice

An enormous difference to the way we live our lives can be created by a shift in perceptions about things we have always taken for granted or never questioned. (Coleridge 1999 p 165)

INTRODUCTION: CONTESTING ASSUMPTIONS

This book began with the following claim: 'Central to the problem of rehabilitation is the failure to address the issue of power and to acknowledge the existence of ideology' (Oliver 1996a p 104). Oliver continued: 'I am not suggesting that we can eradicate the influence and effects of power and ideology in rehabilitation, but that *our failure to even acknowledge their existence gives rise to a set of social relations and a range of therapeutic practices that are disabling for all concerned*' (1996a p 104, emphasis added). As various themes and issues have been explored throughout this book, it has hopefully become clear that a book about disability and rehabilitation is inevitably a book about power and ideology (either implicitly or explicitly); and that acknowledging and addressing these issues can be enabling for all concerned with the practices of the rehabilitation professions.

This final chapter draws together the essential themes that have been developed in the previous pages to suggest future directions for rehabilitation; directions that consciously address issues of power and ideology.

PERSPECTIVES ON DISABILITY AND REHABILITATION

The quantity and quality of theoretical work concerning disability that has arisen in recent years necessitates a critical approach to the assumptions that underpin the theory and practice of rehabilitation. It is apparent from the critiques outlined in this book that many of these assumptions lack a supportive evidence-base. It is also apparent that global rehabilitation services have been disproportionately informed by specific Western ideals and ideas (Schriner 2001). This book has therefore argued for a cross-fertilization of ideas, a critique of established and taken-for-granted ways of thinking and an analysis of how alternative perspectives might inform a renewed vision for rehabilitation practice. This is important work. 'Rather than being of minority interest, the insights of disability studies have the potential to influence many other areas of human life, and force society to reassess questions about normality, independence, the physical body and social environment, suffering and mortality' (Shakespeare 1998b p 257).

Congruent with Said's (1979) demand for a sceptical approach to orthodoxy and a rigorous intellectual commitment to contesting the uncritical acceptance of authoritative ideas, this book has attempted to challenge the inherent assumptions in the field of rehabilitation, raise questions, confront dogma and unmask conventional and received ideas (Said 1996). This sceptical interrogation has raised specific issues about "normality", about the central aim of rehabilitation and about power. These emerging issues will be briefly reviewed and connected with research findings that concern issues of importance to people with impairments.

THE IDEOLOGY OF NORMALITY

Current rehabilitation practice is seen to be value-based and grounded in an ideology of normality. This ideology underpins rehabilitation's attempts to induce conformity in appearance, behaviour and function by "norming" the non-standard. Evidence suggests, however, that while this approach to practice might be useful – even effective – for treating acute injuries and illnesses it is not relevant for people with many forms of impairment and is irrelevant for rehabilitation, which is concerned not with curing but with living.

Furthermore, it is apparent that the assumption of normality is nothing more than an assumption – a human invention – because norms do not exist outside the ideas that create them. It is because "normality" is an ideological construction that the parameters of both normality and abnormality are subject to cultural variations and change over time. Thus, an ideology of normality provides a singularly unstable foundation for practice.

Through their adherence to the ideology of "normality" it is claimed that the rehabilitation professions support and promote specific ableist ideologies and act as agents of the State, protecting the political and social status quo by individualizing problems that are the consequence of environmental factors, justifying the unequal distribution of life opportunities and inducing clients to strive to attain those "norms" of function valued by the dominant population.

Contesting normative ideology

Anthropologists confirm that people with various forms of impairment have always been part of the spectrum of humanity. In our own era, in which enhanced medical knowledge enables people to survive even with very severe degrees of impairment, an increasing proportion of the population currently falls outside the dome of normality's bell curve. It is therefore more useful, and certainly more humane, to think of impairment as a dimension of normal: as one shade of the spectrum of what it means to be human. Indeed, for people who live with many forms of impairment, impairment is a normal dimension of their lives. By recognizing the acceptability of different modes of being, the rehabilitation professions are better positioned to assist their disabled clients in attaining the rights usually accorded those located more centrally under the dome of the 'bell'.

Following his spinal cord injury and subsequent rehabilitation, Neil Slatter mused: 'people sometimes ask me why society should bother with us and I always tell them it's because it's our society as well as theirs' (cited in Hurley 1983 p 137). Therapists can work towards achieving social justice by affirming their clients' fundamental right to be part of their communities and by working with them to ensure this right is upheld. By challenging the diminished life opportunities that normative ideologies justify, therapists encourage their disabled clients to resist the marginal status to which assumptions of "normality/superiority" confine those classified as "abnormal/inferior". By involving as peers those former clients who have successfully transgressed marginality, therapists challenge the cultural script that equates disability with inability and promote counterhegemonic scripts that portray an expanded range of life possibilities for their current clients.

In gauging the success of rehabilitation services, outcome measures could usefully assess the degree to which disabled people are enabled to transcend a minority status and assume the rights and opportunities accorded other citizens. This could be accomplished through assessments of social rather than physical outcomes, such as community participation and integration.

THE CENTRAL AIM OF REHABILITATION

It is claimed that the central aim of rehabilitation is to enhance the quality of lives affected by illness and impairment (e.g. Pain et al 1998). Indeed, this is often viewed as being rehabilitation's raison d'être. Research reviewed throughout the previous chapters demonstrates that this laudable aim is not achievable through minimizing impairments, enhancing physical abilities or increasing physical independence because neither quality of life nor psychological distress correlate with physical function, independence or degree of impairment. While increased function and independence may be useful objectives, they are not sufficient to imbue life with quality and are inadequate responses to the reality of disability.

The rehabilitation professions like to claim that their own goal of enhancing each client's quality of life distinguishes them from other specialties in the healthcare field who focus simply on symptom relief; a comparison that is supported neither by clinical nor research activities (Dijkers et al 2000). Whiteneck (1994) notes that rehabilitation services compile detailed records describing impairments and documenting the degree of assistance required to accomplish various activities of daily living: dimensions with little or no bearing on quality of life. Indeed, because rehabilitation practitioners rarely measure outcomes in terms of their clients' active participation in their community, engagement in productive activities or quality of life (Whiteneck 1994) they have no way of knowing whether their admirable goals have been achieved. So, what does contribute to the experience of a life worth living following impairment?

WHAT IS IMPORTANT? THE RESEARCH EVIDENCE

The reality that depression is considered to be an epidemic in the minority ("developed") world (Murray & Lopez 1996) despite comparative affluence, material comforts and what is termed a 'high standard of living' (Christiansen 1999), suggests that the experience of quality in living is not dependent upon the quantifiable, material conditions of life but upon subjective, qualitative factors: the content of life. A considerable body of qualitative research into the experience of living with impairments has probed the subjective factors perceived to be necessary requisites for a life worth living: a life of 'quality'. By definition, these are also the necessary requisites for relevant and useful rehabilitation services.

Existential philosophy expressed the post-war need to rebuild one's life, the freedom to re-make oneself and a denial of the determinism of circumstances (Lavine 1984), hence its relevance for rehabilitation. Sartre (1956) argued, for example, that although one might not be able to change one's biological, psychological, social or economic circumstances these do not determine who we will become; we are free (and responsible) to choose the meanings we give to these realities and to choose how we will live within our limitations. The existential philosophers asserted that *meaning, purpose, choice* and *self-worth* are fundamentally important to the experience of a life worth living (Lavine 1984, Plahuta et al 2002, Somner & Baumeister 1998). This assertion is supported by the findings of researchers who have explored the experience of living with a variety of impairments and have identified:

- the need for a positive sense of *self-worth*
- a need to establish *continuity* within disrupted 'biographies'
- a need to *belong and contribute* to families and communities
- a need to experience *meaning* and *purpose* in everyday life
- a need to exercise *choice* and exert *control* over their lives (e.g. Hammell 2004h, Pain et al 1998).

These interconnected needs constitute an evidence-based, challenging – but not unattainable – mandate for rehabilitation.

Body/self

Rehabilitation has traditionally attempted to address the *consequences* of impairment – its impact on everyday life activities – while paying little attention to its *significance*: the impact of stigma, cultural norms and ideas of competence and social worth for the individual's sense of self (Bury 1991). Indeed, rehabilitation's allegiance to a biomedical dualism that divides the body from the self has led to a preoccupation with the former and a neglect of the latter (Toombs 1994). This represents a spectacular lack of fit with research evidence.

Autobiographical accounts and a substantial body of research demonstrate that a disruption to one's body/mind is often experienced as a 'biographical disruption' (i.e. of one's routines, habits, roles, lifestyle and life plans); as a disruption to the sense of body/self unity; and as a disruption to one's sense of self, such that loss of certain abilities may be perceived to devalue the whole person (e.g. Becker 1997, Bury 1982, Hill 1997, Keany & Gluekauf 1993, Sparkes & Smith 1999, Toombs 1994). For example, Murphy (1990 p 85) described how when he became paraplegic, 'I had lost much more than the full use of my legs. I had also lost a part of my self'.

The 'self' concept

Within the social sciences and humanities the terms 'self' and 'identity' are used in very specific, yet inconsistent and contested ways. In general, 'identity' is used to refer to one's social 'face' – how one perceives how one is perceived by others. 'Self' is generally used to refer to one's sense of 'who I am and what I am' and is the way the term is employed in this book. However, these are not dualistic constructs. Both the concepts of self and identity evolve out of social interaction (Millward & Kelly 2003), but because we are not merely 'stamped out' by society, we are active participants in our own self/identity construction (Bakhurst & Sypnowich 1995, Sartre 1956).

The importance of a coherent sense of self – of who I am and what I am – is not a uniquely Eurocentric concept. Although many other cultures prize human relations over individual ability, and community over individuality

(Iwama 2003), in every culture people recognize the distinctions between 'self' and 'other'. Iwama (2003) explains that in the Japanese language the word that most closely approximates to 'self' is *jibun* or 'self-part', i.e. one's share of the whole. Thus, when bodily dysfunction disrupts one's ability to enact societal norms and routinized codes of conduct and behaviour, one is unable to maintain one's part in valued social roles and statuses: unable to uphold one's 'self-part'.

Self and self-worth

Research into the experience of impairment has identified the need for a positive sense of self-worth; a sense that may be challenged by an inability to conform to cultural norms of body function or performance (Wendell 1996). Researchers have found that the loss of ability to engage in valued activities of daily life can impact one's sense of self-worth: erasing perceptions of competence and capability and provoking feelings of being useless and worthless (Hammell 2004f, Lyons et al 2002, Reynolds 2003). A young man who sustained a high spinal cord injury playing ice hockey explained it like this: 'There didn't seem to be any value to my life . . . because my value, as I saw it, had been stolen with the injury: because I was a hockey player, an athlete, and my value was physical and that was me. It took a lot of reframing my life and my values before I could see that life was worth it . . . I felt so useless' (Hammell 2004f p 610).

The research evidence therefore implies that the work of rehabilitation includes enabling people to engage in personally valued roles and occupations that enhance their perceptions of being valuable, capable and competent (Bloom 2001, Hammell 2004f, Rebeiro 2004, Vrkljan & Miller-Polgar 2001); and encouraging the rebuilding of a sense of self that is not dependent upon physique or physical abilities but upon other abilities and competencies (Kleiber & Hutchinson 1999). These two dimensions of rehabilitation are worth exploring further.

The importance of 'doing' – of engaging in meaningful and purposeful occupations – is addressed below, and is central to issues of self-worth. Christiansen (1997) proposed that occupation should be understood as a context for appreciation and enjoyment of living, an opportunity for experiencing meaning in everyday endeavours and the basis for establishing self-identity, gaining a sense of control and achieving biographical continuity. It is because ability is of little value without opportunity that the rehabilitation professions also need to address the social, political and physical environments that often restrict opportunities for a range of everyday endeavours to those in the dominant population.

Further, because 'transforming one's self and life is more than a matter of individual resolve; to do so often means challenging prevailing norms, ideals, values and prescriptions that shape both individual action and private self-understanding' (Kleiber & Hutchinson 1999 p 151–2). The ice hockey player mentioned above noted that he learned 'to see [that] value and self-worth are continuing and not tied to physical status' (Hammell 2004f p 612) and that this had been crucial to his desire to live. Another man, who sustained a high spinal cord injury at age 19, explained: 'You have to throw away the way you looked at life. I mean, when you're young everything is how you look, who you're with and how they look . . . and it's all very superficial' (Hammell 2004f p 612). Indeed, for some disabled people, an inability to conform to social norms of function, appearance and lifestyle and the consequent need to live according to their own values is quite liberating (Shakespeare et al 1996)!

Over time, many people undergo a conceptual transformation, enabling them to develop a sense of self that rests on their residual abilities: what they can do, not what they cannot. For example, a participant in the spinal cord injury study advised: 'You've got the rest of your life in front of you . . . you can't spend a lot of time worrying about what you can't do. Figure out what you can do and focus on that' (Hammell 2004f p 614). Indeed, by perceiving themselves as competent and capable – of being an 'able self' (McCuaig & Frank 1991) – many people no longer view themselves as *dis*abled; refusing an identity based on their impairments (Hammell 2004f, Watson 2002). As a Chinese–Canadian man in the same study noted: 'I don't really look at myself any different. I just need somebody to be my hands and feet for me' (Hammell 2004f). 'Normality' can be redefined in terms of the ability to get one's life back on track or of 'just getting on with things' (Watson 2002 p 516). This conceptual transformation can begin during the rehabilitation process as each individual is exposed to a range of possible options for what they might become, as they focus on abilities not inabilities, as they regain the ability to enact their choices and as they are treated as inherently valuable by their service providers.

McCuaig & Frank (1991) demonstrated that the importance of a competent 'able self' lies not solely in self-perception but in the perceptions of others. It is suggested that the ill or injured person looks for clues about the meaning that disability holds for those people who are important in their lives and whether they are able to recognize the 'old me' in the impaired body (Corbin & Strauss 1991). Indeed, Gerhardt (1989 p 141) argued that 'it is through the "looking-glass" effect of others' positive evaluations of one's actions and personal value that the self is constituted'. The 'looking-glass' effect was explained this way by a participant in the spinal cord injury study: 'Your family and friends see you as having value and able to contribute even though you may have written yourself off as having no value. They think you are worth it and you see that you are valued and start to value yourself' (Hammell 2004f p 614). This connects with the idea of belonging (see below).

Body/self unity

Lucke (1997) reported that people with spinal cord injuries defined the 'major work' of the rehabilitation process as 'getting back together', or reintegrating the self. Lucke's study participants described a gradual awareness that they were the same person as before their injury. A reintegration of self occurred as they reconciled their changed physical self (a 'broken body') with an 'inner' self that was perceived as unchanged despite the experience of spinal cord injury. This reintegration reflects a renewed acknowledgement of body/self unity that has been observed by other researchers (e.g. Carpenter 1994).

Biographical disruption and continuity

An inevitable product of the ideology of normality, the idea of *loss* has traditionally held a central place in rehabilitation, notably among psychologists. Despite overwhelming empirical evidence to the contrary, for example, a belief persists that rates of depression and distress will be highest among those whose physical losses (i.e. deviances from the "norm") are the greatest. It has therefore been suggested that for rehabilitation, the concept of 'continuity' is more useful than the traditional preoccupation with change (Boekamp et al 1996).

Research that has explored the experience of impairment suggests that those people who successfully transcend their impairments are those who focus not on their losses but on what remains the same: on *continuity*, and on getting their lives 'back on track' (Carpenter 1994, Hammell 1998a), that is, under some degree of personal control. The term 'continuity' does not imply an uninterrupted life trajectory but a coherence between self and life before and after impairment.

Becker (1993) explored the biographical disruption caused by a stroke and the expressed need of individuals to achieve a continuous and coherent sense of self. This was accomplished, in part, by identifying markers of continuity with former lives and by redefining what sort of life might now be possible. Similarly, Spencer et al (1995) studied the rehabilitation process of a man with a spinal cord injury and his attempts to envision a future life that would relate to his past. Sadly, his therapists overlooked his need to link his future life to his past and failed to assist him in connecting his past competencies, interests and experience to an image of the person he might become in the future. Clearly, one of rehabilitation's mandates is to enable each client to pursue their interests and escape a biographical limbo of dashed hopes and lost ambitions.

Reynolds (2005 p 229) contends that the central objective of rehabilitation is not solely enabling clients to manage their conditions but assisting them to put their lives 'back together'. Research among people following stroke, for example, has demonstrated that return to a meaningful life is of greater importance than the enhancement of functional abilities (Doolittle 1991). This should not be surprising.

Toombs (1994) observed that one does not simply resume life following the onset of an impairment such as multiple sclerosis but integrates one's changed way of being into a new life plan that reflects one's values and priorities (which may have changed). As the former ice hockey player explained: 'the person you were pre-injury is the person you are going to be post-injury – with different values' (Hammell 2004f p 612).

Belonging and contributing

Albrecht & Devlieger (1999) explored the apparent paradox in which people with very severe forms of impairment nonetheless report a high quality of life. They noted that perceptions of quality of life were highest when people were able to contribute – to give as well as take – in reciprocal relationships.

Many researchers have reported consistent findings of the importance to life's quality of being able to contribute to others – partners, assistants, families, friends and communities – in reciprocal relationships that foster perceptions of value and competence, connecting and belonging (e.g. Bloom 2001, Boswell et al 1998, Laliberte-Rudman et al 2000, Rebeiro 2004). This was reflected by several participants in the high spinal cord injury study, one of whom explained that while he was institutionalized: 'I felt so useless, I seemed so dependent. I felt so dependent and the bottom line is that you just felt like you were taking all the time, you weren't giving . . . we need to be able to contribute. We need to be able to give back' (Hammell 2004f p 10).

The ability and opportunity to contribute to others is associated with lower levels of depression and higher self-esteem (Schwartz & Sendor 1999, Stewart & Bhagwanjee 1999). Indeed, a substantial body of research has demonstrated that perceptions of quality of life are significantly influenced by social outcomes: the extent to which people perceive themselves to be active, productive and contributing members of their families and communities (e.g. Dijkers et al 2000, Hammell 2004i). Yet while social outcomes are the most important domains for rehabilitation clients when they return to the community (Dijkers et al 2000), they are only rarely used to gauge the relevance and worth of rehabilitation services.

Meaning and purpose

An Oxfam study into the needs of disabled people in the majority ("third") world found that beyond basic needs such as food and shelter were: 'the need to be creative, to make choices, to exercise judgement, to love others, to have friendships, to contribute something of oneself to the world, to have social function and purpose. These are active needs . . . without them life itself has no meaning. The most basic need of all is the need for meaning' (Coleridge 1993 p 213). Although many people contend that there is no meaning *of* life (e.g. Campbell 1991, Urbanowski & Vargo 1994), it is apparent that people need to experience meaning *in* their lives (Frankl 1959, Taylor 1983) and that this need may be especially apparent when formerly taken-for-granted biographies are disrupted by illness or injury.

Research findings have demonstrated that engagement in personally meaningful occupations restores a sense of value and purpose to life (Bloom 2001, Laliberte-Rudman et al 2000, Ville et al 2001, Vrkljan & Miller-Polgar 2001). For example, in describing those factors that make her life worth living, a university student in the high spinal cord injury study explained: 'I find a lot of meaning in the work that I'm doing at school' (Hammell 2004f p 614). Mee & Sumsion (2001) observed that doing something purposeful is directly associated with the meaning of one's day and that engagement in occupations that are personally meaningful contributes to a sense of purpose. Indeed, 'having things to do that are meaningful fills life with purpose' (Cochran & Laub 1994 p 91). 'Purpose' provides a reason to wake up in the morning and a way to keep busy and may include a pursuit of new opportunities, the opportunity to contribute to others and the ability to envision a meaningful future engaged in valued occupations (Hammell 2004b, 2004f).

However, occupations do not have to be purposeful to be personally meaningful. Research has also identified the importance to the quality of disabled people's lives of time spent in contemplation and appreciation of nature, music, art, being alone or being with special people (Hammell 2004f). These dimensions of 'being' contrast with the Eurocentric preoccupation with 'doing' and have been identified by several researchers as important components of living well with a serious illness or impairment (e.g. Berterö & Ek 1993, Bloom 2001, Young & McNicholl 1998).

Just because someone is 'doing' something does not imply that the activity is personally meaningful or purposeful. While people give different meanings to, and derive different meanings from, their occupations only those that are chosen according to the client's own values and priorities can be deemed 'personally meaningful'. When occupations are dictated by the agendas of occupational therapists, for example, the meaning clients derive from them can be 'humiliating' (Helfrich & Kielhofner 1994). Neither are activities experienced as 'purposeful' when they are selected according to therapists' priorities. Abberley (1997 p 31), for example, contrasts 'productive activity' with 'pseudo-labour, (familiar to many who have undergone occupational therapy)'.

Research findings affirm the importance of engagement in purposeful occupations when these are personally meaningful and valuable to the individual (Gloersen et al 1993, Lyons et al 2002, Vrkljan & Miller-Polgar 2001). Thus, while occupational therapists have traditionally extolled *meaningful* occupations, while focusing in reality on *purposeful*, goal-oriented, socially sanctioned activities (e.g. Wilcock 1998, Yerxa 1998), it is apparent that there is a strong association between these concepts (Hammell 2004h).

It has been suggested that therapists should not only focus on the acquisition of skills to enable people to get out of bed in the morning, but should also assist them in finding their own reasons for so doing (Trieschmann 1988). 'To be meaningful and relevant, rehabilitation must assist each individual to achieve control of his or her life, facilitate the exploration of options and opportunities, encourage the involvement of special people and enable each person to find something meaningful to "do," such that life is filled with both purpose and meaning' (Hammell 2004f p 617). This cannot be accomplished through an individualistic approach to rehabilitation, because as Coleridge (1993) observed, 'active' needs can only be met if political, social and economic forces enable people to have some sort of meaningful control over their own lives.

Choice and control

A recurring theme in the research literature is that the onset of impairment can produce a sense of loss both of autonomy and of control of one's own life: the sense of having choices (opportunities) and of being able to act on those choices may be lost. Yet it is also clear that the experience of a life worth living with a serious illness or impairment is strongly influenced by perceptions of being able to exert control over one's own life (Abresch et al 1998, Hammell 2004f, Laliberte-Rudman et al 2000, Lyons et al 2002, Plahuta et al 2002). Indeed, 'the exercise of choice and the opportunity to take control of the organization of one's own life is one of the first markers of quality [of life]' (Johnstone 1998 p 65).

Disabled people who perceive themselves as having control over their lives experience less depression and less psychological distress (Frank & Elliott 1989). It is therefore perverse that while the onset of impairment can contribute to a sense of powerlessness, the interaction with rehabilitation professionals is often characterized as an experience of powerlessness (Abberley 1995, Corring & Cook 1999, Dalley 1999). Autobiographical and research evidence demonstrates the ways in which occupational therapists, for example, seize control over the decisions that impact their clients' lives, even in such matters as modifications to clients' own homes (Finkelstein 2004, Watson 2003). Indeed, the relationship between disabled people and their service providers has been equated to that of colonized people and their colonizers, with the colonizers determining what services are in the best interests of those who are deemed 'incapable' of determining this for themselves (Hirsch & Hirsch 1995). This has little to do with providing services and everything to do with the expression of power.

Commenting on a study into the provision of services to disabled people in Australia, Kemp (2002) noted the 'ascendancy' (position of dominance and control) of service providers over their disabled clients. For example, clients were unable to make their own lifestyle choices because, as they explained, the service providers 'dictate your lifestyle' (p 211). Achieving control over one's life is inordinately difficult when this must first be wrested from one's 'service' providers.

It has been suggested that people gain a sense of control and of biographical continuity by choosing, shaping and orchestrating their daily occupations (Clark & Jackson 1989). Researchers have noted that people whose lives have been disrupted by illness or injury make a conscious decision to take control of their lives (or 'get back on track'), notably through re-engagement in occupations they find meaningful (Carpenter 1994, Cochran & Laub 1994, Gloersen et al 1993, Hammell 1998a Vrkljan & Miller-Polgar 2001).

Research findings correlating the ability to assert control over one's life with perceptions of quality of life obviously support a client-centred approach to rehabilitation. However, recognition that 'control is dependent on opportunities provided by the environment' (CAOT 1997 p 37) demands an approach to rehabilitation that is informed not solely by *meaning* – individuals' perceptions of the consequences and significance of impairment within their own lives – but also by *context* – the circumstances of each individual within their specific physical, social, cultural, economic, legal and political environments. The power of professionals forms part of this context.

POWER AND IDEOLOGY

It is claimed that the health professions promote those ideologies that strengthen their role and entrench their own power; that they are preoccupied with describing the characteristics of their own 'expertise'; and that their only overtly political actions are undertaken to enhance their own self-interests and protect their 'turf' (e.g. French & Swain 2001, Jongbloed & Crichton 1990a, Oliver 1996a, Schriner 2001). However, because ideologies and power are inseparable, 'the questioning of dominant ideologies can be a starting point for changing power relations' (Swain 2004c p 86).

Said (1979) argued that intellectuals must be on guard against the received ideas handed down in their profession; against being too smug, too insulated, too confident in ideological straitjackets and against being allied with cultural and political dogma. If this is true for intellectuals, then Said's contentions must surely be even more applicable to those professions whose ideas have consequences for people's lives?

However, the rehabilitation professions tend to guard themselves against challenging ideas. Papers achieving publication in professional journals are those that have survived a gauntlet of reviewers and editors: "experts" drawn from among the professions' establishment. Many of the innovative abstracts submitted to professional conferences receive excellent reviews but only those papers that will fit into thematic groupings with other, similar papers are selected for presentation; a format that fosters and rewards 'thinking as usual'. It is therefore unsurprising that first-time conference attenders, unfamiliar with the carefully scripted format, complain of being uninspired and unchallenged, lament the lack of passion or political perspective and condemn the wholehearted acceptance and uncritical promotion of governments' agendas (Pearson & Osgerby 2004).

Knowledge and power are indivisible; indeed, knowledge is 'selected and "shaped" by those in power' (French 1993b p 121) such that the professions are exposed to a narrow range of available ideas. This practice serves to maintain the political status quo and protect professional interests, while 'creating enormous problems for those bent on innovation and challenging conventional ideas' (French 1993b p 121). Perhaps, as hooks (1989 p 16) observed: 'it is silly to think one can challenge and also have approval'.

REHABILITATION'S CONJOINED MANDATES

The critiques and insights explored in this book suggest that if rehabilitation services are to be relevant and accountable to their clients, and effective in enabling them to live rich and fulfilling lives, attention needs to be paid to two inseparable mandates. Clearly, there must be focus at the personal level: enabling clients to achieve biographical continuity and get their lives 'back on track'. Just as clearly, this cannot be achieved through simplistic attempts to enhance physical/mental abilities. Rather, a biographical orientation to rehabilitation is needed to ensure that interventions are relevant to each individual in the context of their lives; with the impairment or illness viewed as just one theme within the context of a life. It has long been observed that when professionals give advice to disabled people they tend to talk as if the illness or impairment is the central issue around which the person's life is organised and it is therefore unsurprising that much of this advice is ignored when it fails to fit with people's everyday lives (Williams & Wood 1988). What clients want is help to manage their impairments or illnesses so they can get on with what really matters: their roles, relationships and valued routines and occupations.

One theme has recurred repeatedly throughout the book: an individualized, function-obsessed, problem-oriented approach to rehabilitation is an inadequate response to the circumstances that confront disabled people in their everyday lives. In conjunction with attention to the personal impact of impairment – the disrupted body/self/biography – rehabilitation practitioners need to focus on the social impact of disability: challenging socially constructed "norms", contesting marginalization and exploitation, striving for equality of opportunity and for respect for human rights. Because disability results from the interplay between an impairment and the environment – and all its cultural, social, physical, political, economic and legal dimensions – a sole focus on impairment fails to address the reality of disability.

It has been argued that professional intervention is a waste of time unless professionals work actively for a society that is accessible to all, that respects everyone's rights and that provides equality of opportunity (Sutherland 1981). Indeed, 'the time is ripe for a thorough evaluation of rehabilitation theory and practice, as well as the possibility for a *transformative rehabilitation practice* that focuses on the societal conditions that create disadvantage for people whose individual characteristics are outside the societal norm' (Schriner 2001 p 653).

THE DEMISE OF THE REHABILITATION PROFESSIONS?

Throughout the book it was noted that many governments are responding to consumers' demands for services that are responsive to their needs and that respect their rights to self-determination (e.g. Groom 2003, Stewart & Bhagwanjee 1999). However, it does not appear as if the rehabilitation professions have acknowledged fully the magnitude of these requirements; a pervasive unresponsiveness that may have serious consequences for the future of these professions. Given the social work profession's failure to meet disabled people's self-articulated needs (Oliver & Sapey 1999), for example, Oliver (2004) predicts the forthcoming demise of that profession's involvement with disabled people.

Reports concerning the public service professions claim these have failed in their mandates because they have been developed to meet the needs of agencies and the professions rather than service users (Hughes, cited in Abberley 2004). For example, rehabilitation therapists have traditionally worked only on weekdays, and then only during the hours that suit their own privileged lifestyles (Hammell 1995, Wigham & Supyk 2001). In addition, the centralized locations of many services, modes of service delivery and agency policies appear to be designed for the benefit of the organization (first) and professionals (second) rather than the service users (Townsend 1998). Further, the ideological underpinnings of the professions are not necessarily relevant to the needs of service users. For instance, Abberley (2004) observed that occupational therapists' claim to professional status has relied upon a disempowering ideology of self-reliance and independence that is out of step with disabled people's articulated needs. None of these practices bode well for the professions' longevity. Traditionally, carefully guarded patterns of referral allowed clients little choice over their rehabilitation services but as service users acquire more rights they will surely opt to see those therapists and seek those services they feel best meet their needs; just as they currently do with practitioners of complimentary or alternative therapies.

Many disabled people claim that the most significant problems they face in their daily lives are a consequence not of their impairments but of a society designed to meet the needs of the dominant population. Indeed, it was the ubiquitous nature of this experience that spawned the original UPIAS declaration and the subsequent social model of disability (Chapter 4). This prompted Williams (1996 p 200) to observe: 'if the problem is not the need of the individual to adapt to the impairment, but rather the complex process of negotiating the interactions out of which daily life is created, then *the role of professional experts as people who do things to the impaired body is clearly limited'* (emphasis added). Witkin (2000 p 205) claims that in the USA social work 'is a profession whose code-of-ethics calls upon its members to work towards a more just social order'. This might be a useful example for the rehabilitation professions to follow in an effort to meet the self-professed needs of their client groups and, perhaps also, to ensure their own longevity.

CHALLENGING ORTHODOXY

Much has been written about the blinkered thinking that is perceived to characterize the healthcare professions and their theorists. Barnes (2004b p 32), for example, observed: 'historically, by their failure to challenge orthodox wisdom on the problems encountered by people with ascribed impairments, academics have been part of the problem rather than the solution'. It is time for rehabilitation professionals to develop a culture of 'healthy scepticism' (Brechin & Sidell 2000 p 12) and to contest the status quo of their own professions (Said 1996).

Groce (1999b) argued that to understand the complexity of disability it is necessary to reach beyond the boundaries of particular disciplines to gain insight and enlightenment from new perspectives, but that this rarely occurs. Martin (2000 p 195) observed that 'the majority of professionals, no matter how well intentioned, have been trained to perceive themselves as experts in their field . . . [their] training has taught them that they should be (or at least appear to be) in control: to diagnose, to prescribe, to treat . . . It can be unnerving to discover that the taken-for-granted principles and values that have guided your life need to be questioned'. Indeed, while it is apparent that 'people feel threatened when their values are attacked or start to disappear' (Coleridge 1999 p 164), this is the necessary foundation for a more sceptical and intellectually rigorous approach to knowledge. We must try to tease apart the ties between knowledge and power.

CONTESTING ASSUMPTIONS; CHALLENGING PRACTICE

It has been argued that the healthcare professions are so much a part of the status quo that they inevitably play a role in the disadvantage and oppression of less powerful people (Brechin 2000). However, if professionals possess the power to reinforce the status quo, they have the power to challenge the status quo by actively contesting hierarchical power structures, dominant ideologies and vested professional interests (Northway 1997).

This book has challenged rehabilitation professionals to contest traditional assumptions about disability and has argued for sustained efforts to reduce power imbalances and professional complacency. It has called for more advocacy with and for disabled people in sociopolitical arenas to attain equality of life opportunities, irrespective of impairments.

Central to its arguments is the belief that ability is of little value without opportunity.

Glossary

Ableism
The belief that disabled people's differences make them inferior; and those social practices resulting from this belief that privilege "normal" ability and serve to marginalize disabled people and to limit their opportunities (Mackelprang & Salsgiver 1999).

Biological determinism
Biological determinism implies that one's life possibilities are wholly dictated – determined – by one's biology. Thus, someone deemed to be biologically "inferior" – on the basis, for example, of "race", gender or ability – is believed to be inherently inferior in physique, intellect and emotions and thus unable to compete in the economic or political life of the community by virtue of biology.

Classificatory practices
Foucault (1977) identified classificatory practices as those techniques that enable the separation of the "normal" from the "deviant".

Critical theory
Critical theories challenge conventional ideologies and contest repressive cultural hegemonies. Acknowledging that no theory can be objective or politically neutral, critical theory highlights the specific positionality, limitations and relations of power underlying "expert" knowledge and critiques the value judgements underpinning seemingly value-free research. 'Inquiry that aspires to the name *critical* must be connected to an attempt to confront the injustice of a particular society or sphere within the society' (Kincheloe & McLaren 1994 p 140).

Cultural imperialism
Cultural imperialism refers to the process by which a defined group is demeaned and devalued by those values of the dominant culture that are established as seemingly universal norms (Young 1990). By perpetuating negative stereotypes, prejudices and discrimination against specific groups of people, cultural imperialism provides the apparent justification for their oppression.

Disabilism
'Discriminatory, oppressive or abusive behaviour arising from the belief that disabled people are inferior to others' (Miller et al 2004 p 9).

Discourse
Foucault employed the term 'discourse' 'to examine how power, language and institutional practices combine at historically significant points in time to determine modes of thought (Fawcett 2000a p 17). Discourses are systems of statements that frame the ways in which, and by which, the world can be known (Ashcroft & Ahluwalia 1999), embodying specific perspectives that a group of people consider to be knowledge. When language is organized into discourses it has 'an immense power to shape the way that people experience and behave in the world' (Humphries et al 2000 p 11). More than simply ways of giving meaning to the world, however, discourses are a phenomenon of social power.

Dominant ideology
A dominant ideology is a set of ideas and values that permeates society due to the cultural power wielded by a dominant population (see below). This ideology is so pervasive as to be largely taken for granted, appearing to be

a 'natural' way of thinking (Barnes 1996a). It operates by legitimizing social inequalities and power relations; establishing what is "normal" (and therefore what is "abnormal") and by defining cultural values and desirable goals (Thompson 1997).

Dominant population
Dominance of a population refers not to numbers, but to power. A dominant population within a society is the group whose members have the power to define themselves as innately superior and to define other populations whose perceived attributes deviate from their own "norms" as inferior. The exercise of this power serves to justify discrimination against the group deemed inferior and abnormal, a practice that leads to disadvantage, marginalization and violations of their fundamental human rights. The dominant population has the power to impose their cultural values (see also cultural imperialism) and wields the political and economic power to control the life destinies of the subordinated populations (Kallen 2004).

Environment
Physiotherapists and occupational therapists acknowledge the importance of the environmental context in their theories of movement (Cott et al 1995) and of occupational performance (CAOT 1997). Any environment has physical, cultural, social, economic, legal and political dimensions (CAOT 1991). The political, legal and economic dimensions of the environment are sometimes referred to as the 'institutional' environment (CAOT 1997): those policies, procedures, political practices, decision-making processes, legislation, funding arrangements, financial priorities, legal processes and government services that exert a strong influence on everyday life (CAOT 1997).

Epistemology
Epistemology is the branch of philosophy concerned with theories of knowledge: beliefs about the nature of knowledge, how knowledge can be acquired and the reliability of claims to knowledge.

Ethnocentrism
Ethnocentrism is the belief that one's own culture is superior to others and is the standard by which all other people should be judged (Leavitt 1999b). Ethnocentrism is often manifest in the assumption that the values, priorities and perspectives of one's own culture are universal, rather than specific.

False consciousness
False consciousness is deemed to constitute any idea or ideology that is held to be inappropriate in light of the "true" or "objective" situation as this is "correctly" perceived by those wielding greater power. Use of the term 'false consciousness' implies that the truth of a given situation is understood correctly and with certitude by someone who is both more enlightened and in possession of a superior consciousness and that those deemed to be inferior are also deemed to be in error (Jary & Jary 1991, Somers & Gibson 1994, Wolf 1996).

Hegemony
Gramsci (1971) developed the concept of hegemony to define the process through which power is exercised by a dominant group over a subordinate group through the diffusion of 'common sense' ideas (Frankenberg 1988).

He observed that the domination of certain ideas is achieved by engineering consensus, such that those ideas and beliefs that benefit the powerful appear "natural", even to the powerless (Bocock 1986). These pervasive ideas serve to legitimate inequality, justify subordination and disguise exploitation and oppression (Frankenberg 1988). Hegemony is successful when inequality – on the basis of "race", gender, class, sexual orientation, [dis]ability, etc. – is accepted by consensus as normal and natural: inevitable. Dominant cultural norms 'always reflect the interests of those within particular social groups or societies who have the power to define situations and the resources with which to ensure that their own definitions are accepted as true' (Swain et al 2003 p 20). Thus, ideologies and beliefs prevail, not due to their intrinsic superiority or inherent "truth", but as a consequence of power (Foucault 1980). This is hegemony.

Heterosexism
Heterosexism is the assumption that everyone's sexuality conforms to specific "norms" (i.e. *heteronormativity*).

Ideology
An ideology is a system of ideas, beliefs and assumptions that operates below one's level of conscious awareness and, by being taken for granted, appears to constitute normal common sense. 'It comprises all the unquestioned preconceptions of the everyday' (Kingwell 1998 p 173). Ideologies play an important role in reinforcing and exercising power (Swain & French 2004). Although not inevitably oppressive, the term 'ideology' is often used to denote 'any system of ideas that justifies or legitimates the subordination of one group by another' (Jary & Jary 1991 p 226).

Liminality
A period in which people are in transition between culturally defined life crises or social states.

Minority and majority worlds
That area of the world self-described as "first" or "developed" constitutes approximately 17% of the global population and is most appropriately termed the 'minority' world. For the same reason, what is often termed the "developing" or "third" world constitutes approximately 83% of the world's population and is therefore described in this book – as elsewhere – as the 'majority' world. More than mere semantics, this acknowledges that the form of 'development' espoused by the minority world is not necessarily a desirable or sustainable goal for the majority of the global population to emulate; and it also recognizes that knowledge, values and ideas should not be made to flow in one direction – from 'us' to 'them' – but that the majority population have much from which the minority could learn (Penn 1999).

Occupation
Anything that people do in their daily lives (McColl et al 1992).

Oppression
Oppression of a specific population – such as disabled people – is said to occur as a consequence of domination; specifically the dominant population's ideologies of superiority and inferiority (Charlton 1998, Oliver 1990).

Young (1990) identified five 'faces' of oppression: marginalization, exploitation, powerlessness, cultural imperialism and violence.

Phenomenology

Phenomenology refers to a philosophical examination of the experience of a phenomenon – such as illness – and of the assumptions underlying the taken-for-granted, routine character of everyday life. A phenomenological inquiry into stroke, for example, would strive to elucidate the existential meaning of stroke as a distinct human experience; the reality of stroke as it is lived through by the individual (Kestenbaum 1982).

Positioning

Positioning, or 'positionality' refers to one's placement within specific axes of differentiation and of access to social power, such as gender, class, caste, "race", ethnicity, sexual orientation, age, religion, (dis)ability, language, nationality, citizenship status, education, professional and employment statuses and material wealth. Different social positions confer unequal access to resources and power and enable different life chances.

Postcolonial theory

Originating in critiques of colonialism – wherein the powerless are controlled, defined, described and represented by the powerful – postcolonial theory is concerned with empowerment of the disempowered and dispossessed, with establishing minorities' human rights and with achieving just and equitable relationships among people. Acknowledging that all theories reflect particular alignments of power and knowledge, postcolonial theory explicitly challenges privilege and power, critiques domination and control, resists all forms of exploitation and oppression and encourages cross-cultural dialogue (Said 1979, Young 2003). Postcolonial theorists examine the ways in which the dominant, powerful social group privileges its own values and norms, defining, marginalizing and excluding others deemed "inferior" on the basis of normative judgements about physical appearance, colour, behaviour, physical ability, etc. (Said 1979). Postcolonialism provides a way to talk about living in a world that seems to exist for others (Young 2003).

Postmodernism

Postmodern perspectives are those theoretical positions that challenge modernity's claims to grand, universal theories of knowledge, progress and truth, contest the myth of the universality of norms and values, and declare instead that all knowledge is partial and that there are multiple positions and perspectives from which reality can be understood (Best & Kellner 1991). Postmodernism disputes the claim that science can be objective or value-neutral, demonstrating that knowledge is always context-specific and a function of social power (Mitchell 1996). At its core, postmodernism is an attack on dogma (Raithatha 1997) and thus on "expertise" and its attempt to monopolize knowledge (Yeatman 1991). Intellectuals reflect a postmodern stance when they challenge received wisdom, engage in sceptical and critical thinking and embrace ideas from a diversity of sources. Although postmodernists usefully challenge authoritarian assumptions, contest the ideology of normality and recognize the possibility of multiple viewpoints (Cheek 2000), they are criticized for undermining the foundation of claims to universal social justice (Watson 2004) and for celebrating difference and diversity while having no committed vision of how things could, or ought to, be (Oliver & Barnes 1998). Thus, while postmodern theory playfully ponders the ambiguity of 'reality', Ashcroft & Ahluwalia (1999 p 46) observe: 'if that reality involves material and emotional deprivation, cultural exclusion and even death, such questions appear self-indulgent and irrelevant'.

Poststructuralism

An important dimension of postmodern theory, poststructuralism highlights the role of language in the workings of power relationships, revealing, for example, how 'discursive practices' – specific ways of using language to define, classify and describe – empower and privilege healthcare professionals and disempower their patients (Mitchell 1996). Poststructuralists deconstruct binary conceptual systems, such as male/female, in which one term is constituted as the privileged norm and in which hierarchies of meaning become socially institutionalized (Jary & Jary 1991). Committed to 'deconstructing' all discursive practices including, for example, ideologies of freedom and justice, poststructuralism – like postmodernism – is apolitical, lacking any commitment to identifying how things might, or should, be different (Oliver & Barnes 1998).

Power/knowledge

French philosopher Michel Foucault (1980) contested the belief that knowledge is ever objective, value free or independent of power, arguing instead that knowledge is tied to power. To conceptualize his argument Foucault referred to power/knowledge, demonstrating that these two concepts are indivisible: two faces of the same coin. Foucault argued, for example, that the dominance of one form of knowledge over another occurs, not because of intrinsic superiority or inherent "truth", but as a consequence of power. He also asserted that 'knowledge . . . authorizes and legitimates the exercising of power' (Danaher et al 2000 p 26). In turn, power legitimates knowledge, determining whose perspectives 'count'; thus knowledge 'is linked in a circular relation with systems of power which produce and sustain it' (Foucault 1980 p 133). Accordingly, Foucault (1980 p 132) claimed that 'the intellectual is not the "bearer of universal values"' but a person occupying a specific position relative to power.

Quality of life

Used by many writers to mean many things, within this book the term 'quality of life' is used to refer to the experience of a life worth living.

Queer theory

Queer theory is a school of thought that interrogates the kaleidoscope of human sex, gender and desire and critiques and destabilizes heteronormativity (Sherry 2004). Queer theory explores the ideological construction and presumed naturalness of "the norm" (McRuer 2003), the processes by which certain people become labelled as deviant (Epstein 1994) and demonstrates the instability of binary oppositions, such as homosexual/heterosexual or male/female (Seidman 1995).

Social constructionism

Social constructionism claims that all knowledge is socially constructed: that 'facts' are not true or real but inventions and interpretations (Berger & Luckmann 1966). 'Constructivist approaches are united by the assumption that all knowledge and all ways of knowing, including the most mathematically rigorous findings of empiricism, are historically confined, ideologically inflected, and culturally specific' (Jeffreys 2002 p 31). Jeffreys contends that constructionism 'can be used to question even the most entrenched assumptions about human nature, by exposing the cultural foundations of those assumptions and by . . . explaining how those assumptions evolved to serve the interests of elite segments of societies and particularly of patriarchal, Eurocentric, colonial, and capitalist societies' (2002 p 31–2). Social constructionists contend that the body, for example, is a 'discursive product of power/knowledge' (Williams 1999 p 813): that the body is produced and shaped by discourse. The experience of being female, for example, will be 'constructed' differently in different societies and cultures, determining the opportunities available to individual women; thus it is argued that gender is 'socially constructed'. However, to argue simplistically that disability is socially constructed – that it is produced through specific discourses and could therefore be deconstructed – is clearly a luxury only for the 'able'.

Theoretical imperialism

Theoretical imperialism is said to occur when academics and researchers (i.e. those wielding more power) frame the experiences of their 'subjects' within their own perspectives, privileging their own understanding and interpretations over those of the researched (Mann 1995). Theoretical imperialism is an expression of power/knowledge.

References

Abberley P 1993 Disabled people and 'normality'. In: Swain J, Finkelstein V, French S, Oliver M (eds) Disabling barriers – enabling environments. Open University and Sage, London p 107–115

Abberley P 1995 Disabling ideology in health and welfare: the case of occupational therapy. Disability and Society 10(2):221–232

Abberley P 1997 The limits of classical social theory in the analysis and transformation of disablement. In: Barton L, Oliver M (eds) Disability studies: past, present and future. The Disability Press, Leeds, p 25–44

Abberley P 2002 Work, disability, disabled people and European social theory. In: Barnes C, Oliver M, Barton L (eds) Disability studies today. Polity, Cambridge, p 120–138

Abberley P 2004 A critique of professional support and intervention. In: Swain J, French S, Barnes C, Thomas C (eds) Disabling barriers – enabling environments, 2nd edn. Sage, London p 239–244

Abbott P 1994 Conflict over the grey areas: district nurses and home helps providing community care. Journal of Gender Studies 3(3):299–306

Abresch RT, Seyden N, Wineinger M 1998 Quality of life. Issues for persons with neuromuscular diseases. Physical Medicine and Rehabilitation Clinics of North America 9:233–248

Abu-Habib L 1997 Gender and disability: women's experiences in the Middle East. Oxfam, Oxford

Acker J, Barry K, Esseveld J 1991 Objectivity and truth. Problems in doing feminist research. In: Fonow MM, Cook JA (eds) Beyond methodology. Feminist scholarship as lived research. Indiana University Press, Bloomington, IN, p 133–153

Ahmad WIV 2000 Introduction. In: Ahmad WIV (ed) Ethnicity, disability and chronic illness. Open University Press, Buckingham, p 1–11

Albrecht GL 1992 The disability business. Sage, Newbury Park, CA

Albrecht GL, Devlieger PJ 1999 The disability paradox: high quality of life against all odds. Social Science and Medicine 48(8):977–988

Alcoff L 1991 The problem of speaking for others. Cultural Critique 23:5–31

Allen S, Strong J, Polatajko H 2001 Graduate-entry master's degrees: launchpad for occupational therapy in this millennium? British Journal of Occupational Therapy 64(11):572–576

Allotey P, Reidpath D, Kouamé A, Cummins R 2003 The DALY, context and the determinants of the severity of disease: an exploratory comparison of paraplegia in Australia and Cameroon. Social Science and Medicine 57:949–958

Amundsen R 1992 Disability, handicap and the environment. Journal of Social Philosophy 23(1):105–118

Anand S, Hanson K 1997 Disability-adjusted life years: a critical review. Journal of Health Economics 16:685–702

Appleby Y 1994 Out in the margins. Disability and Society 9(1):19–32

Armer B 2004 In search of a social model of disability: Marxism, normality and culture. In: Barnes C, Mercer G (eds) Implementing the social model of disability: theory and research. The Disability Press, Leeds, p 48–64

Armstrong D 1983 Political anatomy of the body: medical knowledge in Britain in the twentieth century. Cambridge University Press, Cambridge

Armstrong D, Gosling A, Weinman J, Marteau T 1997 The place of inter-rater reliability in qualitative research: an empirical study. Sociology 31(3):597–606

Armstrong F, Barton L 1999 'Is there anyone there concerned with human rights?' Cross-cultural connections, disability and the struggle for change in England. In: Armstrong F, Barton L (eds) Disability, human rights and education. Cross-cultural perspectives. Open University Press, Buckingham, p 210–229

Arnesen T, Nord E 1999 The value of DALY life: problems with ethics and validity of disability adjusted life years. British Medical Journal 319:1423–1425

Asch A, Fine M 1988 Introduction: beyond pedestals. In: Fine M, Asch A (eds) Women with disabilities. Essays in psychology, culture, and politics. Temple University Press, Philadelphia, p 1–40

Ashcroft B, Ahluwalia P 1999 Edward Said. The paradox of identity. Routledge, New York

Ashcroft B, Griffiths G, Tiffin H 1995 Introduction. In: Ashcroft B, Griffiths G, Tiffin H (eds) The post-colonial studies reader. Routledge, London, p 321–322

Atkin K, Hussain Y 2003 Disability and ethnicity: how young Asian disabled people make sense of their lives. In: Riddel S, Watson N (eds) Disability, culture and identity. Pearson, Harlow, p 161–179

Atwal A 2002 Getting the evidence into practice: the challenges and successes of action research. British Journal of Occupational Therapy 65(7):335–341

Bach JR, Barnett V 1996 Psychosocial, vocational, quality of life, and ethical issues, In: Bach JR (ed) Pulmonary rehabilitation: the obstructive and paralytic conditions. Hanley & Belfus, Philadelphia, p 395–411

Bach JR, Campagnolo DI, Hoeman S, 1991 Life satisfaction of individuals with Duchenne muscular dystrophy using long-term mechanical ventilatory support. American Journal of Physical Medicine and Rehabilitation 70(3):129–135

Badley E 1993 An introduction to the concepts and classifications of the international classification of impairments, disabilities and handicaps. Disability and Rehabilitation 15(4):161–178

Badley EM 1998 Classification of disability. In: McColl MA, Bickenbach JE (eds) Introduction to disability. WB Saunders, London, p 19–28

Bakhurst D, Sypnowich C 1995 The social self. Sage, London

Balibar E, Wallerstein I 1996 Race, nation, class: ambiguous identities. Verso, London

Ballinger C, Wiles R 2001 A critical look at evidence-based practice. British Journal of Occupational Therapy 64(5):253–255

Banja JD 1997 Values and outcomes: the ethical implications of multiple meanings. Topics in Stroke Rehabilitation 4(2):59–70

Barfield T 1997 (ed) The dictionary of anthropology. Blackwell, Oxford

Barnartt S 2001 Using role theory to describe disability. Research in Social Science and Disability 2:53–75

Barnartt S, Altman B 2001 Exploring theories and expanding methodologies: where we are and where we need to go. Research in Social Science and Disability 2:1–7

Barnes C 1991 Disabled people in Britain and discrimination. C.Hurst, London

Barnes C 1994 Images of disability. In: French S (ed) On equal terms. Working with disabled people. Butterworth-Heinemann, Oxford, p 35–46

Barnes C 1996a Theories of disability and the origins of the oppression of disabled people in western society. In: Barton L (ed) Disability and society: emerging issues and insights. Longman, London, p 43–61

Barnes C 1996b Foreword. In: Campbell J, Oliver M, Disability politics. Routledge, London, p ix–xii

Barnes C 1996c Disability and the myth of the independent researcher. Disability and Society 11(1):107–110

Barnes C 1998a Review of: Wendell S. The rejected body. Feminist philosophical reflections on disability. Disability and Society 13(1):145–147

Barnes C 1998b The social model of disability: a sociological phenomenon ignored by sociologists? In: Shakespeare T (ed) The disability reader. Social science perspectives, Cassell, London, p 65–78

Barnes C 2003 Review of: Ustun TB et al (eds) Disability and culture: universalism and diversity. Hogrefe & Huber, Seattle, on behalf of the WHO. Disability and Society 18(6):827–833

Barnes C 2004a Reflections on doing emancipatory disability research. In: Swain J, French S, Barnes C, Thomas C (eds) Disabling barriers – enabling environments, 2nd edn. Sage, London, p 47–53

Barnes C 2004b Disability, disability studies and the academy. In: Swain J, French S, Barnes C, Thomas C (eds) Disabling barriers – enabling environments, 2nd edn. Sage, London, p 28–33

Barnes C, Mercer G (eds) 1996 Exploring the divide. Illness and disability. The Disability Press, Leeds, p 1–16

Barnes C, Mercer G 2003 Disability. Polity Press, Cambridge

Barnes C, Mercer G 2004 Theorising and researching disability from a social model perspective. In: Barnes C, Mercer G (eds) Implementing the social model of disability: theory and research. The Disability Press, Leeds, p 1–17

Barnes C, Mercer G, Shakespeare T 1999 Exploring disability: a sociological introduction. Polity Press, Cambridge

Barnitt R, Partridge C 1999 The legacy of being a research subject: follow-up studies of participants in therapy research. Physiotherapy Research International 4(4):250–261

Barry J 1995 Care-need and care-receivers. Views from the margins. Women's Studies International Forum 18(3):361–374

Basnett I 2001 Health care professionals and their attitudes toward and decisions affecting disabled people. In: Albrecht GL, Seelman KD, Bury M (eds) Handbook of disability studies. Sage, London, p 450–467

Batterham RW, Dunt D, Disler P 1996 Can we achieve accountability for long-term outcomes? Archives of Physical Medicine and Rehabilitation 77(12)1219–1225

Bauby J-D 1997 The diving-bell and the butterfly (trans. R Laffont). Fourth Estate, London

Baylies C 2002 Disability and the notion of human development: questions of rights and capabilities. Disability and Society 17(7):725–739

Beatty PW, Richmond GW, Tepper S, DeJong G 1998 Personal assistance for people with physical disabilities: consumer-direction and satisfaction with services. Archives of Physical Medicine and Rehabilitation 79(6):674–677

Becker G 1993 Continuity after a stroke: implications of life-course disruption in old age. The Gerontologist 33(2):148–158

Becker G 1997 Disrupted lives. How people create meaning in a chaotic world. University of California Press, Berkeley, CA

Becker G, Arnold R 1986 Stigma as a social and cultural construct. In: Ainlay S, Becker G, Coleman LM (eds) The dilemma of difference: a multicultural view of stigma. Plenum, New York, p 39–57

Begum N 1992 Disabled women and the Feminist agenda. Feminist Review 40:70–84

Begum N 1994 Snow white. In: Keith L (ed) Mustn't grumble. Writing by disabled women. Women's Press, London, p 46–51

Bellaby P 1993 The world of illness of the closed head injured. In: Radley A (ed) Worlds of illness. Biographical and cultural perspectives on health and disease. Routledge, London, p 161–178

Bensing J 2000 Bridging the gap. The separate worlds of evidence-based medicine and patient-centred medicine. Patient Education and Counselling 39:17–25

Berger P, Luckmann T 1966 The social construction of reality. Penguin, London

Berterö C, Ek A-C 1993 Quality of life of adults with acute leukaemia. Journal of Advanced Nursing 18:1346–1353

Best S, Kellner D 1991 Postmodern theory. Critical interrogations. The Guildford Press, New York

Bhopal K 2000 Gender, 'race' and power in the research process. In: Truman C, Mertens D, Humphries B (eds) Research and inequality. UCL Press, London, p 67–79

Bibyk B, Day DG, Morris L, et al 1999 Who's in charge here? The client's perspective on client-centred care. OT Now Sept/Oct:11–12

Bickenbach JE 1993 Physical disability and social policy. University of Toronto Press, Toronto

Biklen D 1987 Framed: Print journalism's treatment of disability issues. In: Gartner A, Joe T (eds) Images of the disabled, disabling images. Praeger, New York, p 79–96

Biko S 1978 I write what I like. Heinemann, Oxford

Bithell C 2000 Evidence-based physiotherapy: some thoughts on 'best evidence'. Physiotherapy 86(2):58–61

Bland M 1991 An introduction to medical statistics. Oxford University Press, Oxford

Blank A 2004 Clients' experience of partnership with occupational therapists in community mental health. British Journal of Occupational Therapy 67(3):118–124

Bloom FR 2001 'New beginnings': a case study in gay men's changing perceptions of quality of life during the course of HIV infection. Medical Anthropology Quarterly 15:38–57

Bochel C, Bochel H 1994 Researching disability: insights from and on the social model. International Journal of Rehabilitation Research 17:82–86

Bocock R 1986 Hegemony. Tavistock, London

Bodenhamer E, Achterberg-Lawlis J, Kevorkian G, et al 1983 Staff and patient perceptions of the psychosocial concerns of spinal cord injured persons. American Journal of Physical Medicine 62(4):182–193

Boekamp JR, Overholser JC, Schubet DS 1996 Depression following a spinal cord injury. International Journal of Psychiatry in Medicine 26(3):329–349

Bogdan R 1988 Freak show: presenting human oddities for amusement and profit. University of Chicago Press, Chicago, IL

Bogdan RC, Biklen SK 1992 Qualitative research for education. An introduction to theory and methods, 2nd edn. Allyn & Bacon, Boston, MA

Bonell C 1999 Gay men: drowning (and swimming) by numbers. In: Hood, S, Mayall B, Oliver S (eds) Critical issues in social research. Open University Press, Buckingham, p 111–123

Borlund K 1991 "That's not what I said": Interpretive conflict on oral narrative research. In: Gluck SB, Patai D (eds) Women's words. The feminist practice of oral history. Routledge, New York, p 63–76

Boswell BB, Dawson M, Heininger E 1998 Quality of life as defined by adults with spinal cord injuries. Journal of Rehabilitation 64:27–32

Boswell DM, Wingrove JM (eds) 1974 The handicapped person in the community. Tavistock & Open University Press, London

Bourdieu P 1978 Sport and social class. Social Science Information 17(6):819–840

Bourdieu P 1984 Distinction: a social critique of the judgement of taste. Routledge, London

Bozalek V 2000 Feminist postmodernism in the South African context. In: Fawcett B, Featherstone B, Fook J, Rossiter A (eds) Practice + research in social work. Postmodern feminist perspectives. Routledge, London, p 176–191

Braithwaite DO 1991 'Just how much did that wheelchair cost?': management of privacy boundaries by persons with disabilities. Western Journal of Speech Communication 55:254–274

Brannen J 1993 Research notes: The effects of research on participants: findings from a study of mothers and employment. Sociological Review 41(2):328–346

Brättemark M 1996 International Classification of Impairments, Disabilities and Handicaps (ICIDH). Helios 16:4

Braye S 2000 Participation and involvement in social care. In: Kemshall H, Littlechild R (eds) User involvement and participation in social care. Research informing practice. Jessica Kingsley, London, p 9–28

Brechin A 2000 Introducing critical practice. In: Brechin A, Brown H, Eby MA (eds) Critical practice in health and social care. Sage & Open University, London, p 25–47

Brechin A, Sidell M 2000 Ways of knowing. In: Gomm R, Davies C (eds) Using evidence in health and social care. Sage, London, p 3–25

Brechin A, Liddiard P, Swain J (eds) 1981 Handicap in a social world. Hodder & Stoughton, London

Breckenridge CA, Vogler C 2001 The critical limits of embodiment: disability's criticism. In: Breckenridge CA, Vogler C (eds) The critical limits of embodiment. Reflections on disability criticism. Duke University Press, Durham, NC, p 349–357

Bricher G 2000 Disabled people, health professionals and the social model of disability: can there be a research relationship? Disability and Society 15(5):781–793

Briggs A 1981 Equal Opportunities Commission Report. EOC, Manchester

British Columbia Rehabilitation Society 1990 Keys to freedom. Resource manual for the development of self-managed community living alternatives for quadriplegic persons. BC Rehab. Society, Vancouver

Burke DC, Murray DD 1975 Handbook of spinal cord medicine. Macmillan, Basingstoke

Bury M 1982 Chronic illness as biographical disruption. Sociology of Health and Illness. 4(2):167–182

Bury M 1991 The sociology of chronic illness: a review of research and prospects. Sociology of Health and Illness 13:451–468

Butler J 1997 Against proper objects. In: Weed E, Schor N (eds) Feminism meets queer theory. Indiana University Press, Bloomington, p 1–30

Butler J 1999 Gender trouble: feminism and the subversion of identity. Routledge, New York

Butler R 1999 Double the trouble or twice the fun? Disabled bodies in the gay community. In: Butler R, Parr H (eds) Mind and body spaces. Geographies of illness, impairment and disability. Routledge, London, p 203–220

Butler R, Parr H 1999 Mind and body spaces. Geographies of illness, impairment and disability. Routledge, London

Byzek J 2004 What's in your head? Who put it there? New Mobility 15(128):37–39, 63

Calderbank R 2000 Abuse and disabled people: vulnerability or social indifference? Disability and Society 15(3):521–534

Cambridge P 1999 The first hit: a case study of the physical abuse of people with learning disabilities and challenging behaviours in a residential service. Disability and Society 14(3):285–308

Camilleri J, Callus A-M 2001 Out of the cellars. Disability, politics and the struggle for change: the Maltese experience. In: Barton L (ed) Disability politics and the struggle for change. David Fulton, London, p 79–92

Campbell J 1991 A Joseph Campbell Companion, Harper Collins, New York

Campbell J, Oliver M 1996 Disability politics. Understanding our past, changing our future. Routledge, London

Campbell M, Copeland B, Tate B 1998 Taking the standpoint of people with disabilities in research: experiences with participation. Canadian Journal of Rehabilitation 12(2):95–104

Canadian Association of Occupational Therapists (CAOT) & the Health Services Directorate 1983 Guidelines for the client-centred practice of occupational therapy. Health Services Directorate, Ottawa

Canadian Association of Occupational Therapists (CAOT) 1991 Occupational therapy guidelines for client-centred practice. CAOT, Toronto

Canadian Association of Occupational Therapists (CAOT) 1997 Enabling occupation. An occupational therapy perspective. CAOT, Ottawa

Canadian Association of Occupational Therapists (CAOT) 2000 Enabling occupation. An occupational therapy perspective, 2nd edn. CAOT, Ottawa

Cancian FM 1992 Feminist science: methodologies that challenge inequality. Gender and Society 6(4):623–642

Cant R 1997 Rehabilitation following a stroke: a participant perspective. Disability and Rehabilitation 19(7):297–304

Caplan B, Shechter J 1993 Reflections on the 'depressed', 'unrealistic', 'inappropriate', 'manipulative', 'unmotivated', 'non-compliant', 'denying', 'maladjusted', 'regressed', etc patient. Archives of Physical Medicine and Rehabilitation 74:1123–1124

Carpenter C 1994 The experience of spinal cord injury: The individual's perspective - implications for rehabilitation practice. Physical Therapy 74(7):614–629

Carpenter C 2004a The contribution of qualitative research to evidence-based practice. In: Hammell KW, Carpenter C (eds) Qualitative research in evidence-based rehabilitation. Churchill Livingstone, Edinburgh, p 1–13

Carpenter C 2004b Using qualitative focus groups to evaluate health programmes and service delivery. In: Hammell KW, Carpenter C (eds) Qualitative research in evidence-based rehabilitation. Churchill Livingstone, Edinburgh, p 51–64

Carpenter C, Forman B 2004 Provision of community programs for clients with spinal cord injury: use of qualitative research to evaluate the role of the British Columbia Paraplegic Association. Topics in Spinal Cord Injury Rehabilitation 9(4):57–72

Carpenter C, Hammell K 2000 Evaluating qualitative research. In: Hammell K, Carpenter C, Dyck I (eds) Using qualitative research: a practical introduction for occupational and physical therapists. Churchill Livingstone, Edinburgh, p 107–119

Carricaburu D, Pierret J 1995 From biographical disruption to biographical reinforcement: the case of HIV-positive men. Sociology of Health and Illness 17(1):65–68

Chaleby K 1992 Psychotherapy with Arab patients: towards a culturally oriented technique. Arab Journal of Psychiatry 3(1):16–27

Chambers (1972) Chambers' Twentieth Century Dictionary. Chambers, Edinburgh

Chappell AL 1998 Still out in the cold: people with learning difficulties and the social model of disability. In: Shakespeare T (ed) The disability reader: social science perspectives. Cassell, London, p 211–220

Charles C, Gafni A, Whelan T 1997 Shared clinical decision-making in the medical encounter: what does it mean? (Or it takes at least two to tango). Social Science and Medicine 44(5):681–692

Charlton JI 1998 Nothing about us without us. Disability, oppression and empowerment. University of California Press, Berkeley, CA

Charmé SL 1984 Meaning and myth in the study of lives. A Sartrean perspective. University of Pennsylvania Press, Philadelphia

Chartered Society of Physiotherapy (CSP) 1996 Rules of professional conduct. Physiotherapy 81:460

Cheek J 2000 Postmodern and poststructural approaches to nursing research. Sage, London

Chief Medical Officer 2001 The expert patient – a new approach to chronic disease management for the 21st century. Cited in: More control for patients 2002 Occupational Therapy News February:16

Childs P, Williams P 1997 An introduction to post-colonial theory. Prentice-Hall, London

Christiansen C 1997 Acknowledging a spiritual dimension in occupational therapy practice. American Journal of Occupational Therapy 51(3):169–172

Christiansen C 1999 Defining lives: Occupation as identity: an essay on competence, coherence, and the creation of meaning. American Journal of Occupational Therapy 53:547–558

Chuang Tzu 1964 Basic writings (trans. B Watson). Columbia University Press, New York

Clare E 1999 Exile and pride. Disability, queerness and liberation. South End Press, Cambridge, MA

Clark C, Scott E, Krupa T 1993 Involving clients in programme evaluation and research: a new methodology. Canadian Journal of Occupational Therapy 60(4):192–199

Clark F 1993 Occupation embedded in a real life: interweaving occupational science and occupational therapy. American Journal of Occupational Therapy 47(12):1067–1078

Clark FA, Jackson J 1989 The application of the occupational science negative heuristic in the treatment of persons with human immunodeficiency infection. Occupational Therapy in Health Care 6:69–91

Cochran L, Laub J 1994 Becoming an agent. State University of New York Press, Albany, New York

Coleman LM 1997 Stigma. An enigma demystified. In: Davis LJ (ed) The disability studies reader. Routledge, New York, p 216–231

Coleridge P 1993 Disability, liberation and development. Oxfam, Oxford

Coleridge P 1999 Development, cultural values and disability: the example of Afghanistan. In: Stone E (ed) Disability and development. Disability Press, Leeds, p 149–167

College of Occupational Therapists (COT) 2000 Code of ethics and professional conduct for occupational therapists. COT, London

Consortium for Spinal Cord Medicine 1999 Outcomes following traumatic spinal cord injury: clinical practice guidelines for health care professionals. The Consortium & the Paralyzed Veterans of America, Washington, DC

Cook DW 1981 A multivariate analysis of motivational attributes among spinal cord injured rehabilitation clients. International Journal of Rehabilitation Research 4(1):5–15

Corbet B 2000 Bully pulpit: bound for glory. New Mobility 11(83):4

Corbett J 1994 A proud label: exploring the relationship between disability politics and gay pride. Disability and Society 9(3):343–357

Corbett J 1997 Independent, proud and special: calibrating our differences. In: Barton L, Oliver M (eds) Disability studies: past, present and future. The Disability Press, Leeds, p 90–98

Corbin J, Strauss AL 1987 Accompaniments of chronic illness: changes in body, self, biography and biographical time. Research in the Sociology of Health Care 6:249–281

Corbin J, Strauss A 1991 Comeback: the process of overcoming disability. Advances in Medical Sociology 2:137–159

Corker M 1998a Disability discourse in a postmodern world. In: Shakespeare T (ed) The disability reader: social science perspectives. Cassell, London, p 221–233

Corker M 1998b Deaf and disabled, or deafness disabled? Open University Press, Buckingham

Corker M, French S 1999 Reclaiming discourse in disability studies. In: Corker M, French S (eds) Disability discourse. Open University Press, Buckingham, p 1–11

Cornielje H, Ferrinho P 1999 The sociopolitical context of CBR developments in South Africa. In: Leavitt RL (ed) Cross-cultural rehabilitation. An international perspective. WB Saunders, London, p 217–226

Corring D J 1999 The missing perspective on client-centred care. OT Now Jan-Feb:8–10

Corring D, Cook J 1999 Client-centred care means that I am a valued human being. Canadian Journal of Occupational Therapy 66(2):71–82

Cott CA, Finch E, Gasner D, et al 1995 The movement continuum theory of physical therapy. Physiotherapy Canada 47(2):87–95

Cottingham J 1988 The rationalists. Oxford University Press, Oxford

Craddock J 1996a Responses of the occupational therapy profession to the perspective of the disability movement, Part 1. British Journal of Occupational Therapy 59(1):17–22

Craddock J 1996b Responses of the occupational therapy profession to the perspective of the disability movement, Part 2. British Journal of Occupational Therapy 59(2):73–78

Craig AR, Hancock KM, Dickson HG 1994 Spinal cord injury: a search for determinants of depression two years after the event. British Journal of Clinical Psychology 33:221–230

Craik J, Rappolt S 2003 Theory of research utilization enhancement: a model for occupational therapy. Canadian Journal of Occupational Therapy 70(5):266–275

Crepeau EB 1998 Clinical interpretation of '"My secret life": the emergence of one gay man's authentic identity'. American Journal of Occupational Therapy 52(7):570–572

Crewe NM 1996 Gains and losses due to spinal cord injury: views across 20 years. Topics in Spinal Cord Injury Rehabilitation 2:46–57

Crichton A, Jongbloed L 1998 Disability and social policy in Canada. Captus, North York, ON

Crisp R 1992 The long term adjustment of 60 persons with spinal cord injury. Australian Psychologist 27(1):43–47

Crompton L 2003 Homosexuality and civilization. Harvard University Press, Boston, MA

Cross M 1994 Abuse. In: Keith L (ed) Mustn't grumble. Writing by disabled women. Women's Press, p 163–166

Crouch M 2003 The International Classification of Functioning, Disability and Health. Occupational Therapy News. January:18–19

Crow L 1996 Including all of our lives: renewing the social model of disability. In: Morris J (ed) Encounters with strangers. Feminism and disability. Women's Press, London, p 206–226

Cusack L, Sealey-Lapeš C 2000 Clinical governance and user involvement. British Journal of Occupational Therapy 63(11):539–546

Cushman L, Dijkers M 1990 Depressed mood in spinal cord injured patients: staff perceptions and patient realities. Archives of Physical Medicine and Rehabilitation 71:191–196

d'Aboville E 1991 Social work in an organization of disabled people. In: Oliver M (ed) Social work: disabled people and disabling environments. Jessica Kingsley, London, p 64–85

Dale AE 1995 A research study exploring the patient's view of quality of life using the case study method. Journal of Advanced Nursing 22:1128–1134

Dalley G 1988 Ideologies of caring. Macmillan, London

Dalley J 1999 Evaluation of clinical practice: is a client-centred approach compatible with professional issues? Physiotherapy 85(9):491–497

Dallmeijer AJ, van der Woude LHV 2001 Health related functional status in men with spinal cord injury: relationship with lesion and endurance capacity. Spinal Cord 39(11):577–583

Danaher G, Schirato T, Webb J 2000 Understanding Foucault. Allen & Unwin, St Leonards, NSW, Australia

Darke P 1998 Understanding cinematic representations of disability. In: Shakespeare T (ed) The disability reader: social science perspectives. Cassell, London, p 181–197

Davidson I, Waters K 2000 Physiotherapists working with stroke patients: a national survey. Physiotherapy 86(2):69–80

Davis K 1993 The crafting of good clients. In: Swain J, Finkelstein V, French S, Oliver M (eds) Disabling barriers – enabling environments. Sage, London, p 197–200

Davis LJ 1995 Enforcing normalcy: disability, deafness and the body. Verso, New York

Davis LJ 1997 The encyclopedia of insanity. Harper's Magazine. February:61–66

Davis LJ 2001 Nationality, disability and deafness. In: Aruri N, Shuraydi M (eds) Revising culture. Reinventing peace: the influence of Edward W. Said. Olive Branch Press, New York, p 2–28

Davis LJ 2002a Bending over backwards. Disability, dismodernism and other difficult positions. New York University Press, New York

Davis LJ 2002b Bodies of difference: politics, disability and representation. In: Snyder SL, Brueggemann BJ, Garland-Thomson R (eds) Disability Studies. Enabling the humanities. The Modern Language Association of America. New York, p 100–106

DeLisa JA 2002 Quality of life for individuals with SCI: let's keep up the good work (Editorial). Journal of Spinal Cord Medicine 25(1):1

Department of Health 1997 The new NHS: modern, dependable. The Stationery Office, London

Department of Health 1999 National Service Framework for mental health, modern standards and service models. Department of Health, London

Department of Health 2000 The NHS plan. A plan for investment. A plan for reform. The Stationery Office, London

DePoy E, Gilson SF 2004 Rethinking disability. Principles for professional and social change. Brooks/Cole, Belmont, CA

Deutsch H, Nussbaum F (eds) 2000a 'Defects'. Engendering the modern body. University of Michigan Press, Ann Arbor, MI

Deutsch H, Nussbaum F 2000b Introduction. In: Deutsch H, Nussbaum F (eds) 'Defects'. Engendering the modern body. University of Michigan Press, Ann Arbor, MI, p 1–28

DeVivo MJ, Stover SL 1995 Long-term survival and causes of death. In: Stover SL, DeLisa JA, Whiteneck GG (eds) Spinal cord injury. Clinical outcomes from the model systems. Aspen Publications: Gaithersberg, MD, p 289–316

DeVivo MJ, Black KJ, Richards JS, Stover SL 1991 Suicide following spinal cord injury. Paraplegia 29(9):620–627

Devlieger P, Rusch F, Pfeiffer D 2003 Rethinking disability as same *and* different! Towards a cultural model of disability. In: Devlieger P, Rusch F, Pfeiffer D (eds) Rethinking disability. The emergence of new definitions, concepts and communities. Garant, Antwerp, p 9–16

Dickson HG 1996 Problems with the ICIDH definition of impairment. Disability and Rehabilitation 18:52–54

Dijkers M 1996 Quality of life after spinal cord injury. American Rehabilitation Autumn:18–24

Dijkers M 1997 Measuring quality of life. In: Fuhrer MJ (ed) Assessing medical rehabilitation practices. The promise of outcomes research. Paul Brookes, Baltimore, p 153–179

Dijkers M 1998 Community integration: conceptual issues and measurement approaches in rehabilitation research. Topics in Spinal Cord Injury Rehabilitation 4(1):1–15

Dijkers M 1999 Measuring quality of life: methodological issues. American Journal of Physical Medicine and Rehabilitation 78:286–300

Dijkers M, Whiteneck G, El-Jaroudi R 2000 Measures of social outcomes in disability research. Archives of Physical Medicine and Rehabilitation 81 (Suppl 2) S63–S80

Disability and Society 2004 Editorial on language policy. Disability and Society 19(1):inside back cover

Dockery G 2000 Participatory research. Whose roles, whose responsibilities? In: Truman C, Mertens D, Humphries B (eds) Research and inequality. UCL Press, London, p 95–110

Dombroski RS 1989 Antonio Gramsci. Twayne, Boston, MA

Doolittle ND 1991 Clinical ethnography of lacunar stroke: implications for acute care. Journal of Neuroscience Nursing 23:235–239

Dorn ML 1998 Beyond nomadism. The travel narratives of a 'cripple'. In: Nast NJ, Pile S (eds) Places through the body. Routledge, London, p 183–206

Douard JW 1995 Disability and the persistence of the 'normal'. In: Toombs SK, Barnard D, Carson RA (eds) Chronic illness. From experience to policy. Indiana University Press, Bloomington, IN, p 154–175

Dougherty CJ 1994 Quality-adjusted life years and the ethical values of health care. American Journal of Physical Medicine and Rehabilitation 73:61–65

Driedger D 1989 The last civil rights movement. Disabled Peoples' International. Hurst, London

Drummond MF 1987 Resource allocation decisions in health care: a role for quality of life assessments? Journal of Chronic Diseases 40(6):605–616

Duckett PS, Pratt R 2001 The researched opinions on research: visually impaired people and visual impairment research. Disability and Society 16(6):815–835

Duggan CH, Dijkers M 1999 Quality of life – peaks and valleys: a qualitative analysis of the narratives of persons with spinal cord injuries. Canadian Journal of Rehabilitation 12:181–191

Duggan CH, Lysack C, Dijkers M, Jeji T 2002 Daily life in a nursing home: impact on quality of life after a spinal cord injury. Topics in Spinal Cord Injury Rehabilitation 7(3):112–131

Ear-Dupuy H 2004 You shall go to school . . . tackling the Cinderella syndrome. Guardian Weekly Sept 17–23:34

Edwards R, Ribbens J 1998 Living on the edges. Public knowledge, private lives, personal experience. In: Ribbens J, Edwards R (eds) Feminist dilemmas in qualitative research. Public knowledge and private lives. Sage, London, p 1–23

Eisenberg M, Saltz C 1991 Quality of life among aging spinal cord injured persons: long term rehabilitation outcomes. Paraplegia 29:514–520

Elfström ML, Kreuter M, Rydén A, Persson L-O, Sullivan M 2002 Effects of coping on psychological outcome when controlling for background variables: a study of traumatically spinal cord lesioned persons. Spinal Cord 40(8):408–415

Ellis K 1993 Squaring the circle: user and carer participation in needs assessment. Joseph Rowntree Foundation, London

Ellis-Hill C, Payne S, Ward CD 2000 Self-body split: issues of identity in physical recovery following a stroke. Disability and Rehabilitation 22(6):725–733

Engel GL 1977 The need for a new medical model: a challenge for biomedicine. Science 196(4286):129–136

Epstein S 1994 A queer encounter: sociology and the study of sexuality. Sociological Theory 12(2):188–202

Ernst FA 1987 Contrasting perceptions of distress by research personnel and their spinal cord injured subjects. American Journal of Physical Medicine 66(1):12–15

Fatsiou-Cowan M 1997 State of the arts. New Mobility 8(47):34

Fausto-Sterling A 2000 Sexing the body: gender politics and the construction of sexuality. Basic Books, New York

Fawcett B 2000a Feminist perspectives on disability. Prentice Hall, Harlow, UK

Fawcett B 2000b Researching disability. Meanings, interpretations and analysis. In: Fawcett B, Featherstone B, Fook J, Rossiter A (eds) Practice + research in social work. Postmodern feminist perspectives. Routledge, London, p 62–82

Featherstone M 1991 The body in consumer culture. In: Featherstone M, Hepworth M, Turner B (eds) The body. Social process and cultural theory. Sage, London, p 170–196

Featherstone M, Hepworth M 1991 The mask of ageing and the postmodern life course. In: Featherstone M, Hepworth M, Turner B (eds) The body. Social process and cultural theory. Sage, London, p 371–389

Featherstone M, Hepworth M, Turner BS 1991 The body. Social process and cultural theory. Sage, London

Ferguson I 2003 Challenging a 'spoiled' identity: mental health service users, recognition and redistribution. In: Riddel S, Watson N (eds) Disability, culture and identity. Pearson, Harlow, UK, p 67–87

Ferraro G 1995 Cultural anthropology: an applied perspective, 2nd edn. West Publishing, St Paul, MN

Ferrarotti F 1981 On the autonomy of the biographical method. In: Bertaux D (ed) Biography and society. Sage, Beverley Hills, CA, p 19–27

Field PA, Morse JM 1985 Nursing research. The application of qualitative methods. Chapman and Hall, London

Finch J 1984 Community care: developing non-sexist alternatives. Critical Social Policy 9(Spring):6–18

Finch J, Groves D 1980 Community care and the family: a case for equal opportunities. Journal of Social Policy 9:487–511

Fine M 1994 Working the hyphens: reinventing self and other in qualitative research. In: Denzin NK, Lincoln YS (eds) Handbook of qualitative research. Sage, Thousand Oaks, CA, p 70–82

Fine M, Asch A 1988 Women with disabilities. Essays in psychology, culture and politics. Temple University Press, Philadelphia

Finger A 1995 "Welfare reform" and us. Ragged Edge. Nov/Dec:15, 36

Finkelstein V 1981 Disability and the helper/helped relationship. An historical view. In: Brechin A, Liddiard P, Swain J (eds) Handicap in a social world. Hodder & Stoughton, Sevenoaks, UK, p 59–63

Finkelstein V 1991 Disability: an administrative challenge? In: Oliver M (ed) Social work. Disabled people and disabling environments. Jessica Kingsley, London, p 19–39

Finkelstein V 1993 Disability: a social challenge or an administrative responsibility. In: Swain J, Finkelstein V, French S, Oliver M (eds) Disabling barriers – enabling environments. Open University and Sage, London, p 34–43

Finkelstein V 1999a Extended review: doing disability research. Disability and Society 14(6):859–867

Finkelstein V 1999b A profession allied to the community: The disabled people's trade union. In: Stone E (ed) Disability and development. The Disability Press, Leeds, p 21–24

Finkelstein V 2004 Modernising services? In: Swain J, French S, Barnes C, Thomas C (eds) Disabling barriers – enabling environments, 2nd edn. Sage, London, p 206–211

Finkelstein V, French S 1993 Towards a psychology of disability. In: Swain J, Finkelstein V, French S, Oliver M (eds) Disabling barriers – enabling environments. Sage Publications and the Open University, London, p 26–33

Finkelstein V, Stuart O 1996 Developing new services. In Hales G (ed) Beyond disability. Towards an enabling society. Open University and Sage, London, p 170–187

Fischer D, Stewart A, Bloch D, et al 1999 Capturing the patient's view of change as a clinical outcome measure. Journal of the American Medical Association 282(12):1157–1162

Fonow MM, Cook JA 1991 Back to the future. A look at the second wave of feminist epistemology and methodology. In: Fonow MM, Cook JA (eds) Beyond methodology: feminist scholarship as lived research. Indiana University Press, Bloomington, IN, p 1–15

Fook J 2000 Deconstructing and reconstructing professional expertise. In: Fawcett B, Featherstone B, Fook J, Rossiter A (eds) Practice + research in social work. Postmodern feminist perspectives. Routledge, London, p 104–119

Ford S, Schofield T, Hope T 2003 What are the ingredients for a successful evidence-based patient choice consultation? A qualitative study. Social Science and Medicine 56:589–602

Foster S 2001 Examining the fit between deafness and disability. Research in Social Science and Disability 2:101–123

Foucault M 1963 The birth of the clinic. An archeology of medical perception. Vintage Books, New York

Foucault M 1977 Discipline and punish. Random House, New York

Foucault M 1978 The history of sexuality, Volume 1: an introduction. Random House, New York

Foucault M 1980 Power/knowledge. Pantheon Books, New York

Foucault M 1984 The Foucault Reader. Rabinow P (ed) Pantheon, New York

Fox NJ 1994 Postmodernism, sociology and health. University of Toronto Press, Toronto

Frank AW 1991 For a sociology of the body: an analytical review. In: Featherstone M, Hepworth M, Turner B (eds) The body. Social process and cultural theory. Sage, London, p 36–102

Frank G 1986 On embodiment: a case study of congenital limb deficiency in American culture. Culture, Medicine and Psychiatry 10:189–219

Frank G 2004 Venus on wheels: two decades of dialogue on disability, biography and being female in America. University of California Press, Berkeley, CA

Frank RG, Elliott T 1989 Spinal cord injury and health locus of control beliefs. Paraplegia 27:250–256

Frankenberg R 1988 Gramsci, culture and medical anthropology: Kundry and Parsifal? Or rat's tails to sea serpent? Medical Anthropology Quarterly 2:324–337

Frankl VE 1959 Man's search for meaning. Washington Square Press, New York

Fraser N 1992 The uses and abuses of French discourse theories for feminist politics. Theory, Culture and Society 9:51–71

Fraser N, Nicholson LJ 1990 Social criticism without philosophy: an encounter between feminism and postmodernism. In: Nicholson LJ (ed) Feminism/Postmodernism, Routledge, New York, p 19–38

French S 1993a Disability, impairment or something in between? In: Swain J, Finkelstein V, French S, Oliver M (eds) Disabling barriers – enabling environments. Sage & the Open University, London, p 17–25

French S 1993b Telling. In: Shakespeare P, Atkinson D, French S (eds) Reflecting on research practice. Open University Press, Buckingham, p 119–130

French S 1994a The disabled role. In: French S (ed) On equal terms. Working with disabled people. Butterworth-Heinemann, Oxford, p 47–60

French S 1994b What is disability? In: French S (ed) On equal terms. Working with disabled people. Butterworth-Heinemann, Oxford, p 3–16

French S 1994c Institutional and community living. In: French S (ed) On equal terms. Working with disabled people. Butterworth-Heinemann, Oxford, p 119–135

French S 1994d Disabled people and professional practice. In: French S (ed) On equal terms. Working with disabled people. Butterworth-Heinemann, Oxford, p 103–118

French S 1996 Out of sight, out of mind: the experience and effects of a 'special' residential school. In: Morris J (ed) Encounters with strangers. Feminism and disability. Women's Press, London, p 17–47

French S 2004a Reflecting on ethical decision-making in therapy practice. In: Swain J, Clark J, Parry K, et al, Enabling relationships in health and social care. Butterworth-Heinemann, Oxford, p 29–43

French S 2004b Enabling relationships in therapy practice. In: Swain J, Clark J, Parry K, et al, Enabling relationships in health and social care. Butterworth-Heinemann, Oxford, p 95–107

French S, Swain J 2001 The relationship between disabled people and health and welfare professionals. In: Albrecht GL, Seelman KD, Bury M (eds) Handbook of disability studies. Sage, London, p 734–753

French S, Reynolds F, Swain J, Gillman M 2001 Participatory approaches to research. In: French S, Reynolds F, Swain J (eds) Practical research – a guide for therapists. Butterworth-Heinemann, Oxford, p 234–246

Frost B 1999 Action on Disability and Development: working with disabled people's organisations in developing countries. In: Stone E (ed) Disability and development. The Disability Press, Leeds, p 39–53

Fuhrer MJ, Rintala DH, Hart KA, et al 1992 Relationship of life satisfaction to impairment, disability and handicap among persons with spinal cord injury living in the community. Archives of Physical Medicine and Rehabilitation 73:552–557

Fuhrer MJ, Rintala DH, Hart KA, et al 1993 Depressive symptomatology in persons with spinal cord injury who reside in the community. Archives of Physical Medicine and Rehabilitation 74:255–260

Gabel S, Peters S 2004 Presage of a paradigm shift? Beyond the social model of disability toward resistance theories of disability. Disability and Society 19(6):585–600

Gadacz RR 1994 Re-thinking DisAbility. New structures, new relationships. University of Alberta Press, Edmonton

Gadow S 1982 Body and self. A dialectic. In: Kestenbaum V (ed) The humanity of the ill. Phenomenological perspectives. University of Tennessee Press, Knoxville, TN, p 86–100

Gagnon L 1990 La qualité de vie de paraplégiques et quadriplégiques: analyse relative a l'estime de soi. Revue Canadienne de Recherche en Sciences Infirmières 22(1):6–20

Gaines A 1998, cited in Leavey G 2004 Identity and belief within black Pentecostalism: spiritual encounters with psychiatry. In: Kelleher D, Leavey G (eds) Identity and health. Routledge, London, p 37–58

Gallagher H 1990 By trust betrayed: patients, physicians and the licence to kill in the Third Reich. Henry Holt, New York

Gardner E 1983 The federal role of education. Heritage Foundation, Washington DC

Gerhardt U 1989 Ideas about illness. An intellectual and political history of medical sociology. New York University Press, New York

Gerhart KA 1997 Quality of life: the danger of differing perceptions. Topics in Spinal Cord Injury Rehabilitation 2(3):78–84

Gerhart KA, Corbet B 1995 Uninformed consent: biased decision-making following spinal cord injury. HEC Forum 7(2-3):110–121

Germon P 1998 Activists and academics: part of the same or a world apart? In: Shakespeare T (ed) The disability reader: social science perspectives. Cassell, London, p 247–255

Gerschick TJ 1998 Sisyphus in a wheelchair: men with physical disabilities confront gender domination. In: O'Brien J, Howard J (eds) Everyday inequalities. Critical inquiries. Blackwells, Oxford, p 189–211

Gerschick TJ, Miller AS 1995 Coming to terms. Masculinity and physical disability. In: Sabo D, Gordon D (eds) Men's health and illness. Sage, London, 183–204

Ghai A 2001 Marginalisation and disability: experiences from the Third World. In: Priestley M (ed) Disability and the life course. Global perspectives. Cambridge University Press, Cambridge, p 26–37

Ghai A 2002 Disability in the Indian context: post-colonial perspectives. In: Corker M, Shakespeare T (eds) Disability/postmodernity. Embodying disability theory. Continuum, London, p 88–100

Gibbs KE, Barnitt R 1999 Occupational therapy and the self-care needs of Hindu elders. British Journal of Occupational Therapy 62(3):100–106

Giddens A 1991 Modernity and self-identity. Self and society in the late modern age. Stanford University Press, Stanford, CA

Gill CJ 2001 Divided understandings. The social experience of disability. In: Albrecht GL, Seelman KD, Bury M (eds) Handbook of disability studies. London: Sage, p 351–372

Gill TM, Feinstein AR 1994 A critical appraisal of the quality of quality-of-life measurements. Journal of the American Medical Association 272(8):619–626

Gillman M 2004 Diagnosis and assessment in the lives of disabled people: creating potentials/limiting possibilities? In: Swain J, French S, Barnes C, Thomas C (eds) Disabling barriers – enabling environments, 2nd edn. London, Sage, p 251–257

Gillman M, Heyman B, Swain J 2000 What's in a name? The implications of diagnosis for people with learning difficulties and their family carers. Disability and Society 15(3):389–409

Glass CA 1999 Spinal cord injury: impact and coping. British Psychological Society, Leicester

Gleeson B 1999a Geographies of disability. Routledge, London

Gleeson B 1999b Can technology overcome the disabling city? In: Butler R, Parr H (eds) Mind and body spaces. Geographies of illness, impairment and disability. Routledge, London, p 98–118

Gloersen B, Kendall J, Gray P, et al 1993 The phenomena of doing well in people with AIDS. Western Journal of Nursing Research 15:44–58

Goble C 2003 Controlling life? In: Swain J, French S, Cameron C, Controversial issues in a disabling society. Open University Press, Buckingham, p 45–53

Goble C 2004 Dependence, independence and normality. In: Swain J, French S, Barnes C, Thomas C (eds) Disabling barriers – enabling environments, 2nd edn. Sage, London p 41–46

Goffman E 1959 Presentation of self in everyday life. Penguin, London

Goffman E 1961 Asylums. Penguin, London

Goffman E 1963a Stigma. Notes on the management of spoiled identity. Penguin, London

Goffman E 1963b Behaviour in public places. Free Press, New York

Gold N, Auslander G 1999 Newspaper coverage of people with disabilities in Canada and Israel: an international comparison. Disability and Society 14(6):709–731

Gomm R 2000 Should we afford it? In Gomm R, Davies C (eds) Using evidence in health and social care. Open University and Sage, London, p 192–211

Gomm R, Davies C 2000 Using evidence in health and social care. Open University and Sage, London, Preface

Good BJ 1994 Medicine, Rationality and Experience. University of Cambridge Press, Cambridge

Goodley D, Moore M 2000 Doing disability research: activist lives and the academy. Disability and Society 15(6):861–882

Gramsci A 1971 Selections from the prison notebooks. Lawrence & Wishart, London

Gray DB, Hendershot GE 2000 The ICIDH-2: developments for a new era of outcomes research. Archives of Physical Medicine and Rehabilitation 81 (Supp 2):S10–S14

Greenhalgh T 1997 Assessing the methodological quality of published papers. British Medical Journal 315:305–308

Griffin C, Phoenix A 1994 The relationship between qualitative and quantitative research: lessons from feminist psychology. Journal of Community and Applied Social Psychology 4:287–298

Groce NE 1999a Disability in cross-cultural perspective: rethinking disability. The Lancet 354:756–757

Groce NE 1999b General issues in research on local concepts and beliefs about disability. In: Holzer B, Vreede A, Weigt G (eds) Disability in different cultures. Reflections on local concepts. Transaction, Piscataway, NJ, p 285–295

Groce 1999c Health beliefs and behaviour towards individuals with disability cross-culturally. In: Leavitt RL (ed) Cross-cultural rehabilitation. An international perspective. WB Saunders, London, p 37–47

Groce N, Scheer J 1990 Introduction. Social Science and Medicine 30(8):v–vi

Groom MH 2003 Social cohesion: reflections on European sociopolitical policy concerning professional and disability issues in the European Year of People with Disabilities. British Journal of Occupational Therapy 66(2):82–85

Guadagnoli E, Ward P 1998 Patient participation in decision-making. Social Science and Medicine 47(3):329–339

Guardian Weekly 2003 Electoral shock. October 9–15:23

Guardian Weekly 2003 Curate wins right to contest cleft palate abortion case. December 4–10:9

Guardian Weekly 2004 Pregnant and proud among the pigeons. March 25–31:20

Guardian Weekly 2005 School is a feminist issue. Feb 11–17:31

Guter B 2004 Destination *Bent*: the story behind a cyber community for gay men with disabilities. In: Guter B, Killacky JR (eds) Queer crips. Disabled gay men and their stories. Harrington Park Press, New York, p 217–225

Guyatt GH, Naylor CD, Juniper E, et al for the Evidence-Based Medicine Working Group 1997 Users' guide to the medical literature XII. How to use articles about health-related quality of life. Journal of the American Medical Association 277(15):1232–1237

Hahn H 1988 The politics of physical differences: disability and discrimination. Journal of Social Issues 44(1):39–47

Hahn H 1993 The potential impact of disability studies on political science (as well as vice-versa). Policy Studies Journal 21(4):740–751

Hahn H 2002 Academic debates and political advocacy: the US Disability Movement. In: Barnes C, Oliver M, Barton L (eds) Disability studies today. Polity, Cambridge, p 162–189

Hale S 1991 Feminist method, process and self-criticism: interviewing Sudanese women. In: Gluck SB, Patai D (eds) Women's words. The feminist practice of oral history. Routledge, New York, p 121–136

Hall BL 1992 From margins to center? The development and purpose of participatory research. American Sociologist 23(4):15–28

Hall KM, Harper B, Whiteneck GG 1997 Follow-up study of individuals with high tetraplegia (C1–C4) 10 to 21 years post-injury. Topics in Spinal Cord Injury Rehabilitation 2(3):107–117

Hammell KW 1992 Psychological and sociological theories concerning adjustment to traumatic spinal cord injury: the implications for rehabilitation. Paraplegia 30(5):317–326

Hammell KW 1994a Psychosocial outcome following spinal cord injury. Paraplegia 32:771–779

Hammell KW 1994b Psychosocial outcome following severe closed head injury. International Journal of Rehabilitation Research 17:319–332

Hammell KW 1995 Spinal cord injury rehabilitation. Chapman and Hall, London

Hammell KW 1998a From the neck up: quality in life following high spinal cord injury. PhD thesis. University of British Columbia, Vancouver, Canada

Hammell KW 1998b Client-centered occupational therapy: collaborative planning, accountable intervention, In: Law M (ed) Client-centered occupational therapy. Slack, Thorofare, NJ, p123–143

Hammell KW 2000a High level injury: self-managed care and quality of life. Canadian Paraplegic Association: Total Access 1(3):31–32

Hammell KW 2000b Representation and accountability in qualitative research. In: Hammell KW, Carpenter C, Dyck I (eds) Using qualitative research. A practical introduction for occupational and physical therapists. Churchill Livingstone, Edinburgh, p 59–71

Hammell KW 2001a Intrinsicality: reconsidering spirituality, meaning(s) and mandates. Canadian Journal of Occupational Therapy 68(3):186–194

Hammell KW 2001b Using qualitative research to inform the client-centred, evidence-based practice of occupational therapy. British Journal of Occupational Therapy 64(5):228–234

Hammell KW 2002a Informing client-centred practice through qualitative enquiry: evaluating the quality of qualitative research. British Journal of Occupational Therapy 65(4):175–184

Hammell KW 2002b Graduate-entry master's degrees: benefits to clients? Letter to the editor. British Journal of Occupational Therapy 65(1):37

Hammell KW 2003a Changing institutional environments to enable occupation among people with severe physical impairments. In: Letts L, Rigby P, Stewart D (eds) Using environments to enable occupational performance. Slack, Thorofare, NJ, p 35–53

Hammell KW 2003b Intrinsicality: reflections on meanings and mandates. In: McColl MA (ed) Spirituality and occupational therapy. CAOT Publications, Ottawa, ON, p 67–82

Hammell KW 2004a The rehabilitation process. In: Stokes M (ed) Physical management in neurological rehabilitation, 2nd edn. Elsevier, Edinburgh, p 379–392

Hammell KW 2004b Using qualitative evidence to inform theories of occupation. In: Hammell KW, Carpenter C (eds) Qualitative research in evidence-based rehabilitation. Churchill Livingstone, Edinburgh, p 14–26

Hammell KW 2004c Using qualitative evidence as a basis for evidence-based practice. In: Hammell KW, Carpenter C (eds) Qualitative research in evidence-based rehabilitation. Churchill Livingstone, Edinburgh, p 129–143

Hammell KW 2004d Deviating from the norm: a sceptical interrogation of the ICF. British Journal of Occupational Therapy 67(9):408–411

Hammell KW 2004e Response to 'Deviating from the norm: a response from Pakistan'. British Journal of Occupational Therapy 67(11):515–516

Hammell KW 2004f Quality of life among people with high spinal cord injury living in the community. Spinal Cord 42(11):607–620

Hammell KW 2004g Impaired visions. Guardian Weekly. May 28–June 3:30

Hammell KW 2004h Dimensions of meaning in the occupations of daily life. Canadian Journal of Occupational Therapy 71(5):296–305

Hammell KW 2004i Exploring quality of life following high spinal cord injury: a review and critique. Spinal Cord 42(9):491–502

Hammell KW, Carpenter C 2000 Introduction to qualitative research in occupational therapy and physical therapy. In: Hammell KW, Carpenter C, Dyck I (eds) Using qualitative research. A practical introduction for occupational and physical therapists. Churchill Livingstone, Edinburgh p 1–12

Hammell KW, Carpenter C 2004 Qualitative research in evidence-based rehabilitation. Churchill Livingstone, Edinburgh

Hancock KM, Craig AR, Dickson HG, et al 1993 Anxiety and depression over the first year of spinal cord injury: a longitudinal study. Paraplegia 31:349–357

Haraway D 1988 Situated knowledges. Feminist Studies 14(3):575–599

Haraway D 1990 A manifesto for cyborgs: science, technology and socialist feminism in the 1980s. In: Nicholson L (ed) Feminism/postmodernism. Routledge, New York, p 190–233

Harding S 1986 The science question in feminism. Open University Press, Buckingham

Harding S 1987 Introduction: Is there a feminist method? In: Harding S (ed) Feminism and methodology. Indiana University Press, Bloomington, IN, p 1–14

Harries PA, Harries C 2001 Studying clinical reasoning, Part I: have we been taking the wrong 'track'? British Journal of Occupational Therapy 64(4):164–168

Harris A 1996 Responsibility and advocacy: representing young women. In: Wilkinson S, Kitzinger C (eds) Representing the other. Sage, London, p 152–155

Harris J 1987 QALYfying the value of life. Journal of Medical Ethics 13:117–123

Hartkopp A, Brønnum-Hansen H, Seidenschnur A-M, Biering-Sørensen F 1998 Suicide in a spinal cord injured population: its relation to functional status. Archives of Physical Medicine and Rehabilitation 79(11):1356–1361

Hartsock N 1990 Foucault on power: a theory for women? In: Nicholson LJ (ed) Feminism/postmodernism. Routledge, New York, p 157–175

Hasselkus BR 2002 The meaning of everyday occupation. Slack, Thorofare, NJ

Hawkins R, Stewart S 2002 Changing rooms: the impact of adaptations on the meaning of home for a disabled person and the role of occupational therapists in the process. British Journal of Occupational Therapy 65(2):81–87

Hayashi R, Okuhira M 2001 The Disability Rights Movement in Japan: past, present and future. Disability and Society 16(6):855–869

Hayim GJ 1980 The existential sociology of Jean-Paul Sartre. University of Massachusetts Press, Amherst, MA

Helfrich C, Kielhofner G 1994 Volitional narratives and the meaning of therapy. American Journal of Occupational Therapy 48:319–326

Hendey N, Pascall G 1998 Independent living: gender, violence and the threat of violence. Disability and Society 13(3):415–427

Hershey L 1997 The International Leadership Forum for Women. New Mobility 8(51):30–32

Hevey D 1992 The creatures time forgot: photography and disability imagery. Routledge, London

Hewitt C 2004 Sticks and stones. In: Guter B, Killacky JR (eds) Queer crips. Disabled gay men and their stories. Harrington Park Press, New York, p 13–16

Higgs J, Bithell C 2001 Professional expertise. In: Higgs J, Titchen A (eds) Practice knowledge and expertise in the health professions. Butterworth-Heinemann, Oxford, p 59–68

Higgs J, Jones M 2000 Clinical reasoning in the health professions, 2nd edn. Butterworth-Heinemann, Melbourne, Australia

Hill C 1997 Biographical disruption, narrative and identity in stroke: personal experience in acquired chronic illness. Auto/Biography 5:131–144

Hirsch K, Hirsch J 1995 Self-defining narratives: disability identity in the postmodern era. Disability Studies Quarterly 15(4):21–27

Hockenberry J 1995 Moving violations. Hyperion, New York

Hodge J 1994 The quality of life: a contrast between utilitarian and existentialist approaches. In: Baldwin S, Godfrey C, Propper C (eds) Quality of life. Perspectives and policies. Routledge, London, p 42–54

Hodgkin P 1996 Medicine, postmodernism and the end of certainty. British Medical Journal 313:1568–1569

Holcomb LO 2000 Community reintegration and chronic spinal cord injury. SCI Nursing 17(2):52–58

Holman HR 1993 Qualitative inquiry in medical research. Journal of Clinical Epidemiology 46(1):29–36

hooks b 1981 Ain't I a woman. Black women and feminism. South End Press, Boston, MA

hooks b 1984 Feminist theory: from margin to center. South End Press, Boston, MA

hooks b 1989 Talking back. Thinking feminist, thinking black. South End Press, Boston, MA

hooks b 1990 Yearning: race, gender and cultural politics. South End Press, Boston, MA

hooks b 1995 Killing rage. Ending racism. Henry Holt, New York

Houston S 2004 The centrality of impairment in the empowerment of people with severe physical impairments. Independent living and the threat of incarceration: a human right. Disability and Society 19(4):307–321

Hubbard R 1997 Abortion and disability. Who should and who should not inhabit the world? In: Davis LJ (ed) The disability studies reader. Routledge, New York, p 187–200

Hughes B 1999 The constitution of impairment: modernity and the aesthetic of oppression. Disability and Society 14(2):155–172

Hughes B 2000 Medicine and the aesthetic invalidation of disabled people. Disability and Society 15(4):555–568

Hughes B 2004 Disability and the body. In: Swain J, French S, Barnes C, Thomas C (eds) Disabling barriers – enabling environments, 2nd edn. Sage, London p 63–68

Hughes B, Paterson K 1997 The social model of disability and the disappearing body: towards a sociology of impairment. Disability and Society 12(3):325–340

Hughes G 1998 A suitable case for treatment? Constructions of disability. In: Saraga E (ed) Embodying the social: constructions of difference. Routledge & Open University Press, London, p 44–90

Hughes JL 2002 Illness narrative and chronic fatigue syndrome/myalgic encephalomyelitis: a review. British Journal of Occupational Therapy 65(1):9–14

Hugman R 1991 Power in caring professions. Macmillan, London

Humphries B, Mertens D, Truman C 2000 Arguments for an 'emancipatory' research paradigm. In: Truman C, Mertens D, Humphries B (eds) Research and inequality. UCL Press, London, p 3–23

Hunt J 1996 Joining in the dialogue set by disabled people (letter to the editor). British Journal of Occupational Therapy 59(5):243

Hunt P (ed) 1966 Stigma: the experience of disability. Geoffrey Chapman, London

Hunt P 1981 Settling accounts with the parasite people: a critique of 'A life apart' by EJ Miller and GV Gwynne. Disability Challenge 1:37–50

Hunt P 1998 A critical condition (1966). In: Shakespeare T (ed) The disability reader. Social science perspectives. Cassell, London, p 7–19

Hurley G 1983 Lucky break? Milestone Publications, Hampshire

Hurst R 1995 International perspectives and solutions. In Zarb G (ed) Removing disabling barriers. Policy Studies Institute, London, p 89–95

Hurst R 2000 To revise or not to revise? Disability and Society 15(7):1083–1087

Hyde P 2004 Fool's gold: examining the use of gold standards in the production of research evidence. British Journal of Occupational Therapy 67(2):89–94

Illich I 1976 Limits to medicine. Medical nemesis: the expropriation of health. Penguin, London

Illich I 1977 Disabling professions. Marian Boyars, New York

Ilott I, White E 2001 College of Occupational Therapists' Research and Development Strategic Vision and Action Plan. British Journal of Occupational Therapy 64(6):270–277

Imrie R 1996 Disability and the city: international perspectives. Paul Chapman, London

Imrie R 1997 Rethinking the relationships between disability, rehabilitation and society. Disability and Rehabilitation 19(7):263–271

Ingraham C 1994 The heterosexual imaginary: feminist sociology and theories of gender. Sociological Theory 12(2):203–219

Iwama M 2003 Toward culturally relevant epistemologies in occupational therapy. American Journal of Occupational Therapy 57(5):582–588

Jacob KS, Zachariah K, Bhattacharji S 1995 Depression in individuals with spinal cord injury: methodological issues. Paraplegia 33:377–380

Jagose A 1996 Queer theory. New York University Press, New York

Jarman M, Lamp S, Mitchell D, et al 2002 Theorising disability as political subjectivity: work by the UIC Disability Collective on political subjectivities. Disability and Society 17(5):555–569

Jary D, Jary J 1991 The Harper Collins Dictionary of Sociology. Harper Collins, New York

Jeffreys M 2002 The visible cripple (scars and other disfiguring displays included). In: Snyder SL, Brueggemann BJ, Garland-Thomson R (eds) Disability studies. Enabling the humanities. The Modern Language Association of America, New York, p 31–39

Jensen GM, Gwyer J, Shepard K, Hack L 2000 Expert practice in physical therapy. Physical Therapy 80(1):28–43

Johnson R 1993 'Attitudes don't just hang in the air . . .': disabled people's perceptions of physiotherapists. Physiotherapy 79(9):619–627

Johnston M, Miklos C 2002 Activity-related quality of life in rehabilitation and traumatic brain injury. Archives of Physical Medicine and Rehabilitation 83(Supp 2):S26–S38

Johnston M, Gilbert P, Partridge C, Collins J 1992 Changing perceived control in patients with physical disabilities: an intervention study with patients receiving rehabilitation. British Journal of Clinical Psychology 31:89–94

Johnston M, Nissim E, Wood K, et al 2002 Objective and subjective handicap following spinal cord injury: interrelationships and predictors. Journal of Spinal Cord Medicine 25:11–22

Johnstone D 1998 An introduction to disability studies. David Fulton, London

Jones C, Porter R 1994 Reassessing Foucault. Power, medicine and the body. Routledge, London

Jongbloed L, Crichton A 1990a A new definition of disability: implications for rehabilitation practice and social policy. Canadian Journal of Occupational Therapy 57:32–38

Jongbloed L, Crichton A 1990b Difficulties in shifting from individualistic to socio-political policy regarding disability in Canada. Disability, Handicap and Society 5(1):25–36

Jonsen AR, Siegler M, Winslade W 1998 Clinical ethics, 4th edn. McGraw Hill, New York

Jordan SA, Wellborn W, Kovnik J, Saltzstein R 1991 Understanding and treating motivational difficulties in ventilator dependent SCI patients. Paraplegia 29(7):431–442

Jorgensen P 2000 Concepts of body and health in physiotherapy: the meaning of the social/cultural aspects of life. Physiotherapy Theory and Practice 16:105–115

Juarez E 2002 The autobiography of the aching body in Teresa de Cartagena's *Arboleda de los enfermos*. In: Snyder SL, Brueggemann BJ, Garland-Thomson R (eds) Disability studies. Enabling the humanities. The Modern Language Association of America. New York, p 131–143

Kabzems V, Chimedza R 2002 Development assistance: disability and education in Southern Africa. Disability and Society 17(2):147–157

Kagawa-Singer M 1993 Redefining health: living with cancer. Social Science and Medicine 37:295–304

Kallen E 2004 Social inequality and social justice. A human rights perspective. Palgrave, Basingstoke, UK

Kaminker L 1997 No exceptions made: violence against women with disabilities. New Mobility 8(49):48–55

Kasnitz D, Shuttleworth RP 2001 Anthropology and disability studies. In: Rogers LJ, Swadener BB (eds) Semiotics and dis/ability. Interrogating categories of difference. State University of New York Press, Albany, NY, p 19–41

Katbamna S, Bhakta P, Parker G 2000 Perceptions of disability and care-giving relationships in South Asian communities. In: Ahmad WIV (ed) Ethnicity, disability and chronic illness. Open University Press, Buckingham, p 12–27

Kaufman S 1988a Illness, biography and the interpretation of self following a stroke. Journal of Aging Studies 2(3):217–227

Kaufman S 1988b Stroke rehabilitation and the negotiation of identity. In: Reinharz S, Rowles GD (eds) Qualitative gerontology. Springer, New York, p 82–103

Keany KC, Glueckauf RL 1993 Disability and value change: an overview and reanalysis of acceptance of loss theory. Rehabilitation Psychology 38:199–210

Keith L 1992 Who cares wins? Women, caring and disability. Disability, Handicap and Society 7(2):167–175

Keith L 2001 Take up thy bed and walk. Death, disability and cure in classic fiction for girls. The Women's Press, London

Keith RA 1995 Conceptual basis of outcome measures. American Journal of Physical Medicine and Rehabilitation 74:73–80

Kelly L, Regan L, Burton S 1992 Defending the indefensible? Quantitative methods and feminist research. In: Hinds H, Phoenix A, Stacey J (eds) Working out: new directions for women's studies. Falmer, London, p 149–160

Kelly MP, Field D 1996 Medical sociology, chronic illness and the body. Sociology of Health and Illness 18(2):241–257

Kemp L 2002 Why are some people's needs unmet? Disability and Society 17(2):205–218

Kennedy P, Rogers B 2000 Reported quality of life of people with spinal cord injuries: a longitudinal analysis of the first 6 months post-discharge. Spinal Cord 38:498–503

Kent D 1988 In search of a heroine: images of women with disabilities in fiction and drama. In: Fine M, Asch A (eds) Women with disabilities. Essays in psychology, culture, and politics. Temple University Press, Philadelphia, p 90–110

Kestenbaum V 1982 Preface. In: Kestenbaum V (ed) The humanity of the ill. Phenomenological perspectives. University of Tennessee Press, Knoxville, TN, p vii–x

Khanna T 2004 No choice without rights, say disability campaigners. OT Now 12(8):32

Kielhofner G 2004 Conceptual foundations of occupational therapy, 3rd edn. FA Davis, Philadelphia

Killacky JR 2004 Careening toward Kensho: ruminations on disability and community. In: Guter B, Killacky JR (eds) Queer crips. Disabled gay men and their stories. Harrington Park Press, New York, p 57–62

Kinchloe JL, McLaren PL 1994 Rethinking critical theory and qualitative research. In: Denzin NK, Lincoln YS (eds) Handbook of qualitative research. Sage, Thousand Oaks, CA, p 138–157

King M, McKeown E 2004 Gay and lesbian identities and mental health. In: Kelleher D, Leavey G (eds) Identity and health. Routledge, London, p 149–169

Kingwell M 1998 Better living: in pursuit of happiness from Plato to prozac. Penguin, Toronto

Kirk D, Tinning R 1994 Embodied self-identity, healthy lifestyles and school physical education. Sociology of Health and Illness 16(5):600–625

Kirsch GE 1999 Ethical dilemmas in feminist research. The politics of location, interpretation and publication. State University of New York Press, Albany, NY

Kitchin R 2000 The researched opinions on research: disabled people and disability research. Disability and Society 15(1):25–47

Kittay EF 2001 When caring is just and justice is caring: justice and mental retardation. In: Breckenridge CA, Vogler C (eds) The critical limits of embodiment. Reflections on disability criticism. Duke University Press, Durham, NC, p 557–579

Kitzinger C 1994 Experiential authority and heterosexuality. In: Griffin G (ed) Changing our lives: women in/to women's studies. Pluto, London, p 135–144

Kleiber DA, Hutchinson SL 1999 Heroic masculinity in the recovery from spinal cord injury. In: Sparkes A, Silvennoinen M (eds) Talking bodies: men's narratives of the body and sport. SoPhi, University of Jyväskylä, Jyväskylä, Finland, p 135–155

Kleiber DA, Brock SC, Lee Y, et al 1995 The relevance of leisure in an illness experience: realities of spinal cord injury. Journal of Leisure Research 27(3):283–299

Koch T 2000 Life quality vs the 'quality of life': assumptions underlying prospective quality of life instruments in health care planning. Social Science and Medicine 51:419–427

Krause JS 1992 Life satisfaction after spinal cord injury: a descriptive study. Rehabilitation Psychology 37(1):61–70

Krause JS 1997 Adjustment after spinal cord injury: a 9 year longitudinal study. Archives of Physical Medicine and Rehabilitation 78(6):651–657

Krause JS, Coker J, Charlifue S, Whiteneck G 2000 Health outcomes among American Indians with spinal cord injury. Archives of Physical Medicine and Rehabilitation 81(7):924–931

Krueger DW 1984 Issues in emotional rehabilitation. In: Krueger DW (ed) Rehabilitation psychology. Aspen, Rockville, MD, p 1–13

Kuhn TS 1962 The structure of scientific revolutions. Chicago University Press, London

Kupperman JJ 2001 Classic Asian philosophy. Oxford University Press, Oxford

Kyeong-Hee C 2001 Impaired body as colonial trope: Kang Kyong'ae's 'Underground village'. In: Breckenridge CA, Vogler C (eds) The critical limits of embodiment. Reflections on disability criticism. Duke University Press, Durham, NC, p 431–458

Laliberte-Rudman D, Yu B, Scott E, Pajouhandeh P 2000 Exploration of the perspectives of persons with schizophrenia regarding quality of life. American Journal of Occupational Therapy 54:137–147

Latour B 1987 Science in action. Open University Press, Buckingham, UK

Lavine TZ 1984 From Socrates to Sartre: the philosophic quest. Bantam, New York

Law M 1991 The environment: a focus for occupational therapy. Canadian Journal of Occupational Therapy 58(4):171–180

Law M 1992 Michel Foucault's historical perspective on normality and restrictive environments. Canadian Journal of Rehabilitation 5(4):193–203

Law M 1993 Evaluating activities of daily living: directions for the future. Canadian Journal of Occupational Therapy 47:233–237

Law M 1998 Does client-centered practice make a difference? In: Law M (ed) Client-centered occupational therapy, Slack, Thorofare, NJ, p 19–27

Law M 2002 Introduction to evidence-based practice. In: Law M (ed) Evidence-based rehabilitation: a guide to practice. Slack, Thorofare, NJ, p 3–12

Law M 2004 Building knowledge through participatory research. In: Hammell KW, Carpenter C (eds) Qualitative research in evidence-based rehabilitation. Churchill Livingstone, Edinburgh, p 40–50

Law M, Baum C 1998 Evidence based occupational therapy. Canadian Journal of Occupational Therapy 65(3):131–135

Law M, Baptiste S, Mills J 1995 Client-centered practice: what does it mean and does it make a difference? Canadian Journal of Occupational Therapy 62:250–257

Law M, Baptiste S, Carswell A, et al 1998 The Canadian Occupational Performance Measure, 3rd edn. CAOT Publications, Ottawa, ON

Lawson V 1995 The politics of difference: examining the quantitative/qualitative dualism in post-structuralist feminist research. Professional Geographer 47(4):449–457

Leary MR, Schreindorfer LS 1998 The stigmatization of HIV and AIDS. In: Derlega VJ, Barbee AP (eds) HIV and social interaction. Sage, Thousand Oaks, CA, p 12–29

Leavitt RL 1999a Cross-cultural rehabilitation. An international perspective. WB Saunders, London

Leavitt RL 1999b Moving rehabilitation professionals toward cultural competence: strategies for change. In: Leavitt RL (ed) Cross-cultural rehabilitation. An international perspective. WB Saunders, London, p 375–385

Leavitt RL 1999c Introduction. In: Leavitt RL (ed) Cross-cultural rehabilitation. An international perspective. WB Saunders, London, p 1–7

Leavitt RL 1999d Preface. In: Leavitt RL (ed) Cross-cultural rehabilitation. An international perspective. WB Saunders, London, p ix–x

Le Monde 2001 April 7 Humanity stripped to its bare essence. Reproduced in: Guardian Weekly May 17–23:26

Le Monde 2002 Feb 5 'I thank God I'm gay' says first priest to come out in Spain. Reproduced in: Guardian Weekly: February 14–20:34

Leplège A, Hunt S 1997 The problem of quality of life in medicine. Journal of the American Medical Association 278(1):47–50

Lewis J 1999 Headlights on full beam: disability and education in Hong Kong. In: Armstrong F, Barton L (eds) Disability, human rights and education. Cross-cultural perspectives. Open University Press, Buckingham, p 38–53

Ley P 1988 Communicating with clients. Chapman & Hall, London

Linton S 1998 Claiming disability: knowledge and identity. New York University Press, New York

Lloyd M 2001 The politics of disability and feminism: discord or synthesis? Sociology 35(3):715–728

Loew L, Rapin H 1994 The paradoxes of quality of life and its phenomenologic approach. Journal of Palliative Care 10(1):37–41

Longmore PK 1987 Screening stereotypes: images of disabled people in television and motion pictures. In: Gartner A, Joe T (eds) Images of the disabled, disabling images. Praeger, New York, p 65–78

Lorde A 1984 Sister outsider. Crossing Press, Trumansburg, New York

Lorimer EA 1984 Learned helplessness as a framework for practice in long-term care environments. Australian Occupational Therapy Journal 31(2):62–67

Luborsky M 1993 Sociocultural factors shaping technology usage. Technology and Disability 2(1):71–78

Lucke KT 1997 Knowledge acquisition and decision-making: spinal cord injured individuals' perceptions of caring during rehabilitation. SCI Nursing 14(3):87–95

Lugones MC, Spelman EV 1983 Have we got a theory for you! Feminist theory, cultural imperialism and the demand for the 'woman's voice'. Women's Studies International Forum 6(6):573–581

Lund ML, Nygård L 2004 Occupational life in the home environment: the experiences of people with disabilities. Canadian Journal of Occupational Therapy 71(4):243–251

Lyons M, Orozovic N, Davis J, Newman J 2002 Doing-being-becoming: occupational experiences of persons with life-threatening illnesses. American Journal of Occupational Therapy 56:285–295

MacDonald C, Houghton P, Cox P, Bartlett D 2001 Consensus on physical therapy professional behaviours. Physiotherapy Canada, Summer:212–218, 222

Macfarlane A 1996 Aspects of intervention: consultation, care, help and support. In: Hales G (ed) Beyond disability. Towards an enabling society. Open University and Sage, London, p 6–18

Mackelprang R, Salsgiver R 1999 Disability: a diversity model approach in human service practice. Brooks/Cole, Pacific Grove, CA

Mackelprang R, Salsgiver R 2000 A call to dialogue. SCI Psychosocial Process 13(4):197–199

Macleod L, Macleod G 1998 Control cognitions and psychological disturbance in people with contrasting physically disabling conditions. Disability and Rehabilitation 20(12):448–456

Malleson A 2002 Whiplash and other useful illnesses. McGill-Queen's University Press, Montreal & Kingston

Mann HS 1995 Women's rights versus feminism? Postcolonial perspectives. In: Rajan G, Mohanram R (eds) Postcolonial discourse and changing cultural contexts: theory and criticism. Greenwood Press, Westport, CN, p 69–88

Marks D 1999 Disability. Controversial debates and psychosocial perspectives. Routledge, London

Marquis R, Jackson R 2000 Quality of life and quality of service relationships: experiences of people with disabilities. Disability and Society 15(3):411–425

Martin B 1997 Extraordinary homosexuals and the fear of being ordinary. In: Weed E, Schor N (eds) Feminism meets queer theory. Indiana University Press, Bloomington, p 109–136

Martin M 2000 Critical education for participatory research. In: Truman C, Mertens DM, Humphries B (eds) Research and inequality. UCL Press, London, p 191–204

Mattingly C 1991 What is clinical reasoning? American Journal of Occupational Therapy 45(11):979–986

Mattingly C, Fleming MH 1994 Clinical reasoning: forms of inquiry in a therapeutic practice. FA Davis, Philadelphia

Mattson-Prince J 1997 A rational approach to long-term care: comparing the independent living model with agency-based care for persons with high spinal cord injuries. Spinal Cord 35:326–331

Matysiak B 2001 Interpretive research and people with intellectual disabilities: politics and practicalities. Research in Social Science and Disability 2:185–207

Maynard A 1997 Evidence-based medicine: an incomplete method for informing treatment choices. Lancet 349:126–128

Maynard FM 1993 Changing care needs. In: Whiteneck GG, Charlifue SW, Gerhart KA, et al (eds) Aging with spinal cord injury. Demos, New York, p 191–198

Maynard M 1994 Methods, practice and epistemology: the debate about feminist research. In: Maynard M, Purvis J (eds) Researching women's lives from a feminist perspective. Taylor and Francis, London, p 10–25

McColl MA 2000 Spirit, occupation and disability. Canadian Journal of Occupational Therapy 67(4):217–228

McColl MA, Bickenbach JE 1998a Introduction. In: McColl MA, Bickenbach JE (eds) Introduction to disability. WB Saunders, London, p 3–10

McColl MA, Bickenbach JE 1998b Introduction to disability. WB Saunders, London

McColl MA, Law M, Stewart D 1992 Theoretical basis of occupational therapy. Slack, Thorofare, NJ

McColl MA, Bickenbach J, Johnston J, et al 2000 Changes in spiritual beliefs after traumatic disability. Archives of Physical Medicine and Rehabilitation 81(6):817–823

McCuaig M, Frank G 1991 The able self: adaptive patterns and choices in independent living for a person with cerebral palsy. American Journal of Occupational Therapy 45(3):224–234

McGregor JC 1992 Pressure sores: a personal comment. Paraplegia 30(2):116–117

McKnight J 1981 Professionalised service and disabling help. In: Brechin A, Liddiard P, Swain J (eds) Handicap in a social world. Hodder & Stoughton, Sevenoaks, p 24–33

McMillen JC, Cook CL 2003 The positive by-products of spinal cord injury and their correlates. Rehabilitation Psychology 48:77–85

McMurray R, Heaton J, Sloper P, Nettleton S 2000 Variations in the provision of occupational therapy for patients undergoing primary elective total hip replacement in the United Kingdom. British Journal of Occupational Therapy 63(9):451–455

McRuer R 2002 Compulsory able-bodiedness and queer/disabled existence. In: Snyder S, Brueggemann BJ, Garland-Thomson R (eds) Disability Studies: enabling the humanities. The Modern Language Association of America, New York, p 88–99

McRuer R 2003 As good as it gets. Queer theory and critical disability. In: McRuer R, Wilkerson AL (eds) Desiring disability: queer theory meets disability studies. Duke University Press, Durham, NC, p 79–105

McRuer R, Wilkerson AL 2003 Introduction. In: McRuer R, Wilkerson AL (eds) Desiring disability: queer theory meets disability studies. Duke University Press, Durham, NC, p 1–23

Mead J 1998 Clinical effectiveness: another perspective to evidence-based healthcare. In: Bury T, Mead J (eds) Evidence-based healthcare. A practical guide for therapists. Butterworth-Heinemann, Oxford, p 26–42

Mead J 2000 Patient partnership. Physiotherapy 86(6):282–284

Mee J, Sumsion T 2001 Mental health clients confirm the motivating power of occupation. British Journal of Occupational Therapy 64:121–128

Meekosha H 1998 Body battles: bodies, gender and disability. In: Shakespeare T (ed) The disability reader: social science perspectives. Cassell, London, p 163–180

Mennell S 1991 On the civilizing of appetite. In: Featherstone M, Hepworth M, Turner B (eds) The body. Social process and cultural theory. Sage, London, p 126–156

Menzel P, Dolan P, Richardson J, Olsen JA 2002 The role of adaptation to disability and disease in health state valuation: a preliminary normative analysis. Social Science and Medicine 55:2149–2158

Mercer G 2004 From critique to practice: emancipatory disability research. In: Barnes C, Mercer G (eds) Implementing the social model of disability: theory and research. Disability Press, Leeds, p 118–137

Metts RL 2001 The fatal flaw in the disability adjusted life year. Disability and Society 16(3):449–452

Michalko R 2002 The difference that disability makes. Temple University Press, Philadelphia

Middleton L 1999 Disabled children: challenging social exclusion. Blackwell, Oxford

Miles M 1995 Disability in an Eastern religious context: historical perspectives. Disability and Society 10(1):49–69

Miles M 1996 Community, individual or information development? Dilemmas of concept and culture in South Asian disability planning. Disability and Society 11(4):485–500

Miles M 2000 Disability on a different model: glimpses of an Asian heritage. Disability and Society 15(4):603–618

Miles M, Hossain F 1999 Rights and disabilities in educational provision in Pakistan and Bangladesh: roots, rhetoric, reality. In: Armstrong F, Barton L (eds) Disability, human rights and education. Cross-cultural perspectives. Open University Press, Buckingham, p 67–86

Miles S 1996 Engaging with the disability rights movement: the experience of community-based rehabilitation in southern Africa. Disability and Society 11(4):501–517

Miles-Tapping C, Dyck A, Brunham S, et al 1990 Canadian therapists' priorities for clinical research. Physical Therapy 70(7):448–454

Miller EJ, Gwynne GV 1972 A life apart. Tavistock, London

Miller P, Parker S, Gillinson S 2004 Disabilism. How to tackle the last prejudice. Demos, London

Miller W, Crabtree B 2000 Clinical research. In: Denzin N, Lincoln Y (eds) Handbook of qualitative research, 2nd edn. Sage, Thousand Oaks, CA, p 607–631

Millward LM, Kelly MP 2003 Incorporating the biological. Chronic illness, bodies, selves, and the material world. In: Williams S, Birke L, Bendelow G (eds) Debating biology: sociological reflections on health, medicine and society. Routledge, London, 157–168

Mitchell DP 1996 Postmodernism, health and illness. Journal of Advanced Nursing 23:201–205

Mitchell D, Snyder SL 1997 The body and physical difference. Discourses of disability. University of Michigan Press, Ann Arbor, MI

Mitchell DT, Snyder SL 2000 Narrative prosthesis: disability and the dependencies of discourse. University of Michigan Press, Ann Arbor, MI

Mitchell DT, Snyder SL 2003 The Eugenic Atlantic: race, disability, and the making of an international eugenic science. Disability and Society 18(7):843–864

Mohanty CT 1994 Under Western eyes: feminist scholarship and colonial discourses. In: Williams P, Chrisman L (eds) Colonial discourse and postcolonial theory. Columbia University Press, New York, p 196–220

Moore M, Beazley S, Maelzer J 1998 Researching disability issues. Open University Press, Buckingham

Mor V, Guadagnoli E 1988 Quality of life measurement: a psychometric Tower of Babel. Journal of Clinical Epidemiology 41(11):1055–1058

Morris J 1989 Able lives. Women's experience of paralysis. Women's Press, London

Morris J 1991 Pride against prejudice. Transforming attitudes to disability. The Women's Press, London

Morris J 1992 Personal and political: a feminist perspective on researching physical disability. Disability, Handicap and Society 7(2):157–166

Morris J 1993a Independent lives? Community care and disabled people. Macmillan, Basingstoke, UK

Morris J 1993b Feminism and disability. Feminist Review 43:57–70

Morris J 1993c Gender and disability. In: Swain J, Finkelstein V, French S, Oliver M (eds) Disabling barriers – enabling environments. Sage, London, p 85–92

Morris J 1994 Gender and disability. In: French S (ed) On equal terms. Working with disabled people. Butterworth-Heinemann, Oxford, p 207–219

Morris J 1995 Creating a space for absent voices: disabled women's experience of receiving assistance with daily living activities. Feminist Review 51(Autumn):68–93

Morris J 1996 Encounters with strangers. Feminism and disability. Women's Press, London

Morris J 1997 Care or empowerment? A disability rights perspective. Social Policy and Administration 31(1):54–60

Morrison T 1992 Playing in the dark. Whiteness and the literary imagination. Pan Books, London

Mulkay M, Ashmore M, Pinch T 1987 Measuring the quality of life: a sociological invention concerning the application of economics to health care. Sociology 21(4):541–564

Mulvany J 2000 Disability, impairment or illness? The relevance of the social model of disability to the study of mental disorder. Sociology of Health and Illness 22(5):582–601

Murphy RF 1990 The body silent. New York, WW Norton

Murphy RF, Scheer J, Murphy Y, Mack R 1988 Physical disability and social liminality: a study in the rituals of adversity. Social Science and Medicine 26(2):235–242

Murray CJL, Acharya AK 1997 Understanding DALYs. Journal of Health Economics 16:703–730

Murray CJL, Lopez AD 1996 The global burden of disease. WHO, Geneva

Namsoo AC, Armstrong D 1999 Human rights and the struggle for inclusive education in Trinidad and Tobago. In: Armstrong F, Barton L (eds) Disability, human rights and education. Cross-cultural perspectives. Open University Press, Buckingham, p 24–37

Needham G, Oliver S 1998 Involving service users. In: Bury T, Mead J (eds) Evidence-based healthcare. A practical guide for therapists. Butterworth-Heinemann, Oxford, 85–103

Neistadt M 1995 Methods of assessing clients' priorities: a survey of adult physical dysfunction. American Journal of Occupational Therapy 49(5):428–436

Nettleton S 1994 Inventing mouths: disciplinary power and dentistry. In: Jones C, Porter R (eds) Reassessing Foucault. Power, medicine and the body. Routledge, London, p 73–90

Nettleton S 1995 The sociology of health and illness. Polity Press, Cambridge

Neufeldt AH 1999 'Appearances' of disability, discrimination and the transformation of rehabilitation service practices. In: Leavitt RL (ed) Cross-cultural rehabilitation: an international perspective. WB Saunders, London, p 25–36

New Internationalist 1992 Disabled lives. New Internationalist 233:1–28

Ngugi wa Thiong'o 1986 Decolonizing the mind: the politics of language in African literature. James Currey, London

NHS Executive 1997 Rehabilitation: a guide. Department of Health, Leeds

NHS Executive 1999 Patient and public involvement in the new NHS. Department of Health, London

Nijhof G 1995 Parkinson's disease as a problem of shame in public appearances. Sociology of Health and Illness 17(2):193–205

Norman RJ 1995 Autonomy in applied ethics. In: Honderich T (ed) The Oxford companion to philosophy. Oxford University Press, Oxford, p 70

Northway R 1997 Disability and oppression: some implications for nurses and nursing. Journal of Advanced Nursing 26:736–743

Oakley A 1981 Interviewing women: a contradiction in terms. In: Roberts H (ed) Doing feminist research. Routledge, London, p 30–59

Oliver M 1981 Disability, adjustment and family life – some theoretical considerations. In: Brechin A, Liddiard P, Swain J (eds) Handicap in a social world. Hodder & Stoughton, London, p 49–57

Oliver M 1983 Social work with disabled people. Macmillan, Basingstoke, UK

Oliver M 1987 Re-defining disability: a challenge to research. Research Policy and Planning 5:9–13

Oliver M 1990 The politics of disablement. Macmillan, Basingstoke, UK

Oliver M 1992 Changing the social relations of research production? Disability, Handicap and Society 7(2):101–114

Oliver M 1993 Societal responses to long-term disability. In: Whiteneck GG, Charlifue SW, Gerhart KA, et al (eds) Aging with spinal cord injury. Demos, New York, p 251–262

Oliver M 1996a Understanding disability. From theory to practice. Macmillan, Basingstoke

Oliver M 1996b A sociology of disability or a disablist sociology? In: Barton L (ed) Disability and society. Longman, London, p 18–42

Oliver M 1997 Emancipatory research: realistic goal or impossible dream? In: Barnes C, Mercer G (eds) Doing disability research. The Disability Press, Leeds, p 15–31

Oliver M 1998 Theories of disability in health practice and research. British Medical Journal 317:1446–1449

Oliver M 1999 Final accounts and the parasite people. In: Corker M, French S (eds) Disability discourse. Open University Press, Buckingham, p 183–191

Oliver M 2004 The social model in action: if I had a hammer. In: Barnes C, Mercer G (eds) Implementing the social model of disability: theory and research. The Disability Press, Leeds, p 18–31

Oliver M, Barnes C 1998 Disabled people and social policy: from exclusion to inclusion. Longman, London

Oliver M, Hasler F 1987 Disability and self-help: a case study of the Spinal Injuries Association. Disability, Handicap and Society 2(2):113–125

Oliver M, Sapey B 1999 Social work with disabled people, 2nd edn. Macmillan, Basingstoke, UK

Oliver M, Zarb G, Silver J, Moore M, Salisbury V 1988 Walking into darkness: the experience of spinal cord injury. Macmillan, Basingstoke, UK

Opie A 1992 Qualitative research, appropriation of the 'other' and empowerment. Feminist Review 40:52–69

Pain K, Dunn M, Anderson G, Darrah J, Kratochvil M 1998 Quality of life: what does it mean in rehabilitation? Journal of Rehabilitation 64(2): 5–11

Parker G 1993 A four-way stretch? The politics of disability and caring. In: Swain J, Finkelstein V, French S, Oliver M (eds) Disabling barriers – enabling environments. Sage, London, p 249–256

Parks S 2001 Overcoming the legacy of Nazism. New Mobility 12(93):55–57, 86

Patai D 1991 US academics and third world women: Is ethical research possible? In: Gluck SB, Patai D (eds) Women's words. The feminist practice of oral history. Routledge, New York, p 137–153

Paterson K, Hughes B 2000 Disabled bodies. In: Hancock P (ed) Body, culture and society. Open University Press, Buckingham, p 29–44

Peace S 1993 Negotiating. In: Shakespeare P, Atkinson D, French S (eds) Reflecting on research practice. Issues in health and social welfare. Open University Press, Buckingham, p 25–35

Pearson D, Osgerby C 2004 Letters to the editor: Annual conference. British Journal of Occupational Therapy 67(10):466

Peloquin SM 1990 The patient-therapist relationship in occupational therapy: understanding visions and images. American Journal of Occupational Therapy 44:13–21

Penn H 1999 Children in the majority world: is outer Mongolia really so far away? In: Hood S, Mayall B, Oliver S (eds) Critical issues in social research. Power and prejudice. Open University Press, Buckingham, p 25–39

Peoples J, Bailey G 1994 Humanity. An introduction to cultural anthropology, 3rd edn. West, St Paul, MN

Peters DJ 1995 Human experience in disablement: the imperative of the ICIDH. Disability and Rehabilitation 17(3/4):135–144

Pfeiffer D 1998 The ICIDH and the need for its revision. Disability and Society 13(4):503–523

Pfeiffer D 1999 The categorization and control of people with disabilities. Disability and Rehabilitation 21(3):106–107

Pfeiffer D 2000 The devils are in the details: the ICIDH2 and the disability movement. Disability and Society 15(7):1079–1082

Pfeiffer D 2001 The conceptualization of disability. Research in Social Science and Disability 2:29–52

Pfeiffer D 2003 The disability studies paradigm. In: Devlieger P, Rusch F, Pfeiffer D (eds) Rethinking disability. The emergence of new definitions, concepts and communities. Garant, Antwerp, p 95–106

Philpott S, Washeila S 2001 Disabled children: an emergency submerged. In: Priestley M (ed) Disability and the life course. Global perspectives. Cambridge University Press, Cambridge, p 151–166

Pieters T 1998 Marketing medicines through randomized controlled trials: the case. British Medical Journal 317:1231–1233

Pinder R 1995 Bringing the body back in without the blame? The experience of ill and disabled people at work. Sociology of Health and Illness 17(5):605–631

Plahuta JM, McCulloch BJ, Kasarshis EJ, 2002 Amyotrophic lateral sclerosis and hopelessness: psychosocial factors. Social Science and Medicine 55:2131–2140

Plato 1993 Phaedo (trans. D Gallop). Oxford University Press, Oxford

Pollock N 1993 Client centered assessment. American Journal of Occupational Therapy 47:298–301

Poore C 2002 'No friend of the Third Reich'. Disability as the basis for antifascist resistance in Arnold Zweig's Das Beil von Wandsbek. In: Snyder SL, Brueggemann BJ, Garland-Thomson R (eds) Disability studies. Enabling the humanities. The Modern Language Association of America. New York, p 260–270

Pope C, Mays N 2000 Qualitative research in health care, 2nd edn. BMJ Books, London

Porter JI 1997 Foreword. In: Mitchell D, Snyder SL (eds) The body and physical difference. Discourses of disability. University of Michigan Press, Ann Arbor, MI, p xiii–xiv

Post M, de Witte L, van Asbek F, et al 1998 Predictors of health status and life satisfaction in spinal cord injury. Archives of Physical Medicine and Rehabilitation 78(4):395–402

Pound P, Bury M, Gompertz P, Ebrahim S 1995 Stroke patients views on their admission to hospital. British Medical Journal 311:18–22

Prakash G 1994 Subaltern studies as postcolonial criticism. American Historical Review 99(5):1475–1490

Price J, Shildrick M 1998 Uncertain thoughts on the dis/abled body. In: Shildrick M, Price J (eds) Vital signs: feminist reconfigurations of the bio/logical body. Edinburgh University Press, Edinburgh, p 224–249

Priestley M 1999 Disability politics and community care. Jessica Kingsley, London

Priestley M 2003 Disability. A life course approach. Polity Press, Cambridge

Punch M 1994 Politics and ethics in qualitative research. In: Denzin NK, Lincoln Y (eds) Handbook of qualitative research. Sage, London p 83–97

Purves B, Suto M 2004 In limbo: creating continuity of identity in a discharge planning unit. Canadian Journal of Occupational Therapy 71(3):173–181

Putzke JD, Richards JS, Hicken BL, DeVivo MJ 2002 Predictors of life satisfaction: a spinal cord injury cohort study. Archives of Physical Medicine and Rehabilitation 83(4):555–561

Radnitz CL, Tirch D 1995 Substance misuse in individuals with spinal cord injury. The International Journal of Addictions 30:1117–1140

Raithatha N 1997 Medicine, postmodernism, and the end of certainty. Postmodern philosophy offers a more appropriate system for medicine. British Medical Journal 314:1044

Ransome P 1992 Antonio Gramsci. A new introduction. Harvester Wheatsheaf, Hemel Hempstead, UK

Rawles J 1989 Castigating QALYs. Journal of Medical Ethics 15:143–147

Ray LD, Mayan M 2001 Who decides what counts as evidence? In: Morse J, Swanson J, Kuzel A (eds) The nature of qualitative evidence. Sage, Thousand Oaks, CA, p 50–73

Rebeiro K 2000 Client perspectives on occupational therapy practice: are we truly client-centred? Canadian Journal of Occupational Therapy 67(1):7–14

Rebeiro K 2004 How qualitative research can inform and challenge occupational therapy practice. In: Hammell KW, Carpenter C (eds) Qualitative research in evidence-based rehabilitation. Churchill Livingstone, Edinburgh, p 89–102

Rebeiro KL, Day D, Semeniuk B, et al 2001 Northern Initiative for Social Action: an occupation-based mental health program. American Journal of Occupational Therapy 55:493–500

Reindal SM 1999 Independence, dependence, interdependence: some reflections on the subject and personal autonomy. Disability and Society 14(3):353–367

Reviere R, Hylton K 1999 Poverty and health: an international overview. In: Leavitt RL (ed) Cross-cultural rehabilitation. An international perspective. WB Saunders, London, p 59–69

Reynolds F 2003 Exploring the meanings of artistic occupation for women living with chronic illness: a comparison of template and interpretive phenomenological approaches to analysis. British Journal of Occupational Therapy 66:551–557

Reynolds F 2004a The professional context. In: Swain J, Clark J, Parry K, et al (eds) Enabling relationships in health and social care. Butterworth-Heinemann, Oxford, p 17–27

Reynolds F 2004b Two-way communication. In: Swain J, Clark J, Parry K, et al (eds) Enabling relationships in health and social care. Butterworth-Heinemann, Oxford, p 109–130

Reynolds F 2005 Communication and clinical effectiveness in rehabilitation. Elsevier, Edinburgh

Ribbens J, Edwards R 1998 Feminist dilemmas in qualitative research. Public knowledge and private lives. Sage, London

Richardson B 1999 Professional development. 2. Professional knowledge and situated learning in the workplace. Physiotherapy 85(9):467–474

Richardson L 1990 Narrative and sociology. Journal of Contemporary Ethnography 19(1):116–135

Richardson M 1997 Addressing barriers: disabled rights and the implications for nursing of the social construct of disability. Journal of Advanced Nursing 25:1269–1275

Riger S 1992 Epistemological debates, feminist voices. Science, social values and the study of women. American Psychologist 47:730–740

Rintala DH, Hart KA, Fuhrer MJ 1996 Perceived stress in individuals with spinal cord injury. In: Krotoski DM, Nosek MA, Turk MA (eds) Women with physical disabilities.

Achieving and maintaining health and well-being. Paul H Brookes, Baltimore, MD, p 223–242

Rioux M 1999 Inclusive education in Canada: a piece in the equality puzzle. In: Armstrong F, Barton L (eds) Disability, human rights and education. Cross-cultural perspectives. Open University Press, Buckingham, p 87–99

Rioux M 2001 Bending towards justice. In: Barton L (ed) Disability politics and the struggle for change. David Fulton, London, p 34–47

Ritchie JE 1999 Using qualitative research to enhance the evidence-based practice of health care providers. Australian Journal of Physiotherapy 45:251–256

Ritchie JE 2001 Case series research: a case for qualitative method in assessing evidence. Physiotherapy Theory and Practice 17:127–135

Roberts K 1996 Some observations on the 'Disability Movement'. Forward: Spinal Injuries Association, May:15

Robson C 1993 Real world research. A resource for social scientists and practitioner-researchers. Blackwell, Oxford

Rock M 2000 Discounted lives? Weighing disability when measuring health and ruling on 'compassionate' murder. Social Science and Medicine 51:407–417

Rockhill K 1996 And still I fight. In: Tremain S (ed) Pushing the limits. Disabled dykes produce culture. Women's Press, Toronto, p 172–187

Rogers JC, Holm MB 1994 Accepting the challenge of outcome research: Examining the effectiveness of occupational therapy practice. American Journal of Occupational Therapy 48:871–876

Rogers LJ, Swadener BB 2001 Introduction. In: Rogers LJ, Swadener BB (eds) Semiotics and dis/ability. Interrogating categories of difference. State University of New York Press, Albany, NY, p 1–15

Rohe DE, Athelstan G 1982 Vocational interests of persons with spinal cord injury. Journal of Counseling Psychology 29:283–291

Rose S 2004 Nature's best chat-up lines. Guardian Weekly Sept 17–23:29

Rosenberg W, Donald A 1995 Evidence-based medicine: an approach to clinical problem-solving. British Medical Journal 310:1122–1126

Rossiter A 2000 The postmodern feminist condition. New conditions for social work. In: Fawcett B, Featherstone B, Fook J, Rossiter A (eds) Practice + research in social work. Postmodern feminist perspectives. Routledge, London, p 24–38

Rossiter A, Prilletensky I, Walsh-Bowers R 2000 A postmodern perspective on professional ethics. In: Fawcett B, Featherstone B, Fook J, Rossiter A (eds) Practice + research in social work. Postmodern feminist perspectives. Routledge, London, p 83–103

Rotter JB 1966 Generalized expectancies for internal versus external control of reinforcement. Psychology Monograph 80:1–28

Roughgarden J 2004 Evolution's rainbow: diversity, gender and sexuality in nature and in people. University of California Press, Berkeley, CA

Roy DJ 1992 Editorial. Measurement in the service of compassion. Journal of Palliative Care 8(3):3–4

Rubin G 1997 Sexual traffic. Interview (with Judith Butler). In: Weed E, Schor N (eds) Feminism meets queer theory. Indiana University Press, Bloomington, IN, p 68–108

Ryen A 2000 Colonial methodology? In: Truman C, Mertens D, Humphries B (eds) Research and inequality. UCL Press, London, p 67–79

Sackett DL, Rosenberg W, Gray J, et al 1996 Evidence-based medicine: what it is and what it isn't. British Medical Journal 312:71–72

Sackett D, Strauss S, Richardson W, et al 2000 Evidence-based medicine. How to practice and teach EBM, 2nd edn. Churchill Livingstone, Edinburgh

Sacks O 1991 A leg to stand on. Pan, London

Sacks O 1996 The island of the colour blind. Random House, New York

Safilios-Rothschild C 1981 Disabled persons' self-definitions and their implications for rehabilitation. In: Brechin A, Liddiard P, Swain J (eds) Handicap in a social world. Open University and Hodder & Stoughton, London, p 5–13

Said EW 1976 Interview. Diacritics 6(3):30–47

Said EW 1979 Orientalism. Routledge, London

Said EW 1989 Representing the colonized: anthropology's interlocutors. Critical Inquiry 15:205–225

Said EW 1993 Culture and imperialism. Vintage, New York

Said EW 1996 Representations of the intellectual. Random House, New York

Saleeby D 1994 Culture, theory and narrative: the intersection of meanings in practice. Social Work 39(4):351–359

Salmon N 2003 Service evaluation and the service user: a pluralistic solution. British Journal of Occupational Therapy 66(7):311–317

Sandahl C 2003 Queering the crip or cripping the queer? In: McRuer R, Wilkerson AL (eds) Desiring disability: queer theory meets disability studies. Duke University Press, Durham, NC, p 25–56

Sanders C, Donovan J, Dieppe P 2002 The significance and consequences of having painful and disabled joints in old age: co-existing accounts of normal and disrupted biographies. Sociology of Health and Illness 24:227–253

Sapey B 2004 Disability and social exclusion in the information society. In: Swain J, French S, Barnes C, Thomas C (eds) Disabling barriers – enabling environments, 2nd edn. Sage, London p 273–278

Sartre J-P 1956 Being and nothingness (trans. H Barnes). Washington Square, New York

Scheer J 1994 Culture and disability: an anthropological point of view. In: Trickett EJ, Watts RJ, Birman D (eds) Human diversity: perspectives on people in context. Jossey-Bass, San Francisco, CA, p 244–260

Scheer J, Groce N 1988 Impairment as a human constant: cross-cultural and historical perspectives on variation. Journal of Social Issues 44(1):23–37

Scholnick RJ 2002 "How dare a sick man or an obedient man write poems?" Whitman and the dis-ease of the perfect body. In: Snyder SL, Brueggemann BJ, Garland-Thomson R (eds) Disability studies. Enabling the humanities. The Modern Language Association of America, New York, p 248–259

Schriner K 2001 A disability studies perspective on employment issues and policies for disabled people. In: Albrecht GL, Seelman KD, Bury M (eds) Handbook of disability studies. Sage, London, p 642–662

Schwartz CE, Sendor M 1999 Helping others helps oneself: response shift effects in peer support. Social Science and Medicine 48:1563–1575

Scullion P 1999 'Disability' in a nursing curriculum. Disability and Society 14(4):539–559

Seidman S 1994 Symposium: queer theory/sociology. A dialogue. Sociological Theory 12(2):166–177

Seidman S 1995 Deconstructing queer theory or the under-theorization of the social and the ethical. In: Nicholson L, Seidman S (eds) Social postmodernism. Beyond identity politics. Cambridge University Press, Cambridge, p 116–141

Selden R, Widdowson P 1993 A reader's guide to contemporary literary theory, 3rd edn. University Press of Kentucky, Lexington, KT

Seligman M 1975 Helplessness, on depression, development and death. W.H. Freeman, San Francisco, CA

Seligman M, Abramson L, Semmel A, von Bayer C 1979 Depressive attributional style. Journal of Abnormal Psychology 88:242–247

Serlin D 2003 Crippling masculinity. Queerness and disability in U.S. military culture, 1800–1945. In: McRuer R, Wilkerson AL (eds) Desiring disability: queer theory meets disability studies. Duke University Press, Durham, NC, p 149–179

Seymour W 1989 Bodily alterations. Allen & Unwin, Sydney

Seymour W 1998 Remaking the body. Rehabilitation and change. Routledge, London

Shackelford M, Farley T, Vines CL 1998 A comparison of women and men with spinal cord injury. Spinal Cord 36(5):337–339

Shakespeare T 1994 Cultural representation of disabled people: dustbins for disavowal? Disability and Society 9(3)283–299

Shakespeare T 1996a Rules of engagement: doing disability research. Disability and Society 11(1):115–119

Shakespeare T 1996b Disability, identity and difference. In: Barnes C, Mercer G (eds) Exploring the divide. Illness and disability. The Disability Press, Leeds, p 94–113

Shakespeare T 1996c Power and prejudice: issues of gender, sexuality and disability. In: Barton L (ed) Disability and society: emerging issues and insights. Longman, Harlow, UK, p 191–214

Shakespeare T 1997a Reviewing the past, developing the future. Skill Journal 58:8–11

Shakespeare T 1997b Researching disabled sexuality. In: Barnes C, Mercer G (eds) Doing disability research. The Disability Press, Leeds, p 177–189

Shakespeare T 1998a Introduction. In: Shakespeare T (ed) The disability reader. Social science perspectives. Cassell, London, p 1–3

Shakespeare T 1998b Afterword. In: Shakespeare T (ed) The disability reader. Social science perspectives. Cassell, London, p 256–257

Shakespeare T 1999 When is a man not a man? When he's disabled. In: Wild J (ed) Working with men for change. UCL Press, London, p 47–58

Shakespeare T 2003 Rights, risks and responsibilities. New genetics and disabled people. In: Williams S, Birke L, Bendelow G (eds) Debating biology: sociological reflections on health, medicine and society. Routledge, London, p 198–209

Shakespeare T, Watson N 2001a The social model of disability: an outdated ideology? Research in Social Science and Disability 2:9–28

Shakespeare T, Watson N 2001b Disability, politics and recognition. In: Albrecht GL, Seelman KD, Bury M (eds) Handbook of disability studies. Sage, London, p 546–564

Shakespeare T, Gillespie-Sells K, Davies D 1996 The sexual politics of disability. Cassell, London

Shapiro JP 1993 No pity: people with disabilities forging a new civil rights movement. Times Books, New York

Sharp K, Earle S 2002 Feminism, abortion and disability: irreconcilable differences? Disability and Society 17(2):137–145

Sheldon A 1999 Personal and perplexing: feminist disability politics evaluated. Disability and Society 14(5):643–657

Sherry M 2004 Overlaps and contradictions between queer theory and disability studies. Disability and Society 19(7):769–783

Sherwin S 2002 Towards a feminist ethics of health care. In: Fulford K, Dickenson D, Murray T (eds) Healthcare ethics and human values. Blackwell, London, p 25–28

Shilling C 1993 The Body and social theory. Sage, London

Shuttleworth RP 2001 Symbolic contexts, embodied sensitivities, and the experience of sexually relevant interpersonal encounters for a man with severe cerebral palsy. In: Rogers LJ, Swadener BB (eds) Semiotics and dis/ability. Interrogating categories of difference. State University of New York Press, Albany, NY, p 75–95

Sidell M 1993 Interpreting. In: Shakespeare P, Atkinson D, French S (eds) Reflecting on research practice. Open University Press, Buckingham, p 106–118

Silburn L, Dookum D, Jones C 1994 Innovative practice. In: French S (ed) On equal terms. Working with disabled people. Butterworth-Heinemann, Oxford, p 250–263

Silvers A 1994 'Defective' agents: equality, difference and the tyranny of the normal. Journal of Social Philosophy 25:154–175

Silvers A 2002 The crooked timber of humanity: disability, ideology and the aesthetic. In: Corker M, Shakespeare T (eds) Disability/postmodernity. Embodying disability theory. Continuum, London, p 228–244

Siminski P 2003 Patterns of disability and norms of participation through the life course: empirical support for a social model of disability. Disability and Society 18(6):707–718

Simpson N 1996 Some observations on the 'Disability Movement'. Forward: Spinal Injuries Association May:15

Singer P, McVie J, Kuhse H, Richardson J 1995 Double jeopardy and the use of QALYs in health care allocation. Journal of Medical Ethics 21:144–150

Skeggs B 1995 Introduction. In: Skeggs B (ed) Feminist cultural theory. Process and production. Manchester University Press, Manchester, p 1–29

Slevin ML, Plant H, Lynch D, et al 1988 Who should measure quality of life, the doctor or the patient? British Journal of Cancer 57:109–112

Smith B, Sparkes A 2004 Men, sport, and spinal cord injury: an analysis of metaphors and narrative types. Disability and Society 19(6):613–626

Snyder SL 2002 Infinities of form: disability figures in artistic traditions. In: Snyder SL, Brueggemann BJ, Garland-Thomson R (eds) Disability studies. Enabling the humanities. The Modern Language Association of America. New York, p 173–196

Snyder SL, Mitchell DT 2001 Re-engaging the body: disability studies and the resistance to embodiment. In: Breckenridge CA, Vogler C (eds) The critical limits of embodiment. Reflections on disability criticism. Duke University Press, Durham, NC, p 367–389

Soden RJ, Walsh J, Middleton JW, et al 2000 Causes of death after spinal cord injury. Spinal Cord 38(10):604–610

Solomon A 2001 The noonday demon: an atlas of depression. Simon & Schuster, New York

Somers MR 1994 The narrative construction of identity: a relational and network approach. Theory and Society 23:605–649

Somers MR, Gibson GD 1994 Reclaiming the epistemological 'other': narrative and the social construction of identity. In: Calhoun C (ed) Social theory and the politics of identity. Blackwell, Oxford, p 37–99

Somner KL, Baumeister RF 1998 The construction of meaning from life events. In: Wong PT, Fry PS (eds) The human quest for meaning. Lawrence Erlbaum, Mahwah, NJ, p 143–161

Sparkes A, Smith B 1999 Disrupted selves and narrative reconstructions. In: Sparkes A, Silvennoinen M (eds) Talking bodies: men's narratives of the body and sport. SoPhi, University of Jyväskylä, Jyväskylä, Finland, p 76–92

Spencer J, Krefting L, Mattingly C 1993 Incorporation of ethnographic methods in occupational therapy assessment. American Journal of Occupational Therapy 47(4):303–309

Spencer J, Young ME, Rintala D, Bates S 1995 Socialization to the culture of a rehabilitation hospital: an ethnographic study. American Journal of Occupational Therapy 49(1):53–62

Spiro ME 1993 Is the Western conception of the self 'peculiar' within the context of the world cultures? Ethos 21(2):107–153

Stables J, Smith F 1999 'Caught in the Cinderella trap': narratives of disabled parents and young carers. In: Butler R, Parr H (eds) Mind and body spaces. Geographies of illness, impairment and disability. Routledge, London, p 256–268

Stainton T 2004 Reason's Other: the emergence of the disabled subject in the Northern Renaissance. Disability and Society 19(3):227–243

Stalker K, Jones C 1998 Normalization and critical disability theory. In: Jones D, Blair S, Hartery T, Jones R (eds) Sociology and occupational therapy: an integrated approach. Churchill Livingstone, Edinburgh, p 171–183

Steele DJ, Blackwell B, Guttman M, Jackson T 1987 The activated patient: dogma, dream or desideratum? Patient Education and Counseling 10:3–23

Stein A, Plummer K 1994 'I can't even think straight'. 'Queer' theory and the missing sexual revolution in sociology. Sociological Theory 12(2):178–187

Steinglass P, Temple S, Lisman S, Reiss D 1982 Coping with spinal cord injury: the family perspective. General Hospital Psychiatry 4:359–264

Stenner PHD, Cooper D, Skevington SM 2003 Putting the Q into quality of life; the identification of subjective constructions of health-related quality of life using Q methodology. Social Science and Medicine 57:2161–2172

Stevenson O, Parsloe P 1993 Community care and empowerment. Joseph Rowntree Foundation, London

Stewart D 2002 The new ICF: International Classification of Functioning, Disability and Health. Concepts and implementation issues for occupational therapists. OT Now July/Aug:17–21

Stewart R, Bhagwanjee A 1999 Promoting group empowerment and self-reliance through participatory research: a case study of people with physical disability. Disability and Rehabilitation 21(7):338–345

Stewart W 1985 Counselling in rehabilitation. Croom Helm, London

Stiker H-J 1999 A history of disability (trans. W Sayers). University of Michigan Press, Ann Arbor, MI

Stillman P 1994 The quad squad. New Mobility, September–October:11–15

Stone E 1997 From the research notes of a foreign devil: disability research in China. In: Barnes C, Mercer G (eds) Doing disability research. The Disability Press, Leeds, p 207–227

Stone E 1999 Disability and development in the majority world. In: Stone E (ed) Disability and development. Learning from action and research on disability in the majority world. The Disability Press, Leeds, p 1–18

Stone E 2001 A complicated struggle: survival and social change in the majority world. In: Priestley M (ed) Disability and the life course. Global perspectives. Cambridge University Press, Cambridge, p 50–63

Stone E, Priestley M 1996 Parasites, pawns and partners: disability research and the role of non-disabled researchers. British Journal of Sociology 47(4):699–716

Stratford P, Gill C, Westaway M, Binkley J 1995 Assessing disability and change on individual patients: a report of a patient-specific measure. Physiotherapy Canada 47(4):258–262

Strong J, Gilbert J, Cassidy S, Bennet S 1995 Expert clinicians' and students' views on clinical reasoning in occupational therapy. British Journal of Occupational Therapy 58(3):119–123

Stuart CA 1998 Care and concern: an ethical journey in participatory action research. Canadian Journal of Counselling 32(4):298–313

Stubbs S 1999 Engaging with difference: soul-searching for a methodology in disability and development research. In: Stone E (ed) Disability and development. The Disability Press, Leeds, p 257–279

Sumsion T 1998 The Delphi technique: an adaptive research tool. British Journal of Occupational Therapy 61(4):153–156

Sumsion T 2000 A revised occupational therapy definition of client-centred practice. British Journal of Occupational Therapy 63(7):304–309

Sunday Times 1999 Disabled children will be a 'sin', says scientist. Sunday Times: 4 July, p 28

Sutherland A 1981 Disabled we stand. Souvenir, London

Suto M 2004 Exploring leisure meanings that inform client-centred practice. In: Hammell KW, Carpenter C (eds) Qualitative research in evidence-based rehabilitation. Churchill Livingstone, Edinburgh, p 27–39

Swain J 2004a International perspectives on disability. In: Swain J, French S, Barnes C, Thomas C (eds) Disabling barriers – enabling environments, 2nd edn. Sage, London, p 54–60

Swain J 2004b Challenging walls of discrimination. In: Swain J, Clark J, Parry K, et al (eds) Enabling relationships in health and social care. Butterworth-Heinemann, Oxford, p 151–164

Swain J 2004c From theory to principles. In: Swain J, Clark J, Parry K, et al (eds) Enabling relationships in health and social care. Butterworth-Heinemann, Oxford, p 77–91

Swain J, French S 2000 Towards an affirmation model of disability. Disability and Society 15(4):569–582

Swain J, French S 2004 Understanding inequality and power. In: Swain J, Clark J, Parry K, et al (eds) Enabling relationships in health and social care. Butterworth-Heinemann, Oxford, p 47–59

Swain J, Finkelstein V, French S, Oliver M 1993 Disabling barriers – enabling environments. Sage & The Open University, London

Swain J, French S, Cameron C 2003 Controversial issues in a disabling society. Open University Press, Buckingham

Tate DG, Forchheimer M 1998 Enhancing community reintegration after inpatient rehabilitation for persons with spinal cord injury. Topics in Spinal Cord Injury Rehabilitation 4(1):42–55

Taylor G 1999 Empowerment, identity and participatory research: using social action research to challenge isolation for deaf and hard of hearing people from minority ethnic communities. Disability and Society 14(3):369–384

Taylor L, McGruder J 1996 The meaning of sea kayaking for persons with spinal cord injuries. American Journal of Occupational Therapy 50(1):39–46

Taylor SE 1983 Adjustment to threatening events. American Psychologist 38:1161–1173

Thomas C 1999 Female forms. Experiencing and understanding disability. Open University Press, Buckingham

Thomas C 2001 The body and society: some reflections on the concepts 'disability' and 'impairment'. In: Watson N, Cunningham-Burley S (eds) Reframing the body. Palgrave, Houndmills, Hants, p 47–62

Thomas C 2002 Disability theory: key ideas, issues and thinkers. In: Barnes C, Oliver M, Barton L (eds) Disability studies today. Polity Press, Cambridge, p 38–57

Thomas C 2004 Disability and impairment. In: Swain J, French S, Barnes C, Thomas C (eds) Disabling barriers – enabling environments, 2nd edn. Sage, London, p 21–27

Thomas J 1993 Doing critical ethnography. Sage, Newbury Park, CA

Thompson N 1997 Anti-discriminatory practice, 2nd edn. Macmillan, Houndmills, Hants

Thompson NJ, Coker J, Krause JS, Henry E 2003 Purpose in life as a mediator of adjustment after spinal cord injury. Rehabilitation Psychology 48:100–108

Thomson RG 1996 Freakery: cultural spectacles of the extraordinary body. New York University Press, New York

Thomson RG 1997a Extraordinary bodies: figuring physical disability in American culture and literature. Columbia University Press, New York

Thomson RG 1997b Feminist theory, the body and the disabled figure, In: Davis LJ (ed) The disability studies reader. Routledge, New York, p 279–292

Thomson RG 2002 The politics of staring: visual rhetorics of disability in popular photography. In: Snyder SL, Brueggemann BJ, Garland-Thomson R (eds) Disability studies. Enabling the humanities. The Modern Language Association of America, New York, p 56–75

Time 1996 New hopes, new dreams. Time 26 August:36–48

Titchkosky T 2003 Disability, self and society. University of Toronto Press, Toronto

Tomlinson S, Abdi OA 2003 Disability in Somaliland. Disability and Society 18(7):911–920

Toombs SK 1987 The meaning of illness: a phenomenological approach to the patient-provider relationship. Journal of Medicine and Philosophy 12:219–240

Toombs SK 1988 Illness and the paradigm of lived body. Theoretical Medicine 9:201–226

Toombs SK 1992 The body in multiple sclerosis: a patient's perspective. Philosophy and Medicine. 43:127–137

Toombs SK 1994 Disability and the self. In: Brinthaupt TM, Lipka RP (eds) Changing the self: philosophies, techniques and experiences. SUNY Press, Albany, NY, p 337–357

Toombs SK 1995 The lived experience of disability. Human Studies 18:9–23

Towle A, Godolphin W 1999 Framework for teaching and learning informed shared decision making. British Medical Journal 319:766–769

Townsend E 1998 Good intentions overruled. A critique of empowerment in the routine organization of mental health services. University of Toronto Press, Toronto

Townsend E, Reibero K 2001 Canada's joint position statement on evidence-based occupational therapy. OT Now. January–February: 8–11

Treece A, Gregory S, Ayres B, Mendis K 1999 'I always do what they tell me to do': choice-making opportunities in the lives of two older persons with severe learning difficulties living in a community setting. Disability and Society 14(6):791–804

Tremain S 1996 We're here. We're disabled and queer. Get used to it. In: Tremain S (ed) Pushing the limits. Disabled dykes produce culture. Women's Press, Toronto, p 15–24

Tremain S 2002 On the subject of impairment. In: Corker M, Shakespeare T (eds) Disability/postmodernity. Embodying disability theory. Continuum, London, p 32–47

Trieschmann R 1988 Spinal cord injuries – psychological, social and vocational rehabilitation, 2nd edn. Demos, New York

Turmusani M 1999 Disability policy and provision in Jordan: a critical perspective, In: Stone E (ed) Disability and development. The Disability Press, Leeds, p 193–209

Turmusani M 2001 Work and adulthood: economic survival in the majority world. In: Priestley M (ed) Disability and the life course. Global perspectives. Cambridge University Press, Cambridge, p 192–205

Turner BS 1991 Recent developments in the theory of the body. In: Featherstone M, Hepworth M, Turner BS (eds) The body. Social process and cultural theory. Sage, London, p 1–35

Turner BS 1992 Regulating bodies. Essays in medical sociology. Routledge, London

Turner BS 1995 Medical power and social knowledge, 2nd edn. Sage, London

Turner BS 1996 The body and society, 2nd edn. Sage, London

Turner V 1967 The forest of symbols: aspects of Ndembu ritual. Cornell University Press, Ithaca, NY

Turner V 1969 The ritual process: structure and anti-structure. Aldine, Chicago, IL

Twible R L 1992 Consumer participation in planning health promotion programmes: a case study using the nominal group technique. Australian Occupational Therapy Journal 39(2):13–18

Twigg J 2000 Bathing – the body and community care. Routledge, London

Twigg J 2002 The body in social policy: mapping a territory. Journal of Social Policy 31(3):421–439

Ungerson C 1987 Policy is personal. Tavistock, London

Union of the Physically Impaired Against Segregation (UPIAS) 1976 Fundamental principles of disability. UPIAS, London

United Nations (UN) 1948 Universal declaration of human rights. Resolution 217A III UN General Assembly. UN, New York

Urbanowski R, Vargo J 1994 Spirituality, daily practice, and the occupational performance model. Canadian Journal of Occupational Therapy 61:88–94

Valentine G 1993 (Hetero)sexing space: lesbian perceptions and experiences of everyday spaces. Environment and Planning D: Society and Space 11:395–413

Valentine J 2001 Disabled discourse: hearing accounts of deafness constructed through Japanese television and film. Disability and Society 16(5):707–727

van Bennekom C, Jelles F, Lankhorst G, Kuik D 1996 Value of measuring perceived problems in a stroke population. Clinical Rehabilitation 10:288–294

van Gennep A 1960 The rites of passage. University of Chicago Press, Chicago, IL

van Maanen J 1988 Tales of the field. On writing ethnography. University of Chicago Press, Chicago, IL

Vasey S 2004 Disability culture: the story so far. In: Swain J, French S, Barnes C, Thomas C (eds) Disabling barriers – enabling environments, 2nd edn. Sage, London p 106–110

Vernon A 1996 A stranger in many camps: the experience of disabled black and ethnic minority women. In: Morris J (ed) Encounters with strangers. Feminism and disability. Women's Press, London, p 48–68

Vernon A 1998 Multiple oppression and the disabled people's movement. In: Shakespeare T (ed) The disability reader: social science perspectives. Cassell, London, p 201–210

Vernon A 1999 The dialectics of multiple identities and the disabled people's movement. Disability and Society 14(3):385–398

Vernon A, Swain J 2002 Theorizing divisions and hierarchies: towards a commonality or diversity? In: Barnes C, Oliver M, Barton L (eds) Disability studies today. Polity Press, Cambridge, p 77–97

Ville I, Ravaud J-F 1996 Work, non-work and consequent satisfaction after spinal cord injury. International Journal of Rehabilitation Research 19:241–252

Ville I, Ravaud J-F, Tetrafigap Group 2001 Subjective well-being and severe motor impairments: the Tetrafigap survey on the long-term outcome of tetraplegic spinal cord injured persons. Social Science and Medicine 52:369–384

Vogel B 2004 A life in balance. New Mobility 15(130):29–31

Vogel LC, Klaas SJ, Lubicky JP, Anderson CJ 1998 Long-term outcomes and life satisfaction of adults who had pediatric spinal cord injuries. Archives of Physical Medicine and Rehabilitation 79:1496–1503

von Zweck C 1999 The promotion of evidence-based occupational therapy practice in Canada. Canadian Journal of Occupational Therapy 66(5):208–213

Vrkljan B, Miller-Polgar J 2001 Meaning of occupational engagement in life-threatening illness: a qualitative pilot project. Canadian Journal of Occupational Therapy 68:237–246

Wade D, Halligan P 2003 New wine in old bottles: the WHO ICF as an explanatory model of human behaviour. Clinical Rehabilitation 17(4):349–354

Waldie E 2002 Triumph of the challenged. Conversations with especially able people. Purple Field Press, Ilminster, Somerset, UK

Walker AM 1994 A Delphi study of research priorities in the clinical practice of physiotherapy. Physiotherapy 80(4):205–207

Walker MF, Drummond A, Gatt J, Sackley C 2000 Occupational therapy for stroke patients: a survey of current practice. British Journal of Occupational Therapy 63(8):367–372

Walmsley J 1993 Contradictions in caring: reciprocity and interdependence. Disability, Handicap and Society 8(2)129–142

Walsh P 1993 Tetraplegics and the justice of resource allocation. Paraplegia 31(3):143–146

Wang C 1993 Culture, meaning and disability: injury prevention campaigns and the production of stigma. In: Nagler M (ed) Perspectives on disability, 2nd edn. Health Markets Research, Palo Alto, CA, p 77–90

Ward L 1997 Funding for change: translating emancipatory disability research from theory to practice. In: Barnes C, Mercer G (eds) Doing disability research. The Disability Press, Leeds, p 32–48

Ward L, Flynn M 1994 What matters most: disability, research and empowerment. In: Rioux MH, Bach M (eds) Disability is not measles. New research paradigms in disability. L'Institut Roeher, North York, ONT, p 29–48

Warnock M 1970 Existentialism. Oxford University Press, Oxford

Watson N 1998 Enabling identity: disability, self and citizenship. In: Shakespeare T (ed) The disability reader. Social science perspectives. Cassell, London, p 147–162

Watson N 2002 Well, I know this is going to sound very strange to you, but I don't see myself as a disabled person: identity and disability. Disability and Society 17(5):509–527

Watson N 2003 Daily denials: the routinisation of oppression and resistance. In: Riddell S, Watson N (eds) Disability, culture and identity. Pearson, Harlow, UK, p 34–52

Watson N 2004 The dialectics of disability: a social model for the 21st century? In: Barnes C, Mercer G (eds) Implementing the social model of disability: theory and research. The Disability Press, Leeds, p 101–117

Wax E 2004 Kenyan mothers reject Western baby buggies as 'devices of oppression': 'In Africa we carry our children so they feel loved'. Guardian Weekly, June 18–24, p 17

Weaver F, Guihan M, Pape T, et al 2001 Creating a research agenda in SCI based on provider and consumer input. SCI Psychosocial Process 14(2):77–88

Wehmeyer ML 1998 Self-determination and individuals with significant disabilities: examining meanings and misinterpretations. Journal of the Association for Persons with Severe Handicaps 23(1):5–16

Wendell S 1996 The rejected body. Feminist philosophical reflections on disability. Routledge, London

Westcott H 1994 Abuse of children and adults who are disabled. In: French S (ed) On equal terms. Working with disabled people. Butterworth-Heinemann, Oxford, p 190–206

Westgren N, Levi R 1998 Quality of life and traumatic spinal cord injury. Archives of Physical Medicine and Rehabilitation 79:1433–1439

White GW 2002 Consumer participation in disability research: the golden rule as a guide for ethical practice. Rehabilitation Psychology 47(4):438–446

White GW, Nary DE, Froehlich AK 2001 Consumers as collaborators in research and action. Journal of Prevention and Intervention 21:15–34

Whiteford GE, Wilcock AA 2000 Cultural relativism: occupation and independence reconsidered. Canadian Journal of Occupational Therapy 67(5):324–336

Whiteneck GG 1992 Outcome evaluation and spinal cord injury. Neurorehabilitation 2(4):31–41

Whiteneck GG 1994 Measuring what matters: key rehabilitation outcomes. Archives of Physical Medicine and Rehabilitation 75(10):1073–1076

Whiteneck GG, Charlifue S, Frankel H, et al 1992 Mortality, morbidity and psychosocial outcomes of persons spinal cord injured more than 20 years ago. Paraplegia 30:617–630

Whyte SR 1995 Disability between discourse and experience. In: Ingstad B, Whyte SR (eds) Disability and culture. University of California Press, Berkeley, CA, p 267–291

Whyte SR, Ingstad B 1995 Disability and culture: an overview. In: Ingstad B, Whyte SR (eds) Disability and culture. University of California Press, Berkeley, CA, p 3–32

Widerström-Noga EG, Felipe-Cuervo E, Broton JG, et al 1999 Perceived difficulty in dealing with consequences of spinal cord injury. Archives of Physical Medicine and Rehabilitation 80(5):580–586

Wigham S, Supyk J 2001 Should occupational therapists work shifts? British Journal of Occupational Therapy 64(3):151–152

Wilcock AA 1998 Occupation for health. British Journal of Occupational Therapy 61(8):340–345

Williams A 1985 Economics of coronary artery bypass grafting. British Medical Journal 291:326–329

Williams G 1996 Representing disability: some questions of phenomenology and politics. In: Barnes C, Mercer G (eds) Exploring the divide. Illness and disability. The Disability Press, Leeds, p 194–212

Williams G 1998 The sociology of disability: towards a materialist phenomenology. In: Shakespeare T (ed) The disability reader: social science perspectives. Cassell, London, p 234–244

Williams G 2001 Theorizing disability. In: Albrecht GL, Seelman KD, Bury M (eds) The handbook of disability studies. Sage, Thousand Oaks, CA, p 123–144

Williams GH, Wood P 1988 Coming to terms with chronic illness: the negotiation of autonomy in rheumatoid arthritis. International Disability Studies 10(3):128–133

Williams SJ 1997 Modern medicine and the 'uncertain body': from corporeality to hyperreality? Social Science and Medicine 45(7):1041–1049

Williams SJ 1999 Is anybody there? Critical realism, chronic illness and the disability debate. Sociology of Health and Illness 21(6):797–819

Williams SJ 2000 Chronic illness as biographical disruption or biographical disruption as chronic illness? Reflections on a core concept. Sociology of Health and Illness 22(1):40–67

Williams SJ, Bendelow G 1998a The lived body: sociological themes, embodied issues. Routledge, London

Williams SJ, Bendelow G 1998b In search of the 'missing body'. Pain, suffering and the (post)modern condition. In: Scrambler G, Higgs P (eds) Modernity, health and medicine. Routledge, London, p 125–146

Wilson A, Beresford P 2002 Madness, distress and postmodernity: putting the record straight. In: Corker M, Shakespeare T (eds) Disability/postmodernity. Embodying disability theory. Continuum, London, p 143–158

Wilson JC, Lewiecki-Wilson C 2002 Disability, rhetoric and the body. In: Wilson JC, Lewiecki-Wilson C (eds) Embodied rhetorics: disability in language and culture. Southern Illinois University Press, Carbondale, IL, p 1–24

Wirz SL, Hartley SD 1999 Challenges for universities of the North interested in community based rehabilitation. In: Stone E (ed) Disability and development. Learning from action and research on disability in the majority world. The Disability Press, Leeds, p 89–106

Witkin S 2000 An integrative human rights approach to social research. In: Truman C, Mertens D, Humphries B (eds) Research and inequality. UCL Press, London, p 205–219

Wolbring G 2001 Where do we draw the line? Surviving eugenics in a technological world. In: Priestley M (ed) Disability and the life course. Global perspectives. Cambridge University Press, Cambridge, p 38–49

Wolf DL 1996 Situating feminist dilemmas in fieldwork. In: Wolf DL (ed) Feminist dilemmas in fieldwork. Westview Press, Boulder, CO, p 1–55

Wolfensberger W 1994 Let's hang up 'quality of life' as a hopeless term. In: Godde D (ed) Quality of life for persons with disabilities: international perspectives and issues. Brookline Books, Cambridge, MA, p 285–321

Woodend AK, Nair RC, Tang AS 1997 Definition of life quality from a patient versus health care professional perspective. International Journal of Rehabilitation Research 20:71–80

Woolsey R 1985 Rehabilitation outcome following spinal cord injury. Archives of Neurology 42:116–119

World Health Organization (WHO) 1980 International classification of impairments, disabilities and handicaps. WHO, Geneva

World Health Organization (WHO) 2001 International classification of functioning, disability and health. WHO, Geneva

Wortman C, Silver RC 1989 The myths of coping with loss. Journal of Consulting and Clinical Psychology 57(3):349–357

Wright BA 1983 Physical disability: a psychosocial approach, 2nd edn. Harper & Row, New York

Yeatman A 1991 Postmodernity and revisioning the political. Social Analysis 30:116–130

Yerxa EJ 1998 Health and the human spirit for occupation. American Journal of Occupational Therapy 52:412–418

Yerxa EJ, Locker S 1990 Quality of time use by adults with spinal cord injuries. American Journal of Occupational Therapy 44(4):318–326

Yoshida KK 1993 Reshaping of self: a pendular reconstruction of self and identity among adults with traumatic spinal cord injuries. Sociology of Health and Illness 15(2):217–245

Young IM 1990 Justice and the politics of difference. Princeton University Press, Princeton, NJ

Young JM, McNicholl P 1998 Against all odds: Positive life experiences of people with advanced amyotrophic lateral sclerosis. Health and Social Work 23:35–43

Young RJC 2003 Postcolonialism. Oxford University Press, Oxford

Zandrow LF 2001 Misguided mercy: hastening death in the disability community. Topics in Spinal Cord Injury Rehabilitation 6(4):76–82

Zarb G 1991 Creating a supportive environment: meeting the needs of people who are ageing with disability. In: Oliver M (ed) Social work. Disabled people and disabling environments. Jessica Kingsley, London, p 177–203

Zarb G 1992 On the road to Damascus: first steps towards changing the relations of disability research production. Disability, Handicap and Society 7(2):125–138

Zejdlik C, Forwell S 1993 A PhD in life. Living with SCI. British Columbia Rehabilitation Society and BCPA, Vancouver

Index

Notes: Abbreviations used in the index are: DALY = disability-adjusted life year; ICF = International Classification of Functioning, Disability and Health; ICIDH = International Classification of Impairments, Disabilities and Handicaps; QALY = quality-adjusted life year. Page numbers in **bold** refer to terms in the Glossary.